Solving the Puzzle: Molecular Research in Inflammatory Bowel Diseases

Solving the Puzzle: Molecular Research in Inflammatory Bowel Diseases

Editor

Susanne M. Krug

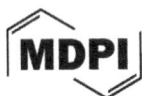

Basel • Beijing • Wuhan • Barcelona • Belgrade • Novi Sad • Cluj • Manchester

Editor
Susanne M. Krug
Clinical Physiology / Nutritional Medicine
Charité–Universitätsmedizin Berlin
Berlin
Germany

Editorial Office
MDPI
St. Alban-Anlage 66
4052 Basel, Switzerland

This is a reprint of articles from the Special Issue published online in the open access journal *International Journal of Molecular Sciences* (ISSN 1422-0067) (available at: www.mdpi.com/journal/ijms/special_issues/IBDs).

For citation purposes, cite each article independently as indicated on the article page online and as indicated below:

Lastname, A.A.; Lastname, B.B. Article Title. *Journal Name* **Year**, *Volume Number*, Page Range.

ISBN 978-3-0365-9864-2 (Hbk)
ISBN 978-3-0365-9863-5 (PDF)
doi.org/10.3390/books978-3-0365-9863-5

Cover image courtesy of Susanne M. Krug

© 2023 by the authors. Articles in this book are Open Access and distributed under the Creative Commons Attribution (CC BY) license. The book as a whole is distributed by MDPI under the terms and conditions of the Creative Commons Attribution-NonCommercial-NoDerivs (CC BY-NC-ND) license.

Contents

Susanne M. Krug
Solving the Puzzle: Molecular Research in Inflammatory Bowel Diseases
Reprinted from: *Int. J. Mol. Sci.* 2023, 24, 13389, doi:10.3390/ijms241713389 1

Jenisha Ghimire, Rida Iftikhar, Harrison M. Penrose, Patricia Snarski, Emmanuelle Ruiz and Suzana D. Savkovic
FOXO3 Deficiency in Neutrophils Drives Colonic Inflammation and Tumorigenesis
Reprinted from: *Int. J. Mol. Sci.* 2023, 24, 9730, doi:10.3390/ijms24119730 5

Christopher T. Capaldo
Claudin Barriers on the Brink: How Conflicting Tissue and Cellular Priorities Drive IBD Pathogenesis
Reprinted from: *Int. J. Mol. Sci.* 2023, 24, 8562, doi:10.3390/ijms24108562 20

Kun He, Xiaxiao Yan and Dong Wu
Intestinal Behcet's Disease: A Review of the Immune Mechanism and Present and Potential Biological Agents
Reprinted from: *Int. J. Mol. Sci.* 2023, 24, 8176, doi:10.3390/ijms24098176 33

Francesca Lombardi, Francesca Rosaria Augello, Paola Palumbo, Laura Bonfili, Serena Artone and Serena Altamura et al.
Bacterial Lysate from the Multi-Strain Probiotic SLAB51 Triggers Adaptative Responses to Hypoxia in Human Caco-2 Intestinal Epithelial Cells under Normoxic Conditions and Attenuates LPS-Induced Inflammatory Response
Reprinted from: *Int. J. Mol. Sci.* 2023, 24, 8134, doi:10.3390/ijms24098134 48

Yasmina Rodríguez-Sillke, Michael Schumann, Donata Lissner, Federica Branchi, Fabian Proft and Ulrich Steinhoff et al.
Analysis of Circulating Food Antigen-Specific T-Cells in Celiac Disease and Inflammatory Bowel Disease
Reprinted from: *Int. J. Mol. Sci.* 2023, 24, 8153, doi:10.3390/ijms24098153 66

Nguyen Phan Khoi Le, Markus Jörg Altenburger and Evelyn Lamy
Development of an Inflammation-Triggered In Vitro "Leaky Gut" Model Using Caco-2/HT29-MTX-E12 Combined with Macrophage-like THP-1 Cells or Primary Human-Derived Macrophages
Reprinted from: *Int. J. Mol. Sci.* 2023, 24, 7427, doi:10.3390/ijms24087427 77

Leonie Wittner, Lukas Wagener, Jakob J. Wiese, Iris Stolzer, Susanne M. Krug and Elisabeth Naschberger et al.
Proteolytic Activity of the Paracaspase MALT1 Is Involved in Epithelial Restitution and Mucosal Healing
Reprinted from: *Int. J. Mol. Sci.* 2023, 24, 7402, doi:10.3390/ijms24087402 96

Junsuke Uwada, Hitomi Nakazawa, Ikunobu Muramatsu, Takayoshi Masuoka and Takashi Yazawa
Role of Muscarinic Acetylcholine Receptors in Intestinal Epithelial Homeostasis: Insights for the Treatment of Inflammatory Bowel Disease
Reprinted from: *Int. J. Mol. Sci.* 2023, 24, 6508, doi:10.3390/ijms24076508 117

Nathalie Britzen-Laurent, Carl Weidinger and Michael Stürzl
Contribution of Blood Vessel Activation, Remodeling and Barrier Function to Inflammatory Bowel Diseases
Reprinted from: *Int. J. Mol. Sci.* **2023**, *24*, 5517, doi:10.3390/ijms24065517 . . . . **132**

Andrey V. Markov, Innokenty A. Savin, Marina A. Zenkova and Aleksandra V. Sen'kova
Identification of Novel Core Genes Involved in Malignant Transformation of Inflamed Colon Tissue Using a Computational Biology Approach and Verification in Murine Models
Reprinted from: *Int. J. Mol. Sci.* **2023**, *24*, 4311, doi:10.3390/ijms24054311 . . . . **161**

Sarah Lemire, Oana-Maria Thoma, Lucas Kreiss, Simon Völkl, Oliver Friedrich and Markus F. Neurath et al.
Natural NADH and FAD Autofluorescence as Label-Free Biomarkers for Discriminating Subtypes and Functional States of Immune Cells
Reprinted from: *Int. J. Mol. Sci.* **2022**, *23*, 2338, doi:10.3390/ijms23042338 . . . . **183**

Editorial

Solving the Puzzle: Molecular Research in Inflammatory Bowel Diseases

Susanne M. Krug

Clinical Physiology/Nutritional Medicine, Charité—Universitätsmedizin Berlin, 12203 Berlin, Germany; susanne.m.krug@charite.de

Inflammatory bowel disease (IBD) encompasses chronic idiopathic relapsing and remitting gastrointestinal autoimmune diseases characterized by chronic inflammatory disorders of complex etiology, posing clinical challenges due to their often therapy-refractory nature. The primary disorders within the IBD classification are ulcerative colitis (UC) and Crohn's disease (CD), sharing similarities but exhibiting distinct differences, sometimes making their discrimination challenging.

A prominent feature of IBD is the inflammation of the intestinal mucosa, characterized by the robust and persistent infiltration of immune cells and compromised intestinal barrier integrity, leading to the phenomenon known as "leaky gut." The inflammation can manifest acutely or chronically relapsing and can increase in severity over time, thereby causing life-long morbidities and reduced quality of life for affected individuals, underscoring the need for a deeper comprehension of the molecular contributors to disease pathogenesis and progression.

Despite extensive research, the etiology of IBD is still not fully understood, and so far, existing treatments are inadequate to effect a complete cure. The disease's multifactorial nature implicates genetic, environmental, infectious, and immunologic factors as key contributors. The dysregulation of both transcellular and paracellular intestinal barriers, along with the activation of mucosal immune responses, either as a consequence or a trigger, play pivotal roles in the pathological manifestations.

Recent developments in IBD research are broadening our overall understanding of the disease enabling the discovery of novel molecular predictive indicators and facilitating the creation of cutting-edge therapeutic approaches. This Special Issue presents a comprehensive compilation of diverse facets that contribute to the advancement of solving the puzzle of IBD.

In general, impaired homeostasis is known to be critical for the development of IBD. A multitude of factors and components are involved in the physiological maintenance of homeostasis and are found to be affected or to be an effector in IBD. For example, muscarinic acetylcholine receptors (mAChRs) play a significant role in maintaining intestinal epithelial homeostasis, and their activation is essential for the maintenance and reinforcement of epithelial function. Non-neuronal acetylcholine systems are also recognized to be involved in mAChR activation in epithelial cells. A review in this Special Issue summarizes recent advances in research on mAChRs and non-neuronal acetylcholine systems as potential targets for therapy in treating IBD [1].

Shifts in the oxidative status of the intestinal epithelium may not only affect the epithelium but also gut-microbiota homeostasis. Hypoxia-inducible factor-1α (HIF-1α) is one of the central players for that. The lysate from the probiotic formulation SLAB51 was found to increase HIF-1α levels in human intestinal epithelium under normoxic conditions, leading to higher glycolytic metabolism and protection from lipopolysaccharide (LPS)-induced inflammatory response. The probiotic treatment stabilized HIF-1α via the activation of the PI3K/AKT pathway, resulting in an inhibition of NF-κB, nitric oxide synthase 2 (NOS2), and an increase in the IL-1β triggered via LPS treatment [2].

Another key player for mucosal inflammation has been discussed to be the paracaspase MALT1, particularly in the context of IBD. MALT1's proteolytic activity was shown to be involved in inhibiting ferroptosis and promoting STAT3 signaling, which is essential for regulating immune and inflammatory responses as well as mucosal healing. These mechanisms might be used for the identification of novel therapeutic targets for the treatment not only of IBD but also other inflammatory diseases [3].

Immune cells are one main group of important players in the development and progression of inflammatory processes in IBD. In this Special Issue, for example, the role of polymorphonuclear neutrophils (PMNs) and their significance in promoting colonic pathobiology IBD and colon cancer, which can develop from IBD, is discussed. Special focus was laid on intracellular lipid droplets (LDs) and transcription factor FOXO3 in PMNs. The presence of FOXO3-deficient PMNs could be associated with increased transmigratory activity, differentially expressed genes linked to metabolism, inflammation, and tumorigenesis, and predicts colon cancer invasion and poor survival [4].

Food antigen-specific effector T-cells that may respond to barrier disruption and antigen in patients with celiac disease (CeD) were also found in comparable levels in active CD patients. The frequency and phenotype of nutritional antigen-specific T-cells in these two patient groups correlated with the presence of small intestinal inflammation, indicating that active inflammation in the small intestine plays a crucial role in the development of peripheral food antigen-specific T-cell responses in CD as well as in CeD and could be a key factor [5].

A new and innovative methodical approach to identifying immune cells is a label-free optical technology, which utilizes autofluorescence using NADH and FAD signals. These can be utilized to classify and characterize different immune cell subtypes and their activation states in the context of IBD. This study demonstrates the value of autofluorescence as a tool for identifying innate and adaptive immune cells, determining their relative amounts, and distinguishing their functional states, which could lead to a label-free clinical classification of IBD in the future [6].

Besides the intestinal immune system, another major factor in IBD is the epithelial barrier. The claudin family of tight junction proteins is a crucial component of intestinal barriers, and their altered expression and localization in IBD may lead to intestinal barrier dysfunction and worsen immune hyperactivity and disease. While claudins are known to control the passage of ions and water between cells, emerging evidence suggests additional non-canonical functions during mucosal homeostasis and healing after injury, leaving the question open whether claudins play adaptive or pathological roles in IBD responses. Analyzing current research, it is hypothesized that claudins' versatility might come at the cost of specialized mastery, potentially leading to conflicts between maintaining a robust claudin barrier and facilitating tissue repair, thereby exposing vulnerabilities in the barrier's integrity and compromising overall tissue healing during IBD [7].

To study the epithelial barrier in joint context with immune cells Le and colleagues developed an advanced in vitro inflammation-triggered triple-culture model involving the human intestinal epithelial cell line Caco-2, mucus-producing goblet cell line HT29-MTX-E12, and macrophages of different origin. This model demonstrated characteristics of a "leaky gut" upon an inflammatory stimulus and could be valuable for screening and evaluating therapeutic drugs for the treatment of IBD, including potential IL-23 inhibitors that were analyzed in that model [8].

In IBD, there is significant activation and remodeling of mucosal micro-vessels. The role of the gut vasculature in inducing and persisting mucosal inflammation is increasingly recognized, where endothelial cell activation and angiogenesis are thought to promote inflammation. On the other hand, the vascular barrier may offer protection against bacterial translocation and sepsis, which indicates that other barriers besides the intestinal epithelial one are of importance in IBD. One review of this Special Issue focuses on examining the different phenotypical changes observed in the microvascular endothelium during IBD and presents potential vessel-specific targeted therapy options for the treatment of IBD [9].

Another review focuses on diseases other than IBD, which affect the intestine. These may give insights of general importance and could link symptoms and treatments of more than one disease. Behçet's disease (BD) is a chronic and recurrent systemic vasculitis involving almost all organs and tissues. Intestinal BD may have severe gastrointestinal complications and share similarities with classical IBD, particularly active CD. The review highlights the dysregulation of immune function as one of the main pathogenes in both, intestinal BD and IBD. It emphasizes the potential of biological agents, particularly anti-tumor necrosis factor agents, as effective treatment options for patients with refractory intestinal BD, a therapy that is also employed in IBD [10].

IBD is often associated with the development of colorectal cancer. Despite extensive studies of IBD pathogenesis, the molecular mechanism of how IBD is promoting tumorigenesis is not yet fully understood. Through a comprehensive bioinformatics analysis of transcriptomics data from mouse models of acute colitis and colitis-associated cancer (CAC), a set of key genes involved in the regulation of colitis and CAC was identified. These genes, particularly matrix metalloproteinases (MMPs), can potentially serve as novel prognostic markers and therapeutic targets for controlling IBD and IBD-associated colorectal neoplasia. Additionally, a translational bridge connecting these genes with the pathogenesis of UC, CD, and CAC was established [11].

Taken together, this Special Issue brings together new research and reviews covering various aspects of IBD. It includes studies by joining functional, genetic, and molecular research as well as innovative methods. By doing so, it helps piece together multiple aspects of the complex puzzle of understanding IBD.

Funding: The research of the author is funded by the Deutsche Forschungsgemeinschaft DFG TRR 241-375876048 (B06).

Conflicts of Interest: The author declares no conflict of interest.

References

1. Uwada, J.; Nakazawa, H.; Muramatsu, I.; Masuoka, T.; Yazawa, T. Role of Muscarinic Acetylcholine Receptors in Intestinal Epithelial Homeostasis: Insights for the Treatment of Inflammatory Bowel Disease. *Int. J. Mol. Sci.* **2023**, *24*, 6508. [CrossRef] [PubMed]
2. Lombardi, F.; Augello, F.R.; Palumbo, P.; Bonfili, L.; Artone, S.; Altamura, S.; Sheldon, J.M.; Latella, G.; Cifone, M.G.; Eleuteri, A.M.; et al. Bacterial Lysate from the Multi-Strain Probiotic SLAB51 Triggers Adaptative Responses to Hypoxia in Human Caco-2 Intestinal Epithelial Cells under Normoxic Conditions and Attenuates LPS-Induced Inflammatory Response. *Int. J. Mol. Sci.* **2023**, *24*, 8134. [CrossRef] [PubMed]
3. Wittner, L.; Wagener, L.; Wiese, J.J.; Stolzer, I.; Krug, S.M.; Naschberger, E.; Jackstadt, R.; Beyaert, R.; Atreya, R.; Kühl, A.A.; et al. Proteolytic Activity of the Paracaspase MALT1 Is Involved in Epithelial Restitution and Mucosal Healing. *Int. J. Mol. Sci.* **2023**, *24*, 7402. [CrossRef]
4. Ghimire, J.; Iftikhar, R.; Penrose, H.M.; Snarski, P.; Ruiz, E.; Savkovic, S.D. FOXO3 Deficiency in Neutrophils Drives Colonic Inflammation and Tumorigenesis. *Int. J. Mol. Sci.* **2023**, *24*, 9730. [CrossRef] [PubMed]
5. Rodríguez-Sillke, Y.; Schumann, M.; Lissner, D.; Branchi, F.; Proft, F.; Steinhoff, U.; Siegmund, B.; Glauben, R. Analysis of Circulating Food Antigen-Specific T-Cells in Celiac Disease and Inflammatory Bowel Disease. *Int. J. Mol. Sci.* **2023**, *24*, 8153. [CrossRef] [PubMed]
6. Lemire, S.; Thoma, O.-M.; Kreiss, L.; Völkl, S.; Friedrich, O.; Neurath, M.F.; Schürmann, S.; Waldner, M.J. Natural NADH and FAD Autofluorescence as Label-Free Biomarkers for Discriminating Subtypes and Functional States of Immune Cells. *Int. J. Mol. Sci.* **2022**, *23*, 2338. [CrossRef] [PubMed]
7. Capaldo, C.T. Claudin Barriers on the Brink: How Conflicting Tissue and Cellular Priorities Drive IBD Pathogenesis. *Int. J. Mol. Sci.* **2023**, *24*, 8562. [CrossRef] [PubMed]
8. Le, N.P.K.; Altenburger, M.J.; Lamy, E. Development of an Inflammation-Triggered In Vitro "Leaky Gut" Model Using Caco-2/HT29-MTX-E12 Combined with Macrophage-like THP-1 Cells or Primary Human-Derived Macrophages. *Int. J. Mol. Sci.* **2023**, *24*, 7427. [CrossRef] [PubMed]
9. Britzen-Laurent, N.; Weidinger, C.; Stürzl, M. Contribution of Blood Vessel Activation, Remodeling and Barrier Function to Inflammatory Bowel Diseases. *Int. J. Mol. Sci.* **2023**, *24*, 5517. [CrossRef] [PubMed]

10. He, K.; Yan, X.; Wu, D. Intestinal Behcet's Disease: A Review of the Immune Mechanism and Present and Potential Biological Agents. *Int. J. Mol. Sci.* **2023**, *24*, 8176. [PubMed]
11. Markov, A.V.; Savin, I.A.; Zenkova, M.A.; Sen'kova, A.V. Identification of Novel Core Genes Involved in Malignant Transformation of Inflamed Colon Tissue Using a Computational Biology Approach and Verification in Murine Models. *Int. J. Mol. Sci.* **2023**, *24*, 4311. [CrossRef] [PubMed]

Disclaimer/Publisher's Note: The statements, opinions and data contained in all publications are solely those of the individual author(s) and contributor(s) and not of MDPI and/or the editor(s). MDPI and/or the editor(s) disclaim responsibility for any injury to people or property resulting from any ideas, methods, instructions or products referred to in the content.

FOXO3 Deficiency in Neutrophils Drives Colonic Inflammation and Tumorigenesis

Jenisha Ghimire, Rida Iftikhar, Harrison M. Penrose, Patricia Snarski, Emmanuelle Ruiz and Suzana D. Savkovic *

Department of Pathology and Laboratory Medicine, Tulane University School of Medicine, New Orleans, LA 70112, USA
* Correspondence: ssavkovi@tulane.edu; Tel.: +1-504-988-1409

Abstract: Inflammatory bowel disease (IBD), characterized by infiltration of polymorphonuclear neutrophils (PMNs), increases the risk of colon cancer. PMN activation corresponds to the accumulation of intracellular Lipid Droplets (LDs). As increased LDs are negatively regulated by transcription factor Forkhead Box O3 (FOXO3), we aim to determine the significance of this regulatory network in PMN-mediated IBD and tumorigenesis. Affected tissue of IBD and colon cancer patients, colonic and infiltrated immune cells, have increased LDs' coat protein, PLIN2. Mouse peritoneal PMNs with stimulated LDs and FOXO3 deficiency have elevated transmigratory activity. Transcriptomic analysis of these FOXO3-deficient PMNs showed differentially expressed genes (DEGs; FDR < 0.05) involved in metabolism, inflammation, and tumorigenesis. Upstream regulators of these DEGs, similar to colonic inflammation and dysplasia in mice, were linked to IBD and human colon cancer. Additionally, a transcriptional signature representing FOXO3-deficient PMNs (PMN-FOXO3$_{389}$) separated transcriptomes of affected tissue in IBD ($p = 0.00018$) and colon cancer ($p = 0.0037$) from control. Increased PMN-FOXO3$_{389}$ presence predicted colon cancer invasion (lymphovascular $p = 0.015$; vascular $p = 0.046$; perineural $p = 0.03$) and poor survival. Validated DEGs from PMN-FOXO3$_{389}$ (*P2RX1, MGLL, MCAM, CDKN1A, RALBP1, CCPG1, PLA2G7*) are involved in metabolism, inflammation, and tumorigenesis ($p < 0.05$). These findings highlight the significance of LDs and FOXO3-mediated PMN functions that promote colonic pathobiology.

Keywords: IBD; colon cancer; PMNs; LDs; FOXO3

1. Introduction

Inflammatory bowel disease (IBD), a chronic inflammation of the intestinal tract, includes two distinct clinical entities, Crohn's disease (CD) and ulcerative colitis (UC) [1]. Both CD and UC are linked to genetic predisposition, impaired barrier function, aberrant microbiota, and dysregulation in the immune system [2,3]. One of the hallmarks of IBD is an excessive infiltration of polymorphonuclear leukocytes (PMNs), also known as neutrophils [4,5]. Moreover, chronic inflammation within IBD may lead to dysplasia, and patients with a history of UC are more predisposed to colon cancer than their healthy counterparts [6,7]. Although PMNs contribute to this inflammation-induced colonic tumorigenesis [8,9], the mechanisms involved in the processes are not fully understood.

PMNs, accounting for ~60% of circulating immune cells, are the first and most rapidly migrating cells to the sites of tissue damage and microbial invasion, where they neutralize microorganisms, recruit other immune cells, and remodel damaged tissues to resolve injury [10,11]. In the intestine, hyperactivation of PMNs results in abnormal immune responses, tissue damage, and aberrant barrier function leading to chronic inflammation [12,13]. Furthermore, in inflamed tissue, PMNs release reactive oxygen and nitrogen species in intestinal epithelial cells, causing DNA mutations that consequently drive tumorigenesis [14,15]. Additionally, augmented PMNs mediate the breakdown of barrier function in the intestine, allowing for the presence of microbiota products [16,17], which can further foster tumorigenic processes in colonic cells. Recent studies have demonstrated that intracellular lipid metabolism is critical in driving PMN activity. Specifically, lipid droplets (LDs), intracellular lipid-storing organelles, are crucial for the development and differentiation of PMNs. Their increase in PMNs is associated with inflammation and bacterial infection [18–21]. Inflammatory mediators that activate PMNs are also shown to elevate their LDs accumulation [22,23]. Additionally, PMNs in the tumorigenic environment have elevated LDs, which act as an energy source for cancer cell growth and survival, as well as release oxidized lipids that can activate dormant tumor cells and promote metastasis [24,25].

In mouse models of colonic inflammation and inflammatory tumors, LDs are elevated in colonic cells and infiltrated immune cells [26–30]. Our lab demonstrated the existence of a self-regulating negative loop between LDs and transcription factor Forkhead Box O3 (FOXO3) in colonic cells that drive inflammatory and tumorigenic processes [27,29–31]. Further, FOXO3 deficiency in the liver leads to hyperlipidemia in mice, with increased hepatic lipid secretion and elevated serum triacylglycerol and cholesterol levels [32]. In addition, FOXO3 cellular function is associated with inflammation and tumorigenesis in the colon [33–36]. Genome-wide association studies (GWAS) have linked the polymorphism of *FOXO3* (leading to its reduced levels) to the severity of inflammation in IBD [37]. Additionally, FOXO3 can act as a tumor suppressor, and its loss correlates with advanced human colon cancer [33,36]. Given this line of evidence, we hypothesize that this LDs and FOXO3 negative regulatory network in PMNs acts as a promoter of inflammatory tumorigenesis in the colon. These findings provide conceptual advances in understanding mechanisms in PMNs linked to IBD and IBD-facilitated colon cancer.

2. Results

2.1. Levels of PLIN2 Are Increased in Affected Tissue in IBD and Human Colon Cancer

We have previously demonstrated in the inflamed mouse colon elevated levels of LDs in colonic and infiltrating immune cells [27]. To determine the significance of increased LDs in human intestinal pathobiology, we assessed the levels of PLIN2, the LDs coat protein, in affected tissue obtained from UC and CD patients and in tumor tissue from colon cancer patients. In normal human colonic tissue, immunohistostaining for PLIN2 showed the presence of the protein in the cytosol of colonic epithelial cells along the crypts. In UC and CD, PLIN2 levels were increased by more than 2-fold in the affected tissue, which is significant in both intestinal epithelial cells and infiltrated immune cells (Figure 1A–C). Similar increased PLIN2 levels were found in human colonic tumor tissue (adenocarcinoma, Stage IIB, and Stage IIIC) relative to adjacent normal tissue (Figure 1D,E). These findings demonstrated that LDs are elevated in affected tissue of IBD and human colon cancer as well as in infiltrated immune cells.

2.2. Increased Migratory Activity of PMNs Is Associated with Elevated LDs and FOXO3 Deficiency

We have demonstrated the critical role of elevated LDs and loss of FOXO3, an established regulatory network in colonic cells, in driving inflammation and tumorigenesis in the colon, the role of which in immune cells is not well understood. As PMNs are critical players in inflammatory and tumorigenic processes in the colon [5,9,38,39], we investigated the significance of increased LDs and loss of FOXO3 in PMNs' activity. Intraperitoneal PMNs were obtained from wild type (WT) and FOXO3 knock-out (KO) mice following casein injection [40,41]. After PMNs enrichment, the final fraction contained more than 90% PMNs (FACS assessment of surface marker Ly6G), and peritoneal PMNs in FOXO3 KO mice were increased compared to WT. PMNs were seeded in the upper compartment of a transwell system, and migration activity toward bacterial fMLP or chemokine KC was assessed by quantification of the activity of myeloperoxidase (MPO), an enzyme released by activated PMNs. Oleic acid (OA) stimulation of LDs accumulation in PMNs from WT mice significantly increased their migration, basally stimulated by fMLP and KC (Figure 2A, $p < 0.05$). Further, FOXO3 KO PMNs, relative to WT, had significantly increased migration in response to fMLP, as shown by the MPO activity (Figure 2B, $p < 0.05$). These findings demonstrate that PMNs migration is increased with LDs accumulation and FOXO3 deficiency, suggesting that LDs and FOXO3 regulatory networks in PMNs may play a role in driving inflammation and tumorigenesis.

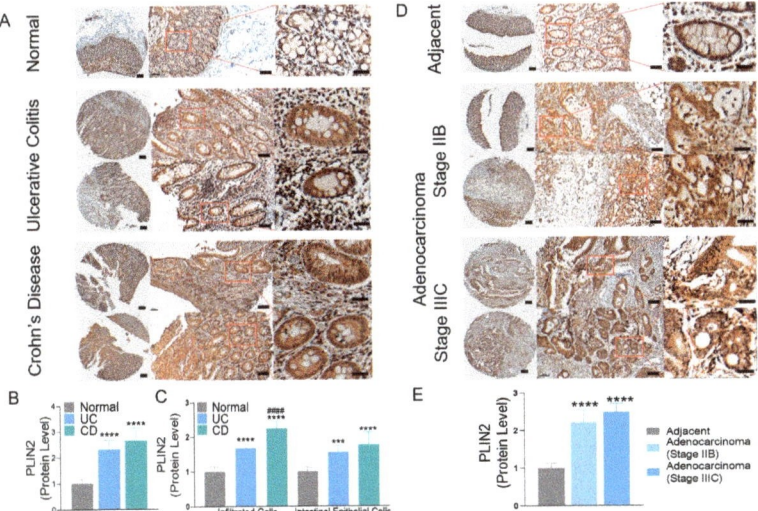

Figure 1. LDs' coat protein PLIN2 levels are increased in affected human colonic tissue obtained from (**A**) Ulcerative Colitis (UC), Crohn's Disease (CD), and (**D**) Colon Cancer patients. PLIN2 levels in tissue were determined by immunohistostaining (IHC) (tissue array). Areas selected in red boxes are further magnified sections (scale bar 800 μM, 100 μM, 20 μM) (**B,C,E**) Graphs represent the quantification of IHC of PLIN2 using ImageJ/Fiji 2.1.0, performing spectrum deconvolution for separation of DAB color spectra. Total number of patients ($n = 10$) included normal ($n = 2$), UC ($n = 2$), CD ($n = 2$), tumor-adjacent mucosa ($n = 2$), and adenocarcinoma ($n = 2$). Quantification included 5–8 separate areas/samples (**** $p < 0.0001$, *** $p < 0.001$ vs. normal control, #### $p < 0.0001$ vs. UC samples).

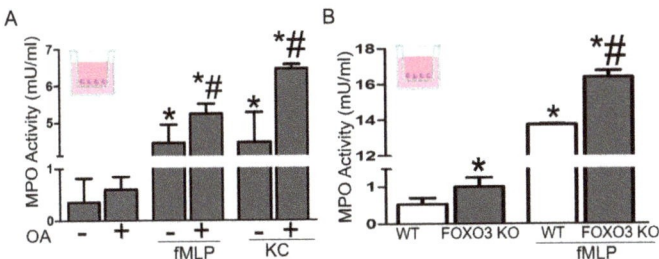

Figure 2. Increased LDs and FOXO3 deficiency in PMNs facilitate their migratory activity. (**A**) MPO activity showing transmigration of mouse peritoneal PMNs with Oleic acid (OA) stimulated LDs. fMLP and KC are used as PMNs chemoattractants. ($n = 6$ mice per group, $n = 3$ wells per mouse, * $p < 0.05$ vs. control, # $p < 0.05$ vs. fMLP or KC without OA) (**B**) MPO activity showing transmigration of peritoneal PMNs from FOXO3 KO mouse relative to wild type (WT) in response to fMLP. ($n = 6$ mice per group, $n = 3$ wells per mouse, * $p < 0.05$ vs. WT, # $p < 0.05$ vs. WT treated with fMLP).

2.3. FOXO3 Deficiency in PMNs Is Associated with Mouse Colonic Inflammation and Dysplasia

Next, we determined in FOXO3-deficient PMNs systemic transcriptional changes and associated molecular pathways driving their activity in the colon. Transcriptional assessment of intraperitoneal PMNs from FOXO3 KO mice showed 212 increased and 242 decreased differentially expressed genes (DEGs) relative to WT (> |0.5|-fold change, FDR < 0.05). The diseases and functions associated with these DEGs include gastrointestinal disorders, metabolic diseases, lipid metabolism, immune responses, immune cell trafficking, inflammatory pathways, and cancer (Figure 3A). To determine the contribution of loss of FOXO3 in PMNs to colonic pathobiology, their upstream regulators of DEGs were identified and compared to transcriptomes from the total colonic tissue of FOXO3-deficient mice, which has exacerbated inflammatory and tumorigenic processes [27,35,42]. We found substantial similarities in upstream regulators of DEGs associated with FOXO3 KO PMNs and total FOXO3 KO colon, which were related to lipid metabolism (eicosapentenoic acid, LEP), immune response (CD40LG, CpG oligonucleotide), inflammatory pathways (SIRT1, HNF-4α), and tumorigenesis (NUPR1, ID1, CREB1, CBFB) (Figure 3B). Next, we determined the significance of FOXO3 KO PMNs in mouse intestinal pathobiology by comparing FOXO3-dependent DEGs in PMNs with publicly available transcriptomes obtained from mouse colons with inflammation and dysplasia (GSE31106). Upstream regulators of FOXO3 KO-dependent DEGs in PMNs were similar to those related to both inflammation and high-grade dysplasia in mouse colon (Figure 3C,D). These shared regulators were linked to metabolism (LDL, FOS, PPAR-γ), immune response (BTK, CD3, BCL6), inflammation (SIRT1, MMP9, TRAF2), and tumorigenesis (MAPK1, CDKN2A, KLF5, Sp1, TGFbeta). These findings revealed the significance of the loss of FOXO3 in PMNs in driving metabolic, inflammatory, and tumorigenic processes in mouse colon.

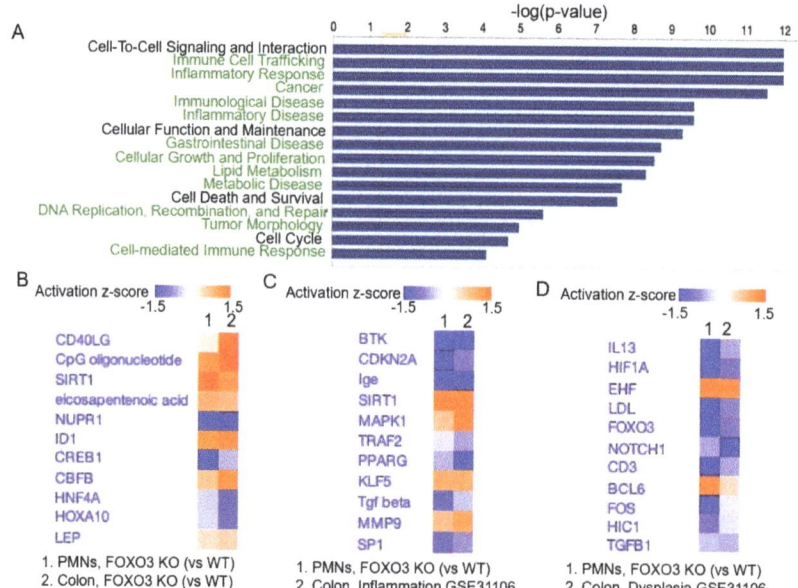

Figure 3. FOXO3 deficiency in PMNs is linked to mouse colonic pathobiology. (**A**) Top diseases and pathways associated with FOXO3 KO in PMNs relative to control ($p < 0.05$, IPA). (**B**) Top upstream regulators of DEGs mediated by FOXO3 deficiency in PMNs, shared with FOXO3 KO mouse colon (IPA, n = 3–5 mice per group, $p < 0.05$). (**C,D**) Top regulators of FOXO3 KO-dependent DEGs in PMNs shared with regulators in mouse colon with inflammation and high-grade dysplasia (n = 3 mice per group, IPA, $p < 0.05$, IPA, GSE31106).

2.4. FOXO3 Deficiency in PMNs Is Associated with Metabolic, Inflammatory, and Tumorigenic Processes in IBD and Human Colon Cancer

Based on our above findings, we sought to determine the significance of the loss of FOXO3 in PMNs in IBD and human colon cancer. The transcriptomes from PMNs of FOXO3 KO mouse have shared regulators with those representing publicly available transcriptomes of affected tissue of different patient cohorts with UC (GSE36807, GSE53306, GSE59071) and CD (GSE59071, GSE95095, GSE102133) (Figure 4A,B). Similar upstream regulators included those involved in metabolism (LEP, NR1H4, PLCG2), immune response (CpG oligonucleotide), inflammatory pathways (C5AR1), and tumorigenesis (NFAT5, RHOA, PTEN, MAPK8). Moreover, DEGs for FOXO3 KO PMNs shared upstream regulators with publicly available transcriptomes from several human colon cancer patient cohorts (GSE141174, GSE8671, GSE9348). These regulators had roles in metabolism (ACOX1, NR1H4), immune response (butyric acid, HIC1), inflammation (ETV5, HNF4-α), and tumorigenesis (Mek, RHOA, EHF, MAPK8, PTEN, LEF1) (Figure 4C). These data demonstrated that loss of FOXO3 in PMNs is important in driving metabolic, inflammatory, and tumorigenic processes in affected tissue of IBD and human colon cancer patients.

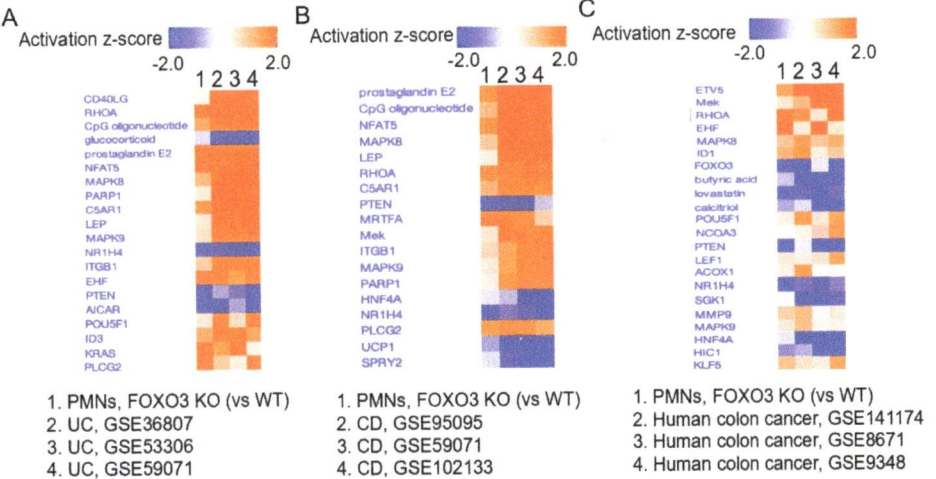

Figure 4. FOXO3 deficiency in PMNs is linked to drivers of IBD and human colon cancer. Top regulators of DEGs in FOXO3 KO PMNs similar to regulators in (**A**) UC, (**B**) CD, and (**C**) human colon cancer. Publicly available data from three different patient cohorts for each, UC (GSE36807, GSE53306, GSE59071, total n = 132), CD (GSE59071, GSE95095, GSE102133, total n = 91), and human colon cancer (GSE141174, GSE8671, GSE9348; total n = 162) were utilized (IPA, $p < 0.05$).

2.5. Transcriptomic Signature Representing FOXO3-Deficient PMNs Is Highly Prevalent in Transcriptomes of IBD and Human Colon Cancer

To further determine the significance of the FOXO3-deficient PMNs in colonic pathobiology, we established their transcriptional signature, which represents a panel of 389 DEGs (PMN-FOXO3$_{389}$), with stringent differential expression and statistical thresholds relative to WT (log2 fold-change > |1.5| and an adjusted p-value < 0.001). Unsupervised hierarchical clustering demonstrated that the PMN-FOXO3$_{389}$ signature separated transcriptomes (publicly available data, GSE4183) of affected IBD tissue (UC and CD) and colon cancer samples (adenomas and adenocarcinomas) from the control (unaffected) group (Figure 5A). Additionally, principal component analysis (PCA) showed that in the transcriptome of patients with IBD and colon cancer, the PMN-FOXO3$_{389}$ signature stratified samples of the affected colon from the normal (Figure 5B,C). The PCA index score indicated that PMN-FOXO3$_{389}$-dependent differentiation of the two groups was strongly significant, with

$p = 1.8 \times 10^{-4}$ for IBD (vs. normal) and $p = 3.7 \times 10^{-3}$ for colon cancer (vs. normal) (Figure 5D,E).

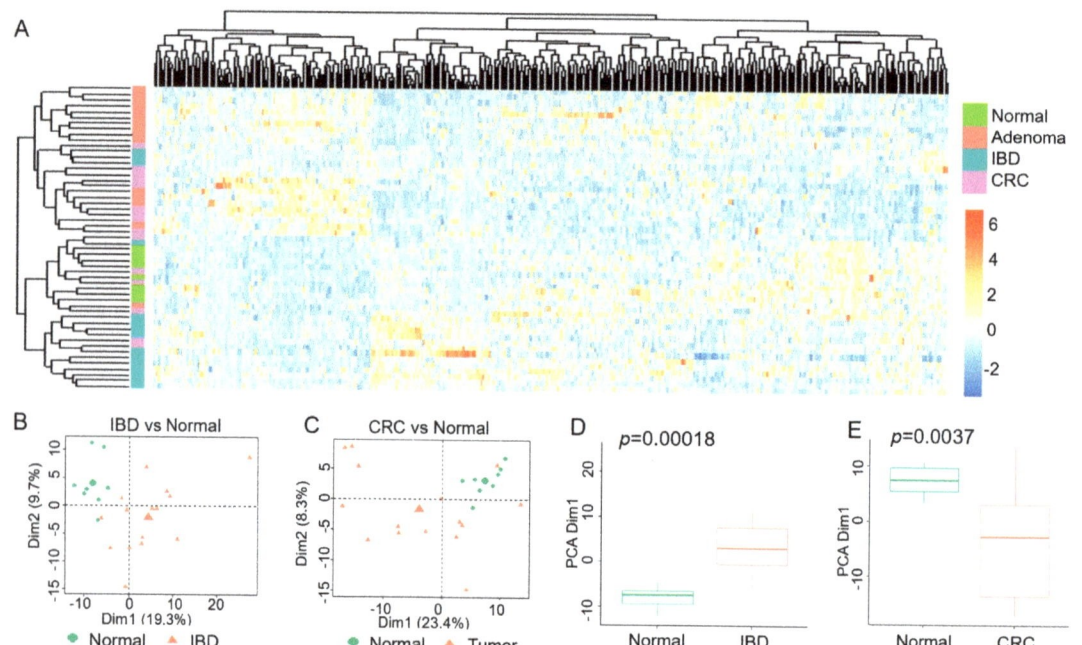

Figure 5. Transcriptional signature for FOXO3-dependent PMNs in IBD and human colon cancer. (**A**) Hierarchical clustering, as shown by a heatmap, revealing the separation of transcriptomes representing IBD (blue) and colon cancer (adenomas (pink) and adenocarcinomas (CRC, violet)) from normal (green) by the PMNs-FOXO3$_{389}$ signature. PMN-FOXO3$_{389}$ signature on x-axis and human samples on y-axis. (**B**,**C**) FOXO3$_{389}$ signature was used to perform principal component analysis (PCA) of active IBD and matched control transcriptomes, as well as human colon cancer and control transcriptomes, to estimate variation between samples. (**D**,**E**) Two-axis values of the PCA showed that PMN-FOXO3$_{389}$ significantly differentiated IBD from matched control tissue ($p = 0.00018$) and colon cancer tissue from control ($p = 0.0037$) ($n = 53$, GSE4183).

Moreover, we determined the significance of PMN-FOXO3$_{389}$ in a large number of colon cancer patients using publicly available transcriptomes from the TCGA database. In unsupervised hierarchal clustering, PMN-FOXO3$_{389}$ signature separated transcriptomes of colon cancer samples from normal, which was further quantified by PCA index score between two groups ($p = 2 \times 10^{-16}$) (Figure 6A,B). In addition, PMN-FOXO3$_{389}$ signature separated colon cancer samples according to the probability for invasions in the vasculature (PCA, $p = 0.046$), lymphovasculature (PCA, $p = 0.015$), and perineural space (PCA, $p = 0.03$) (Figure 6C–E). Moreover, Kaplan–Meier estimates showed that the increased presence of PMN-FOXO3$_{389}$ signature in transcriptomes of colon cancer is linked to poor 5-year patient survival rates of 47% (28–65%) when compared to 65% (55–74%) for lower presence ($p = 8.2 \times 10^{-4}$) (TCGA) (Figure 6F). Together, these data demonstrated that the loss of FOXO3 in PMNs is associated with human colon cancer progression, metastasis, and survival.

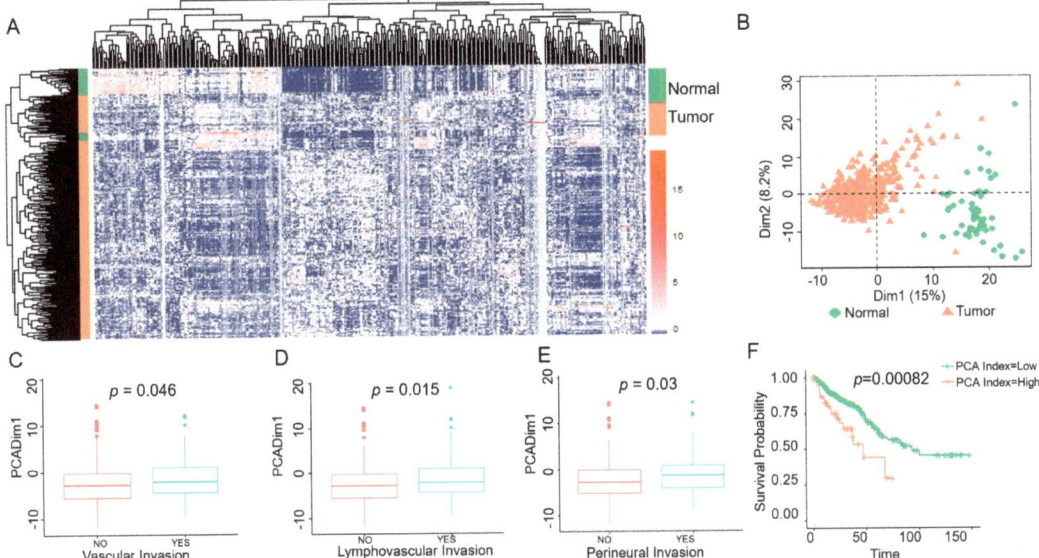

Figure 6. Transcriptional signature for FOXO3-dependent PMNs in human colon cancer. (**A,B**) Hierarchical clustering, shown by heatmap, revealed distinct clusters separated by the PMN-FOXO3$_{389}$ signature differentiating human colon cancer (pink) from matched normal (green) transcriptomes (n = 432, TCGA). PMN-FOXO3$_{389}$ signature on x-axis and human samples on y-axis. PMN-FOXO3$_{389}$ stratify the colon tumor samples from normal. (**C–E**) Increased PMN-FOXO3$_{389}$ signature presence in colon cancer patients is associated with metastasis (lymphovascular invasion, vascular invasion, perineural invasion. (**F**) Increased PMN-FOXO3$_{389}$ signature presence in transcriptomes of colon cancer patients revealed worse overall 5-year survival with a high PCA index score (pink)) compared to low score (green) ($p = 0.00082$).

2.6. FOXO3-Dependent Genes Regulate Metabolic, Inflammatory, and Tumorigenic Processis in PMNs

We identified the top FOXO3 KO-dependent DEGs in PMNs, as shown in the heatmap (Figure 7A) and Table 1. Among these DEGs, we selected for validation genes involved in diverse PMN functions, such as signaling receptors important for their recruitment, adhesion molecules essential for their tissue infiltration and expansion, as well as genes involved in lipid metabolism in PMNs. These DEGs were validated in FOXO3 deficient PMNs (vs. WT) by qPCR (Figure 7B). Specifically, the genes included purinergic receptor P2X 1 (*P2RX1*), which belongs to G-protein-coupled receptors, RalA-binding protein 1 (*RALBP1*), which plays a role in receptor-mediated endocytosis, and melanoma cell adhesion molecule (*MCAM*), as well as cell cycle progression gene 1 (*CCPG1*), which is involved in the immune response to endoplasmic reticulum stress and cyclin-dependent kinase inhibitor 1A (*CDKN1A*). Further, Phospholipase A2 Group VII (*PLA2G7*) is responsible for phospholipid metabolism, and Monoacylglycerol lipase (*MGLL*) catalyzes the conversion of monoacylglycerides to free fatty acids and glycerol. In addition to *MGLL*, adipose triglyceride lipase (*ATGL*) and hormone-sensitive lipase (*HSL*) were lowered in DEGs from FOXO3 KO PMNs (NS). These lipases are responsible for the breakdown of triacylglycerols from LDs [43], suggesting that loss of FOXO3 in PMNs may regulate LDs utilization. These findings establish the importance of FOXO3-mediated gene expression in PMNs that regulate human colonic inflammatory and tumorigenic pathobiology linked to lipid metabolism.

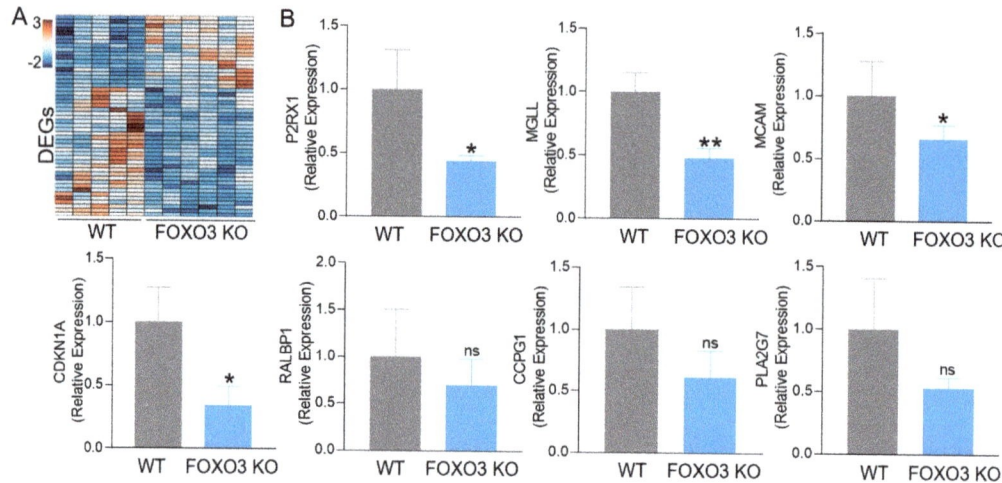

Figure 7. FOXO3-mediated differentially expressed genes in PMNs. (**A**) A heatmap of the top DEGs specific to FOXO3-deficient PMNs relative to control (>|0.5|-fold change, FDR < 0.05). (**B**) Validation of select FOXO3 dependent *P2RX1, MGLL, MCAM, CDKN1A, RALBP1, CCPG1* and *PLA2G7* transcripts in peritoneal PMNs (qPCR, $n = 3$ mice per group, * $p < 0.05$, ** $p < 0.01$, ns = not significant).

Table 1. Differentially expressed genes in FOXO3-deficient mouse PMNs relative to control ($n = 5$–6, FC $\geq |1.5|$, $p < 0.5$).

	Gene	Gene Name	FC	*p*-Value
1	UBE2D2A	Ubiquitin-conjugating enzyme E2D 2A	4.98	8.9×10^{-3}
2	CATSPERE2	Cation channel sperm associated auxiliary subunit epsilon 2	4.77	1.4×10^{-2}
3	LALBA	Lactalbumin alpha	3.58	4.8×10^{-2}
4	DLL3	Delta-like canonical Notch ligand 3	3.31	1.2×10^{-2}
5	ANO2	Anoctamin 2	3.30	4.2×10^{-2}
6	ASCL4	Achaete-scute family bHLH transcription factor 4	3.24	4.9×10^{-2}
7	HIST1H3B	Histone cluster 1, H3b	3.17	2.4×10^{-2}
8	CCDC85A	Coiled-coil domain containing 85A	3.12	1.7×10^{-2}
9	FAM198A	Family with sequence similarity 198 member A	3.05	1.9×10^{-2}
10	CDKL1	Cyclin-dependent kinase-like 1	3.00	2.0×10^{-2}
11	GBP2B	Guanylate binding protein 2b	2.56	3.0×10^{-2}
12	MYRFL	Myelin regulatory factor-like	2.47	5.3×10^{-2}
13	MRAP2	Melanocortin 2 receptor accessory protein 2	2.43	1.6×10^{-2}
14	SYNPO2	Synaptopodin 2	2.37	4.4×10^{-3}
15	RNF183	Ring finger protein 183	2.37	1.4×10^{-2}
16	CACNA1H	Calcium voltage-gated channel subunit alpha1 H	2.35	2.6×10^{-2}
17	DLG2	Discs large MAGUK scaffold protein 2	2.26	4.9×10^{-2}
18	LRIG3	Leucine-rich repeats and immunoglobulin-like domains 3	2.25	5.7×10^{-3}
19	MAP3K19	Mitogen-activated protein kinase kinase kinase 19	2.22	1.7×10^{-2}
20	TECTA	Tectorin alpha	2.14	2.1×10^{-2}
21	CUBN	Cubilin	1.98	1.0×10^{-2}
22	LDHD	Lactate dehydrogenase D	1.92	1.8×10^{-2}
23	IQCN	IQ motif containing N	1.87	4.0×10^{-2}
24	AMD2	S-adenosylmethionine decarboxylase 2	1.82	7.8×10^{-4}
25	SNORD15A	Small nucleolar RNA, C/D box 15A	1.78	2.7×10^{-2}
26	ASTN2	Astrotactin 2	1.67	7.0×10^{-3}

Table 1. Cont.

	Gene	Gene Name	FC	p-Value
27	MIR146	MicroRNA 146	1.65	3.8×10^{-4}
28	GBP11	Guanylate binding protein 11	1.65	4.3×10^{-2}
29	GUCY2C	Guanylate cyclase 2C	1.64	6.0×10^{-6}
30	MDRL	Mitochondrial dynamic related lncRNA	1.59	4.8×10^{-2}
31	ADAMTS13	ADAM metallopeptidase with thrombospondin type 1 motif 13	1.56	4.1×10^{-2}
32	RAPGEF4	Rap guanine nucleotide exchange factor 4	1.56	3.4×10^{-2}
33	STX1A	Syntaxin 1A	1.55	1.0×10^{-2}
34	NECTIN3	Nectin cell adhesion molecule 3	1.54	3.9×10^{-2}
35	SLC22A1	Solute carrier family 22 member 1	1.54	7.1×10^{-3}
36	MEX3A	Mex−3 RNA binding family member A	1.52	5.0×10^{-2}
37	RALBP1	RalA-binding protein 1	−0.44	9.0×10^{-5}
38	CDKN1A	Cyclin-dependent kinase inhibitor 1A	−0.55	1.0×10^{-3}
39	PLA2G7	Phospholipase A2 Group VII	−0.6	1.0×10^{-3}
40	TLR9	Toll Like Receptor 9	−0.8	1.7×10^{-2}
41	CCPG1	Cell cycle progression gene 1	−1.12	2.0×10^{-3}
42	MGLL	Monoacylglycerol lipase	−1.29	3.0×10^{-3}
43	GFI1B	Growth factor independent 1B transcriptional repressor	−1.50	2.1×10^{-3}
44	HGF	Hepatocyte growth factor	−1.52	6.1×10^{-3}
45	BATF2	Basic leucine zipper ATF-like transcription factor 2	−1.52	2.2×10^{-2}
46	P2RX1	Purinergic receptor P2X 1	−1.53	1.4×10^{-3}
47	ZFP469	Zinc finger protein 469	−1.56	1.0×10^{-2}
48	TMEM26	Transmembrane protein 26	−1.56	7.0×10^{-3}
49	HUNK	Hormonally up-regulated Neu-associated kinase	−1.58	2.2×10^{-2}
50	SIGLECF	Sialic acid binding Ig-like lectin F	−1.58	7.4×10^{-3}
51	FAIM2	Fas apoptotic inhibitory molecule 2	−1.59	2.0×10^{-2}
52	MCAM	Melanoma cell adhesion molecule	−1.61	1.9×10^{-3}
53	MYLK3	Myosin light chain kinase 3	−1.62	1.2×10^{-2}
54	IL4	Interleukin 4	−1.65	5.0×10^{-3}
55	CCR3	C-C motif chemokine receptor 3	−1.67	8.4×10^{-3}
56	POM121L2	POM121 transmembrane nucleoporin like 2	−1.85	1.1×10^{-2}
57	PLA2G3	Phospholipase A2 group III	−2.12	7.6×10^{-3}
58	SLC27A2	Solute carrier family 27 member 2	−2.35	3.6×10^{-3}
59	IL13	Interleukin 13	−2.54	5.4×10^{-3}
60	PDK4	Pyruvate dehydrogenase kinase 4	−2.54	1.1×10^{-2}
61	CTSG	Cathepsin G	−2.80	3.3×10^{-3}
62	TNXB	Tenascin XB	−2.85	3.6×10^{-3}
63	VSNL1	Visinin like 1	−3.16	1.7×10^{-2}
64	MPO	Myeloperoxidase	−3.37	2.0×10^{-3}
65	TDG-PS	Thymine DNA glycosylase, pseudogene	−3.38	5.6×10^{-4}
66	BPI	Bactericidal permeability-increasing protein	−3.40	2.2×10^{-2}
67	ELANE	Elastase, neutrophil expressed	−3.54	5.2×10^{-3}
68	CAPN1	Calpain 1	−24.1	1.3×10^{-15}

3. Discussion

Chronic inflammation in IBD, characterized by massive infiltration of PMNs, is associated with increased risk and progression of colon cancer [4–7]. Here, we demonstrated that PMNs promote inflammation and inflammatory tumorigenesis in the colon via the LDs and FOXO3 negative regulatory network. Further, we identified the PMN-FOXO3$_{389}$ transcriptional signature, which is increased in IBD and human colon cancer and is highly significant in their pathobiology. Ultimately, we identified FOXO3-dependent differentially expressed genes in PMNs with roles in metabolism, inflammation, and tumorigenesis. Together, these findings establish a novel mechanism in PMNs involving LDs and FOXO3, driving inflammatory and tumorigenesis processes in the colon.

Aberrant PMN function exacerbates inflammation and tumorigenesis in the colon [8,9,14,38]. In DSS-induced colitis in mice, depletion of PMN leads to lowered inflammation and colitis-associated tumorigenesis [9]. In humans, impaired PMN function during chronic inflammation can promote tumorigenesis, as demonstrated in lung and pancreatic cancer [44–46]. PMNs can also cluster with cancer cells, aiding tumor growth and metastasis [47,48]. Altered lipid metabolism in PMNs is linked to inflammatory conditions. Accumulation of LDs facilitates early innate response to viral infection through modulation of interferon signaling, in part via TLR7 and TLR9 pathways [23,49]. Similarly, our data showed in FOXO3-deficient PMNs increased *TLR9*, suggesting their sensitivity to viral components. Moreover, this LDs and FOXO3-mediated immune sensitivity to infection is shown in FOXO3 KO colon with increased bacterial LPS sensing *TLR4* [35]. Additionally, LDs accumulation in PMNs is accompanied by elevated inflammatory mediators, which in turn promotes PMN activity [22]. Further, increased LDs in PMNs, due to deficiency of adipose triglyceride lipase (ATGL), also increase PMN activity [19]. For instance, in metastatic breast cancer in the lung, reduced ATGL elicits LDs accumulation in PMNs, promoting the invasive capacity of cancer [24]. Moreover, PMNs can release oxidized lipids that reactivate dormant cancer cells and facilitate tumor recurrence [25]. Hence, PMNs with elevated LDs can facilitate inflammatory and tumorigenic processes in various tissue, including the colon.

Moreover, we demonstrated that in PMNs, a negative regulatory network of LDs and FOXO3 might be one of the mechanisms of colonic inflammation and tumorigenesis within IBD and colon cancer. We have previously demonstrated that this regulatory network drives pathobiological processes in human colonic cells [27,29–31]. In mice, global FOXO3 deficiency increases PMNs in the spleen, bone marrow, blood, and colon [35,50]. Similarly, FOXO3 inactivation results in elevated PMNs and aberrant immune response in bronchial epithelia [51]. We speculate that the increased infiltration and elevated transmigration of these PMNs are supported by their FOXO3-dependent metabolic reprogramming. Further, our findings revealed, in FOXO3 deficient PMNs, decreased farnesoid X receptor (FXR; *NR1H4*), a sensor of intracellular bile acid levels. FXR protects against bile acid toxicity, and it is reduced in CD patients [52].

Further, we identified several FOXO3-dependent differentially expressed genes in PMNs involved in metabolism, inflammation, and tumorigenesis. Specifically, *MGLL* is involved in fatty acid metabolism and plays roles in tumorigenesis and metastasis [53]. *P2RX1* is linked to the modulation of microbiota and the alleviation of inflammation in colitis [54]. *PLA2G7*, which is shown to be reduced in FOXO3 KO PMNs, is associated with inflammation [55]. Two other DEGs, *MCAM* and *CDKN1A*, in FOXO3 KO PMNs, are involved in tumorigenesis [56,57]. *RALBP1* has a key effector function in cancer cell survival [58]. Moreover, we found several DEGs in FOXO3 KO PMNS involved in lipid metabolisms linked to LDs utilization. *MGLL*, *ATGL*, and *HSL* lipase, critical for the breakdown of triacylglycerols stored in LDs [43], are decreased in FOXO3 KO PMNs. ATGL deficiency in PMNs leads to increased LDs and hyperactivation [19]. These findings suggest that although FOXO3 deficiency in colonic epithelial cells leads to increased LDs biosynthesis [27,30,31,35], in PMNs, it may lead to increased LDs by lowering their utilization. In addition, the significance of the loss of FOXO3 in driving PMN function is at least multifactorial, and while multiple differentially expressed genes were insignificantly altered, their synergistic effects on the transcriptomic and metabolic remodeling of PMN drive colonic inflammation and tumorigenesis.

One of the hallmarks of IBD is excessive infiltration of PMNs that intensify the inflammatory pathobiology, leading to tumorigenesis [4,5,12,13,15], the mechanisms of which are poorly understood. Here, we showed that PMNs drive colonic inflammation and tumorigenesis by facilitating a self-reinforced LDs and FOXO3 negative regulatory network. Additionally, we demonstrated the significance of this mechanism in both IBD and colon cancer. It is important to highlight that, in addition to LDs and FOXO3 in PMNs, complex processes drive IBD and colonic tumorigenesis that include multiple cells, different pathways, and regulators. Further, this network altered the expression of multiple genes, which, even if insignificant, may orchestrate systemic changes in PMNs functions. As PMNs are highly sensitive cells to multiple stimuli and may initially be protective to infiltrated tissue, it is required to further delineate these mechanisms in context to other cells and regulators. Together, our findings establish an important mechanism that drives PMN activity, bringing us one step closer to solving the complex puzzle of IBD and inflammatory colon cancer.

4. Materials and Methods

4.1. Human IBD and Colon Cancer Samples

Tissue microarray samples included human intestinal tissue representing normal, Inflammatory Bowel Diseases (Ulcerative Colitis and Crohn's Disease), and colon adenocarcinoma with tumor-adjacent colonic mucosa (tissuearray.com LLC). These tissues were obtained from different individuals, males and females, aged 20 to 66 (total $n = 10$, $n = 2$ of each for normal, UC, CD, tumor-adjacent mucosa, and adenocarcinoma).

Publicly available transcriptomes were obtained for control and affected tissue from three different patient cohorts of UC (total $n = 132$; GSE36807, GSE53306, GSE59071) and CD (total $n = 91$; GSE59071, GSE95095, GSE102133). Publicly available transcriptomic data from tumor tissue obtained from three colon cancer patient cohorts (total $n = 162$; GSE141174, GSE8671, GSE9348) were used. Moreover, publicly available transcriptomic data of colon cancer patients, including normal controls, were also utilized ($n = 498$, TCGA). These data were acquired by using NCBI's GEO2R.

4.2. Mice

Mice, strain C57BL/6, male and female, were housed under pathogen-free conditions at Tulane University School of Medicine. Both wild type (WT) and FOXO3 knock-out (FOXO3 KO) mice had free access to a standard chow diet and water. All littermates were genotyped to identify homozygous WT and FOXO3 KO, according to the guidelines of Tulane Institutional Animal Care and Use Committee [34]. Transcriptomic data from the colon of FOXO3 KO and WT mice were acquired as described before ($n = 5$–6 mice per group) [35].

Moreover, publicly available transcriptomes obtained from mice with colonic inflammation ($n = 3$) and dysplasia ($n = 3$) were utilized (GSE31106) [59].

4.3. Histological Analysis

Immunohistostaining against antibody PLIN2 (LS Bio, Seattle, WA, USA) of tissue microarray with samples from IBD and human colon cancer patients was performed by The Pathology Core Laboratory at Tulane University Health Sciences Center as described previously [35]. Images were obtained using the PhenoImager fusion slide scanner (Akoya, Menlo Park, CA, USA) and Phenochart 1.2.0 software. Images were quantified utilizing ImageJ/Fiji 2.1.0 by performing spectrum deconvolution for the separation of DAB (diaminobenzidine) color spectra. The DAB image was then analyzed pixel by pixel for immunohistochemistry quantification.

4.4. Mouse Peritoneal Polymorphonuclear Neutrophils (PMNs)

Experimental mice (six to eight weeks old) were injected intraperitoneally with 1 mL of sterile casein (Sigma, St. Louis, MO, USA) solution, followed by a second injection the next day, which caused a response of peritoneal PMNs [41]. Three hours after the second injection, mouse peritoneal cells were harvested from the abdominal cavity and pelleted ($200 \times g$ for 3 times). Next, PMNs were isolated from the peritoneal fluid using histopaque separation media using a density gradient centrifugation method [40].

4.5. Transmigration Assay

Mice peritoneal PMNs, 10×10^6 cells in assay buffer, HEPES containing 10 mM glucose, 0.1% BSA, pH 7.4, and 1% penicillin/streptomycin, was incubated with oleic acid (OA) (50 µM), for 2 h, and were placed on the top of transwells, an 8 mM pore size polycarbonate filter. In the lower compartments of transwells, 1 mL of the assay media with

N-Formylmethionyl-leucyl-phenylalanine (fMLP) (1 mM) or chemokine KC (29 ng/mL) was added. After 30 min, at 37 °C, assay media from the lower compartment was collected and centrifuged at 400× g for 5 min to assess for migrated PMNs.

4.6. Myeloperoxidase (MPO) Colorimetric Activity Assay

Enzymatic activity of the activated PMN's marker, known as myeloperoxidase (MPO), was quantified in PMNs from WT ($n = 6$) and FOXO3 KO ($n = 6$) mice ($n = 3$ wells per mouse) using MPO Colorimetric Activity Assay Kit according to the manufacturer's protocol (Sigma, St. Louis, MO, USA). Briefly, collected PMN samples were rapidly homogenized in MPO assay buffer and centrifuged at 13,000× g for 10 min at 4 °C to remove insoluble material. These samples were then plated in a 96-well plate, further assessed, and used for colorimetric detection of MPO activity at 412 nm.

4.7. RNA Isolation and cDNA Synthesis

Total RNA from harvested PMNs ($n = 5$–6 mice per group) was isolated using the miRNeasy kit (Zymo Research, Irvine, CA, USA), following the manufacturer's instructions. First, RNA was evaluated for quality using Agilent Bioanalyzer (Agilent Technologies, Santa Clara, CA, USA). Samples having RNA integrity numbers (RIN) of more than 8 were utilized. RNA was then reverse transcribed to cDNA with qScript cDNA Super-Mix (Quantabio, Beverly, MA, USA) and used for qPCR as described previously [35]. The primers used for the amplification of mouse cDNA are as follows: (mP2RX1-FOR 5′-GACAAACCGTCGTCACCTCT-3′, mP2RX1-REV 5′-TCACGTTCACCCTCCCCA-3′, mMGLL-FOR 5′-TTTCCTTCCCTAAGCGGTCG-3′, mMGLL-REV 5′-GGGGTCTTTAGGCC CTGTTT-3′, mMCAM-FOR 5′-CGGGTGTGCCAGGAGAG-3′, mMCAM-REV 5′-GGTTCCT CTGGGGCTTTGAA-3′, mCDKN1A-FOR 5′-GCAGAATAAAAGGTGCCACAGG-3′, mCDKN1A-REV 5′-AGAGTGCAAGACAGCGACAA-3′, mRALBP1-FOR 5′-CTCGTCCTGTTCTGTCCC AA-3′, mRALBP1-REV 5′-ACCTATCCATTACACCAGTGCC-3′, mCCPG1-FOR 5′-AGAAA GCAGCGCAAACAACA-3′, mCCPG1-REV 5′-CTAGGCTGAGATGAAAAGACGGG-3′, mPLA2G7-FOR 5′-TCCCTGGAGCTAGTGTTGTG-3′, mPLA2G7-REV 5′-TGGCTTCAGTTT GATGTTCTGGT-3′. The comparative Ct method was used to determine mRNA expression with actin as a housekeeping control. cDNA was quantified using the C1000 Thermal Cycler system (Bio-Rad, Hercules, CA, USA) and PerfeCTa SYBR Green FastMix (Quantabio, Beverly, MA, USA).

4.8. RNA Sequencing and Differential Expression Testing

RNA sequencing (RNAseq) was performed as described previously [35]. Sequencing data are submitted in NCBI's Sequence Read Archive and are available under GSE234072 study accession number. Transcriptomic analysis for RNAseq was performed using Ingenuity Pathway Analysis (IPA) (Qiagen, Germantown, MD, USA). Differentially expressed genes (DEGs) with an expression threshold of >|0.5|-fold change relative to control and a false discovery rate (FDR) of less than 0.05 were evaluated in IPA. Clustered heatmaps of z-scaled transcripts per million (TPM) values for the top DEGs across all samples were obtained using a Python data visualization package (Seaborn v0.12.0).

4.9. Hierarchical Clustering

Hierarchical clustering of transcriptomes among experimental groups was performed using an uncentered correlation as a symmetric matrix, as described before [28].

4.10. Principal Component Analysis

Principal component analysis (PCA) of FOXO3-deficient PMNs' signatures with IBD (GSE4183) and human colon cancer (TCGA) transcriptomes was performed with the FactoMineR R package with the PCA function, as described before [28].

4.11. Statistical Analysis

All results are represented as mean ± SD. The statistical analysis of experiments was carried out by Student's unpaired *t*-test or through ANOVA for one-way analysis of variance in Graph Pad Software. A *p*-value of <0.05 was considered significant.

Author Contributions: Conceptualization, S.D.S.; methodology, J.G., R.I. and H.M.P.; software, E.R.; validation, J.G. and P.S.; formal analysis, J.G. and S.D.S.; investigation, J.G., R.I. and H.M.P.; resources, S.D.S.; data curation, S.D.S., J.G. and R.I.; writing—original draft preparation, J.G. and S.D.S.; writing—review and editing, S.D.S., J.G. and P.S.; visualization, S.D.S. and J.G.; supervision, S.D.S.; project administration, S.D.S.; funding acquisition, S.D.S. All authors have read and agreed to the published version of the manuscript.

Funding: This work is supported by NIH R01 (CA252055) and the Crohn's & Colitis Foundation (663445).

Institutional Review Board Statement: The study was conducted according to the guidelines approved by the Institutional Review Board (or Ethics Committee) of Tulane University (Protocol number 867, approved on 25 August 2021).

Informed Consent Statement: Patient consent was waived because the tissue array was commercially obtained and the transcriptomes were publicly available.

Data Availability Statement: The data presented in this study are available on request from the corresponding author. RNA sequencing of experimental PMNs will be submitted to NCBI's Archive to be publicly available.

Conflicts of Interest: The authors declare no conflict of interest. The funders had no role in the design of the study; in the collection, analyses, or interpretation of data; in the writing of the manuscript, or in the decision to publish the results.

References

1. Guan, Q. A Comprehensive Review and Update on the Pathogenesis of Inflammatory Bowel Disease. *J. Immunol. Res.* **2019**, *2019*, 7247238. [CrossRef] [PubMed]
2. Baumgart, D.C.; Carding, S.R. Inflammatory bowel disease: Cause and immunobiology. *Lancet* **2007**, *369*, 1627–1640. [CrossRef]
3. Zhang, Y.-Z. Inflammatory bowel disease: Pathogenesis. *World J. Gastroenterol.* **2014**, *20*, 91. [CrossRef] [PubMed]
4. Zhou, G.X.; Liu, Z.J. Potential roles of neutrophils in regulating intestinal mucosal inflammation of inflammatory bowel disease. *J. Dig. Dis.* **2017**, *18*, 495–503. [CrossRef] [PubMed]
5. Fournier, B.M.; Parkos, C.A. The role of neutrophils during intestinal inflammation. *Mucosal Immunol.* **2012**, *5*, 354–366. [CrossRef] [PubMed]
6. Kim, E.R. Colorectal cancer in inflammatory bowel disease: The risk, pathogenesis, prevention and diagnosis. *World J. Gastroenterol.* **2014**, *20*, 9872. [CrossRef] [PubMed]
7. Lakatos, P.L.; Lakatos, L. Risk for colorectal cancer in ulcerative colitis: Changes, causes and management strategies. *World J. Gastroenterol.* **2008**, *14*, 3937. [CrossRef]
8. Mazaki, J.; Katsumata, K.; Kasahara, K.; Tago, T.; Wada, T.; Kuwabara, H.; Enomoto, M.; Ishizaki, T.; Nagakawa, Y.; Tsuchida, A. Neutrophil-to-lymphocyte ratio is a prognostic factor for colon cancer: A propensity score analysis. *BMC Cancer* **2020**, *20*, 922. [CrossRef]
9. Wang, Y.; Wang, K.; Han, G.-C.; Wang, R.-X.; Xiao, H.; Hou, C.-M.; Guo, R.-F.; Dou, Y.; Shen, B.-F.; Li, Y.; et al. Neutrophil infiltration favors colitis-associated tumorigenesis by activating the interleukin-1 (IL-1)/IL-6 axis. *Mucosal Immunol.* **2014**, *7*, 1106–1115. [CrossRef]
10. Kraus, R.F.; Gruber, M.A. Neutrophils-From Bone Marrow to First-Line Defense of the Innate Immune System. *Front. Immunol.* **2021**, *12*, 767175. [CrossRef]
11. Borregaard, N. Neutrophils, from Marrow to Microbes. *Immunity* **2010**, *33*, 657–670. [CrossRef] [PubMed]
12. Chen, H.; Wu, X.; Xu, C.; Lin, J.; Liu, Z. Dichotomous roles of neutrophils in modulating pathogenic and repair processes of inflammatory bowel diseases. *Precis Clin. Med.* **2021**, *4*, 246–257. [CrossRef] [PubMed]
13. Wéra, O.; Lancellotti, P.; Oury, C. The Dual Role of Neutrophils in Inflammatory Bowel Diseases. *J. Clin. Med.* **2016**, *5*, 118. [CrossRef] [PubMed]
14. Bui, T.M.; Butin-Israeli, V.; Wiesolek, H.L.; Zhou, M.; Rehring, J.F.; Wiesmuller, L.; Wu, J.D.; Yang, G.Y.; Hanauer, S.B.; Sebag, J.A.; et al. Neutrophils Alter DNA Repair Landscape to Impact Survival and Shape Distinct Therapeutic Phenotypes of Colorectal Cancer. *Gastroenterology* **2021**, *161*, 225–238.e15. [CrossRef] [PubMed]

15. Canli, Ö.; Nicolas, A.M.; Gupta, J.; Finkelmeier, F.; Goncharova, O.; Pesic, M.; Neumann, T.; Horst, D.; Löwer, M.; Sahin, U.; et al. Myeloid Cell-Derived Reactive Oxygen Species Induce Epithelial Mutagenesis. *Cancer Cell* **2017**, *32*, 869–883.e5. [CrossRef] [PubMed]
16. Tlaskalová-Hogenová, H.; Štěpánková, R.; Kozáková, H.; Hudcovic, T.; Vannucci, L.; Tučková, L.; Rossmann, P.; Hrnčíř, T.; Kverka, M.; Zákostelská, Z.; et al. The role of gut microbiota (commensal bacteria) and the mucosal barrier in the pathogenesis of inflammatory and autoimmune diseases and cancer: Contribution of germ-free and gnotobiotic animal models of human diseases. *Cell. Mol. Immunol.* **2011**, *8*, 110–120. [CrossRef]
17. Michielan, A.; D'Incà, R. Intestinal Permeability in Inflammatory Bowel Disease: Pathogenesis, Clinical Evaluation, and Therapy of Leaky Gut. *Mediat. Inflamm.* **2015**, *2015*, 628157. [CrossRef]
18. Zhang, W.; Xu, L.; Zhu, L.; Liu, Y.; Yang, S.; Zhao, M. Lipid Droplets, the Central Hub Integrating Cell Metabolism and the Immune System. *Front Physiol* **2021**, *12*, 746749. [CrossRef]
19. Schlager, S.; Goeritzer, M.; Jandl, K.; Frei, R.; Vujic, N.; Kolb, D.; Strohmaier, H.; Dorow, J.; Eichmann, T.O.; Rosenberger, A.; et al. Adipose triglyceride lipase acts on neutrophil lipid droplets to regulate substrate availability for lipid mediator synthesis. *J. Leukoc. Biol.* **2015**, *98*, 837–850. [CrossRef]
20. Jiang, J.; Tu, H.; Li, P. Lipid metabolism and neutrophil function. *Cell. Immunol.* **2022**, *377*, 104546. [CrossRef]
21. Bozza, P.T.; Magalhães, K.G.; Weller, P.F. Leukocyte lipid bodies—Biogenesis and functions in inflammation. *Biochim. Et Biophys. Acta (BBA)-Mol. Cell Biol. Lipids* **2009**, *1791*, 540–551. [CrossRef] [PubMed]
22. Monson, E.A.; Crosse, K.M.; Duan, M.; Chen, W.; O'Shea, R.D.; Wakim, L.M.; Carr, J.M.; Whelan, D.R.; Helbig, K.J. Intracellular lipid droplet accumulation occurs early following viral infection and is required for an efficient interferon response. *Nat. Commun.* **2021**, *12*, 4303. [CrossRef] [PubMed]
23. Monson, E.A.; Crosse, K.M.; Das, M.; Helbig, K.J. Lipid droplet density alters the early innate immune response to viral infection. *PLoS ONE* **2018**, *13*, e0190597. [CrossRef] [PubMed]
24. Li, P.; Lu, M.; Shi, J.; Gong, Z.; Hua, L.; Li, Q.; Lim, B.; Zhang, X.H.-F.; Chen, X.; Li, S.; et al. Lung mesenchymal cells elicit lipid storage in neutrophils that fuel breast cancer lung metastasis. *Nat. Immunol.* **2020**, *21*, 1444–1455. [CrossRef] [PubMed]
25. Perego, M.; Tyurin, V.A.; Tyurina, Y.Y.; Yellets, J.; Nacarelli, T.; Lin, C.; Nefedova, Y.; Kossenkov, A.; Liu, Q.; Sreedhar, S.; et al. Reactivation of dormant tumor cells by modified lipids derived from stress-activated neutrophils. *Sci. Transl. Med.* **2020**, *12*, eabb5817. [CrossRef]
26. Accioly, M.T.; Pacheco, P.; Maya-Monteiro, C.M.; Carrossini, N.; Robbs, B.K.; Oliveira, S.S.; Kaufmann, C.; Morgado-Diaz, J.A.; Bozza, P.T.; Viola, J.P. Lipid bodies are reservoirs of cyclooxygenase-2 and sites of prostaglandin-E2 synthesis in colon cancer cells. *Cancer Res.* **2008**, *68*, 1732–1740. [CrossRef] [PubMed]
27. Heller, S.; Cable, C.; Penrose, H.; Makboul, R.; Biswas, D.; Cabe, M.; Crawford, S.E.; Savkovic, S.D. Intestinal inflammation requires FOXO3 and prostaglandin E2-dependent lipogenesis and elevated lipid droplets. *Am. J. Physiol. Gastrointest Liver Physiol.* **2016**, *310*, G844–G854. [CrossRef] [PubMed]
28. Iftikhar, R.; Penrose, H.M.; King, A.N.; Kim, Y.; Ruiz, E.; Kandil, E.; Machado, H.L.; Savkovic, S.D. FOXO3 Expression in Macrophages Is Lowered by a High-Fat Diet and Regulates Colonic Inflammation and Tumorigenesis. *Metabolites* **2022**, *12*, 250. [CrossRef]
29. Penrose, H.; Heller, S.; Cable, C.; Makboul, R.; Chadalawada, G.; Chen, Y.; Crawford, S.E.; Savkovic, S.D. Epidermal growth factor receptor mediated proliferation depends on increased lipid droplet density regulated via a negative regulatory loop with FOXO3/Sirtuin6. *Biochem. Biophys. Res. Commun.* **2016**, *469*, 370–376. [CrossRef]
30. Qi, W.; Fitchev, P.S.; Cornwell, M.L.; Greenberg, J.; Cabe, M.; Weber, C.R.; Roy, H.K.; Crawford, S.E.; Savkovic, S.D. FOXO3 growth inhibition of colonic cells is dependent on intraepithelial lipid droplet density. *J. Biol. Chem.* **2013**, *288*, 16274–16281. [CrossRef]
31. Iftikhar, R.; Penrose, H.M.; King, A.N.; Samudre, J.S.; Collins, M.E.; Hartono, A.B.; Lee, S.B.; Lau, F.; Baddoo, M.; Flemington, E.F.; et al. Elevated ATGL in colon cancer cells and cancer stem cells promotes metabolic and tumorigenic reprogramming reinforced by obesity. *Oncogenesis* **2021**, *10*, 82. [CrossRef] [PubMed]
32. Zhang, K.; Li, L.; Qi, Y.; Zhu, X.; Gan, B.; DePinho, R.A.; Averitt, T.; Guo, S. Hepatic suppression of Foxo1 and Foxo3 causes hypoglycemia and hyperlipidemia in mice. *Endocrinology* **2012**, *153*, 631–646. [CrossRef] [PubMed]
33. Bullock, M.D.; Bruce, A.; Sreekumar, R.; Curtis, N.; Cheung, T.; Reading, I.; Primrose, J.N.; Ottensmeier, C.; Packham, G.K.; Thomas, G.; et al. FOXO3 expression during colorectal cancer progression: Biomarker potential reflects a tumour suppressor role. *Br. J. Cancer* **2013**, *109*, 387–394. [CrossRef] [PubMed]
34. Lin, L.; Hron, J.D.; Peng, S.L. Regulation of NF-κB, Th Activation, and Autoinflammation by the Forkhead Transcription Factor Foxo3a. *Immunity* **2004**, *21*, 203–213. [CrossRef] [PubMed]
35. Penrose, H.M.; Cable, C.; Heller, S.; Ungerleider, N.; Nakhoul, H.; Baddoo, M.; Hartono, A.B.; Lee, S.B.; Burow, M.E.; Flemington, E.F.; et al. Loss of Forkhead Box O3 Facilitates Inflammatory Colon Cancer: Transcriptome Profiling of the Immune Landscape and Novel Targets. *Cell. Mol. Gastroenterol. Hepatol.* **2019**, *7*, 391–408. [CrossRef] [PubMed]
36. Savkovic, S.D. Decreased FOXO3 within advanced human colon cancer: Implications of tumour suppressor function. *Br. J. Cancer* **2013**, *109*, 297–298. [CrossRef] [PubMed]
37. Lee, J.C.; Espeli, M.; Anderson, C.A.; Linterman, M.A.; Pocock, J.M.; Williams, N.J.; Roberts, R.; Viatte, S.; Fu, B.; Peshu, N.; et al. Human SNP Links Differential Outcomes in Inflammatory and Infectious Disease to a FOXO3-Regulated Pathway. *Cell* **2013**, *155*, 57–69. [CrossRef] [PubMed]

38. Mizuno, R.; Kawada, K.; Itatani, Y.; Ogawa, R.; Kiyasu, Y.; Sakai, Y. The Role of Tumor-Associated Neutrophils in Colorectal Cancer. *Int. J. Mol. Sci.* **2019**, *20*, 529. [CrossRef]
39. Muthas, D.; Reznichenko, A.; Balendran, C.A.; Böttcher, G.; Clausen, I.G.; Kärrman Mårdh, C.; Ottosson, T.; Uddin, M.; Macdonald, T.T.; Danese, S.; et al. Neutrophils in ulcerative colitis: A review of selected biomarkers and their potential therapeutic implications. *Scand. J. Gastroenterol.* **2017**, *52*, 125–135. [CrossRef]
40. Swamydas, M.; Luo, Y.; Dorf, M.E.; Lionakis, M.S. Isolation of Mouse Neutrophils. *Curr. Protoc. Immunol.* **2015**, *110*, 3–20. [CrossRef]
41. Van Epps, D.E.; Bankhurst, A.D.; Williams, R.C. Casein-mediated neutrophil chemotaxis. *Inflammation* **1977**, *2*, 115–123. [CrossRef] [PubMed]
42. Snoeks, L.; Weber, C.R.; Wasland, K.; Turner, J.R.; Vainder, C.; Qi, W.; Savkovic, S.D. Tumor suppressor FOXO3 participates in the regulation of intestinal inflammation. *Lab. Investig.* **2009**, *89*, 1053–1062. [CrossRef] [PubMed]
43. Grabner, G.F.; Xie, H.; Schweiger, M.; Zechner, R. Lipolysis: Cellular mechanisms for lipid mobilization from fat stores. *Nat. Metab.* **2021**, *3*, 1445–1465. [CrossRef] [PubMed]
44. Hedrick, C.C.; Malanchi, I. Neutrophils in cancer: Heterogeneous and multifaceted. *Nat. Rev. Immunol.* **2022**, *22*, 173–187. [CrossRef] [PubMed]
45. Di Mitri, D.; Toso, A.; Chen, J.J.; Sarti, M.; Pinton, S.; Jost, T.R.; D'Antuono, R.; Montani, E.; Garcia-Escudero, R.; Guccini, I.; et al. Tumour-infiltrating Gr-1+ myeloid cells antagonize senescence in cancer. *Nature* **2014**, *515*, 134–137. [CrossRef]
46. Houghton, A.M.; Rzymkiewicz, D.M.; Ji, H.; Gregory, A.D.; Egea, E.E.; Metz, H.E.; Stolz, D.B.; Land, S.R.; Marconcini, L.A.; Kliment, C.R.; et al. Neutrophil elastase–mediated degradation of IRS-1 accelerates lung tumor growth. *Nat. Med.* **2010**, *16*, 219–223. [CrossRef]
47. Szczerba, B.M.; Castro-Giner, F.; Vetter, M.; Krol, I.; Gkountela, S.; Landin, J.; Scheidmann, M.C.; Donato, C.; Scherrer, R.; Singer, J.; et al. Neutrophils escort circulating tumour cells to enable cell cycle progression. *Nature* **2019**, *566*, 553–557. [CrossRef]
48. Iriondo, O.; Yu, M. Unexpected Friendship: Neutrophils Help Tumor Cells En Route to Metastasis. *Dev. Cell* **2019**, *49*, 308–310. [CrossRef]
49. Saitoh, T.; Satoh, T.; Yamamoto, N.; Uematsu, S.; Takeuchi, O.; Kawai, T.; Akira, S. Antiviral Protein Viperin Promotes Toll-like Receptor 7- and Toll-like Receptor 9-Mediated Type I Interferon Production in Plasmacytoid Dendritic Cells. *Immunity* **2011**, *34*, 352–363. [CrossRef]
50. Kang, H.; Corr, M.; Mansson, R.; Welinder, E.; Hedrick, S.M.; Stone, E.L. Loss of Murine FOXO3 in Cells of the Myeloid Lineage Enhances Myelopoiesis but Protects from K/BxN-Serum Transfer-Induced Arthritis. *PLoS ONE* **2015**, *10*, e0126728. [CrossRef]
51. Di Vincenzo, S.; Heijink, I.H.; Noordhoek, J.A.; Cipollina, C.; Siena, L.; Bruno, A.; Ferraro, M.; Postma, D.S.; Gjomarkaj, M.; Pace, E. SIRT1/FoxO3 axis alteration leads to aberrant immune responses in bronchial epithelial cells. *J. Cell. Mol. Med.* **2018**, *22*, 2272–2282. [CrossRef] [PubMed]
52. Vavassori, P.; Mencarelli, A.; Renga, B.; Distrutti, E.; Fiorucci, S. The bile acid receptor FXR is a modulator of intestinal innate immunity. *J. Immunol.* **2009**, *183*, 6251–6261. [CrossRef] [PubMed]
53. Zhang, J.; Song, Y.; Shi, Q.; Fu, L. Research progress on FASN and MGLL in the regulation of abnormal lipid metabolism and the relationship between tumor invasion and metastasis. *Front. Med.* **2021**, *15*, 649–656. [CrossRef] [PubMed]
54. Wang, X.; Yuan, X.; Su, Y.; Hu, J.; Ji, Q.; Fu, S.; Li, R.; Hu, L.; Dai, C. Targeting Purinergic Receptor P2RX1 Modulates Intestinal Microbiota and Alleviates Inflammation in Colitis. *Front. Immunol.* **2021**, *12*, 696766. [CrossRef] [PubMed]
55. Candels, L.S.; Becker, S.; Trautwein, C. PLA2G7: A new player in shaping energy metabolism and lifespan. *Signal Transduct. Target. Ther.* **2022**, *7*, 195. [CrossRef] [PubMed]
56. Kramer, H.B.; Lai, C.F.; Patel, H.; Periyasamy, M.; Lin, M.L.; Feller, S.M.; Fuller-Pace, F.V.; Meek, D.W.; Ali, S.; Buluwela, L. LRH-1 drives colon cancer cell growth by repressing the expression of the CDKN1A gene in a p53-dependent manner. *Nucleic Acids Res.* **2016**, *44*, 582–594. [CrossRef] [PubMed]
57. Wu, Z.; Wu, Z.; Li, J.; Yang, X.; Wang, Y.; Yu, Y.; Ye, J.; Xu, C.; Qin, W.; Zhang, Z. MCAM is a novel metastasis marker and regulates spreading, apoptosis and invasion of ovarian cancer cells. *Tumor Biol.* **2012**, *33*, 1619–1628. [CrossRef]
58. Mollberg, N.; Steinert, G.; Aigner, M.; Hamm, A.; Lin, F.-J.; Elbers, H.; Reissfelder, C.; Weitz, J.; Buchler, M.W.; Koch, M. Overexpression of RalBP1 in colorectal cancer is an independent predictor of poor survival and early tumor relapse. *Cancer Biol. Ther.* **2012**, *13*, 694–700. [CrossRef]
59. Tang, A.; Li, N.; Li, X.; Yang, H.; Wang, W.; Zhang, L.; Li, G.; Xiong, W.; Ma, J.; Shen, S. Dynamic activation of the key pathways: Linking colitis to colorectal cancer in a mouse model. *Carcinogenesis* **2012**, *33*, 1375–1383. [CrossRef]

Disclaimer/Publisher's Note: The statements, opinions and data contained in all publications are solely those of the individual author(s) and contributor(s) and not of MDPI and/or the editor(s). MDPI and/or the editor(s) disclaim responsibility for any injury to people or property resulting from any ideas, methods, instructions or products referred to in the content.

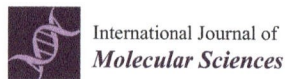

Review

Claudin Barriers on the Brink: How Conflicting Tissue and Cellular Priorities Drive IBD Pathogenesis

Christopher T. Capaldo

College of Natural and Computer Sciences, Hawai'i Pacific University, Honolulu, HI 96813, USA; ccapaldo@hpu.edu

Abstract: Inflammatory bowel diseases (IBDs) are characterized by acute or chronic recurring inflammation of the intestinal mucosa, often with increasing severity over time. Life-long morbidities and diminishing quality of life for IBD patients compel a search for a better understanding of the molecular contributors to disease progression. One unifying feature of IBDs is the failure of the gut to form an effective barrier, a core role for intercellular complexes called tight junctions. In this review, the claudin family of tight junction proteins are discussed as they are a fundamental component of intestinal barriers. Importantly, claudin expression and/or protein localization is altered in IBD, leading to the supposition that intestinal barrier dysfunction exacerbates immune hyperactivity and disease. Claudins are a large family of transmembrane structural proteins that constrain the passage of ions, water, or substances between cells. However, growing evidence suggests non-canonical claudin functions during mucosal homeostasis and healing after injury. Therefore, whether claudins participate in adaptive or pathological IBD responses remains an open question. By reviewing current studies, the possibility is assessed that with claudins, a jack-of-all-trades is master of none. Potentially, a robust claudin barrier and wound restitution involve conflicting biophysical phenomena, exposing barrier vulnerabilities and a tissue-wide frailty during healing in IBD.

Keywords: claudin; tight junctions; barrier function; gut; colitis; inflammatory bowel disease; ZO-1; actin; cell migration; cell division

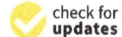

Citation: Capaldo, C.T. Claudin Barriers on the Brink: How Conflicting Tissue and Cellular Priorities Drive IBD Pathogenesis. *Int. J. Mol. Sci.* **2023**, *24*, 8562. https://doi.org/10.3390/ijms24108562

Academic Editor: Susanne M. Krug

Received: 31 March 2023
Revised: 8 May 2023
Accepted: 9 May 2023
Published: 10 May 2023

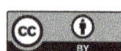

Copyright: © 2023 by the author. Licensee MDPI, Basel, Switzerland. This article is an open access article distributed under the terms and conditions of the Creative Commons Attribution (CC BY) license (https://creativecommons.org/licenses/by/4.0/).

1. Barrier Loss in IBD

Inflammatory bowel diseases (IBDs) encompass Crohn's disease (CD) and ulcerative colitis (UC). Both diseases are progressive, characterized by abdominal pain, diarrhea, occult blood in the stool, anemia, and weight loss, incurring significant lifelong morbidities and decreased quality of life for patients [1,2]. IBDs have unclear etiologies and are believed to be initiated by genetic abnormalities combined with environmental factors such as diet and smoking. While the primary causes of IBDs are unclear, a maladaptive inflammatory response to enteric bacteria and/or mucosal barrier dysfunction have been implicated in disease initiation. Early studies of IBD pathogenesis demonstrated penetration of small tracer molecules in IBD patients when compared with healthy relatives, indicating some degree of intestinal barrier loss [3–5]. More recently, genome-wide association studies (GWAS) identified a host of genes linked to IBD, many of which are involved in either maintenance of the mucus barrier or epithelial integrity [6–8]. This has led to the supposition that a subset of IBD patients likely have an intestinal barrier deficiency as a root cause of their disease [1–3]. Furthermore, aberrant inflammation is known to compromise the mucosal barrier. Therefore, the inability to maintain an effective barrier to luminal antigens is a unifying pathological feature of IBDs, regardless of initiating events [9–11]. Such studies add support to calls for increased attention to the development of therapies aimed at supporting mucosal barrier integrity to resolve IBD [1,4–6].

IBD-associated barrier dysfunction falls into two categories, loss of the barrier or degradation of the barrier quality. For example, barrier failure would be expected in highly ulcerated regions due to epithelial cell loss. This should be contrasted with increased leak, which refers to a decrease in the ability of the epithelial cells to exclude disease causing luminal antigens [7,8]. Studies in animal models of colitis suggest bacterial products induce IBD, including lipopolysaccharides, N-formyl-L-methionyl-L-leucyl-L-phenylalanine (fMLP), and flagellin [12–15]. However, the role of barrier leak in IBD initiation and progression remains in question given our understanding of immune tolerance mechanisms and some conflicting evidence provided by laboratory models of colitis (reviewed here [16]). This review attempts to bring some clarity by discussing the functions of the claudin family of transmembrane proteins. Claudins act within tight junction structures to regulate material passage through the paracellular space (see Figure 1). The ability of claudins to regulate barrier permeability comes in large part through complex differential gene expression. Importantly, claudin expression and localization are altered in IBD, and these alterations are believed to play a role in IBD pathogenesis [17–21].

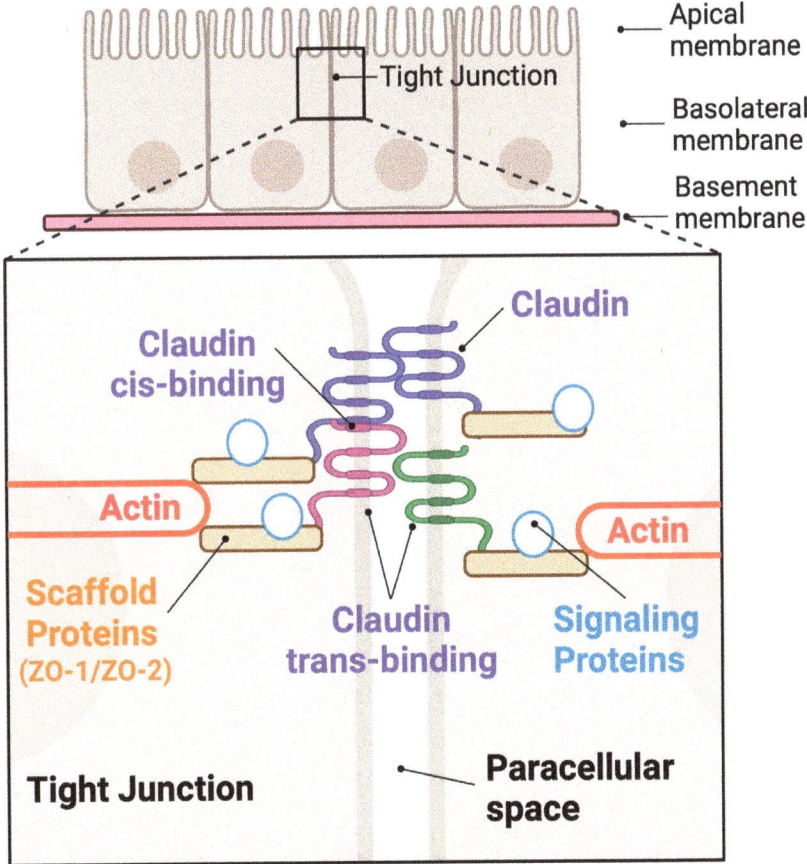

Figure 1. Schematic showing tight junction localization in an epithelial monolayer. Paracellular claudin proteins form both cis and trans interactions, thereby sealing the paracellular space. Claudins anchor scaffolding and signaling proteins at the junction. Scaffolds also connect the claudins to the actin network.

2. Claudin Expression in Health and Disease

Claudins are required components of intercellular tight junctions: multiprotein structures that occlude the paracellular space and prevent antigens from the gut lumen penetrating into the body. In most studies, tight junction complexity correlates strongly with "tight" barrier function in a number of tissues [22–24]. With a "tight" barrier characterized by limited antigen and/or ion penetration. Claudin-based tight junctions have a number of canonical functions in intestinal tissues: they physically occlude the paracellular space, create ion pores between cells, and maintain cell polarity [9]. Of these, the antigen barrier function of junctions is the best connected to IBD pathogenesis. Ion dysregulation correlates with disease but has not been directly linked to IBD, and cell polarity defects are thought to be involved in later stage IBD-linked carcinogenesis [4,10,11]. Therefore, a distinction has been made in discussing the quality of epithelial barrier regulation with regard to ion permeability (pore pathway) and antigen leak (leak pathway) [25]. Both categories of barrier function relate to claudin expression, with claudin isoform expression linked to solute size and charge restricted paracellular flux. Indeed, claudins 2, 7, 10, 15, 16, and 19 have all been shown to form ion pores within the junction [26,27]. Claudins exhibit differential capacity for antigen exclusion as well, although the molecular details are less apparent than for ion pore formation. For example, claudins 3 and 4 have inverse effects on material flux when overexpressed in alveolar cells [28]. Additionally, mice transgenically modified to express claudin 2 in the gut show increased mucosal penetration of small molecule tracers [12].

Under physiological conditions, claudins show dramatic spatial diversity in the gut, with differential claudin expression in the stomach, small intestine, and colon [13]. Additionally, claudin gene expression varies within intestinal tissues. For example, in the colon, ion pore forming "leaky" claudins are restricted to the crypt base (2, 5, 10, and 15), whereas "tight" sealing claudins accumulate near the surface of the lumen (3, 4, 7, and 23) (Figure 2). Current theories of IBD development hold that inflammation increases gut leakiness in part through alterations in claudin expression and, therefore, barrier function [10]. This leakiness increases the probability that gut antigens will penetrate into the body, further perpetuate inflammation, and exacerbate disease. RNAseq studies of UC and CD patient biopsies revealed altered claudin levels, with increases in claudins 1, 2, and 18 and decreases in 3, 4, 5, 7, 8, and 12 (reviewed in [14], Figure 2). Recent single-cell RNAseq surveys and antibody-based techniques largely confirm these findings, ameliorating concerns that patient biopsies contain a confounding mix of cell types [15]. In general, these changes represent an increase in pore-forming "leaky" claudins and a decrease in sealing claudins. Indeed, increased claudin 2 is commonly found in inflamed tissues and frequently corelates with increased disease severity [17,29]. Importantly, claudin expression is disturbed during inflammatory episodes, driven in part by exposure of mucosal cells to proinflammatory cytokines [18]. Cytokines such as Tumor Necrosis Factor Alpha (TNF-α) and Interferon Gamma (IFN-γ) are considered key drivers of a degradative feedback system. Indeed, these cytokines are commonly found in inflamed IBD patient samples and are known to lead to claudin switching (e.g., replacement of "tight" claudins with "leaky" ones) and tight junction re-structuring [19–21]. Indeed, a host of cytokines that are elevated in IBD have been shown to alter epithelial barrier as well as claudin levels in vitro (reviewed [14,18]). These studies provide abundant evidence that claudin switching in IBD is secondary to proinflammatory cytokine production. In theory, this switching leads to a subsequent increase in antigen leak, further increasing cytokine production.

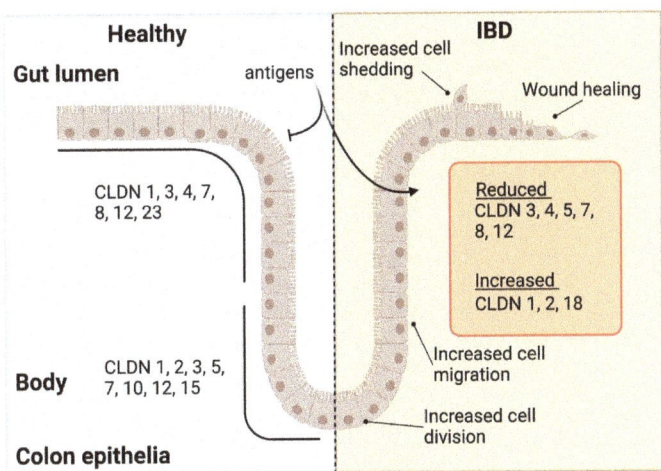

Figure 2. Claudin expression changes in IBD. Claudins are differentially expressed within healthy colonic epithelia. This distribution changes in IBD are coincident with increased antigen flux, cell proliferation, cell migration, cell shedding, and wound healing processes.

Just such a feedback loop is illustrated by studies in claudin-knockout mice (reviewed in [22,23]). Claudin-7-knockout mice experience antigen leak from the gut and succumb to severe spontaneous lethal colitis soon after birth [24,30]. Lethality in this model was secondary to the presence of intestinal microflora and at minimum, the bacterial antigen N-formyl-L-methionyl-L-leucyl-L-phenylalanine (fMLP). These studies clearly demonstrate the potential of a leaky gut as an initiator of severe colitis. However, not all claudins protect against colitis, as demonstrated by claudin 7 deletion. For example, colitis resistance was shown in mice transgenically modified to produce high levels of claudin 2, presenting the possibility that the increased claudin 2 levels found in human disease are beneficial [12]. Indeed, claudin 2 was shown to be protective in chemically induced and pathogen-induced colitis but not in immune-mediated T-cell-transfer-induced colitis [12,31,32]. In this later study, Raju et al. show increased disease in animals where colitis is induced by an overactive immune response; high claudin 2 levels exacerbate disease, whereas claudin 2 deletion is beneficial [32]. Therefore, even after intense study with sophisticated tools, there remains an unclear distinction between potentially beneficial claudin responses and pathobiological ones. The question remains: are changes in claudin part of natural wound repair or part of the pathobiology of IBD?

3. Claudin Family Proteins and the Hierarchy of Tight Junction Structure

Given the centrality of claudin proteins in constricting the paracellular space against antigens, extensive structural/functional studies have been pursued that may help resolve this conundrum. Claudins, first discovered by Furuse et al., are small transmembrane proteins that act at intercellular tight junctions to seal adjacent cells together [33]. The claudin gene family is large, with around 27 known members, producing proteins of a stereotyped domain structure [27,34]. All claudins have three functionally distinct protein domains (see Figure 1 [35]). Firstly, extracellular loop domains protrude from the plasma membrane into the paracellular space, allowing for interactions with claudins on adjacent cells (trans-binding). Trans interactions of extracellular loop domains for a given claudin pair are functionally important and are responsible for either sealing the paracellular space or, with select claudin pairings, creating an ion pore [36,37]. For example, a claudin 2-claudin 2 pairing across the paracellular space produces a sodium pore, whereas claudin 3 pairs do not [38,39]. Second, claudins contain four plasma membrane spanning domains that facilitate stability within the membrane. Interactions between claudins within both plasma membranes (cis binding) combined with trans interactions allow for self-assembly into strands: claudin oligomers so large that they form circumnavigating fibrils embedded in the membrane [40,41]. This strand formation is a requirement for all tight junction core functions listed above. Lastly, cytoplasmic-facing claudin domains bind to a host of scaffolding proteins and, through them, to both the actin cytoskeleton and intercellular signaling proteins. Almost all claudin C-terminal domains contain PDZ motifs (PSD95 (postsynaptic density protein), Dlg1 (*Drosophila* disc large tumor suppressor), and ZO-1 (zonula occludens-1 protein) or PDZ) that stabilize PDZ-domain-containing scaffolding proteins [42,43]. The number and diversity of potential cytoplasmic interactors is immense, and this region is frequently referred to as the tight junction "plaque" [44]. This review touches on two abundant plaque proteins, Zonula occludens 1 and 2 (ZO-1 and ZO-2), which have been shown to form a functionally important bridge between claudins and the actin cytoskeleton [45–49]. Adding to this complexity are additional transmembrane proteins, junctional adhesion molecules (JAMs), occludin, and tricellulin, as well as signaling proteins sequestered on the scaffolding plaque [50–52]. Signaling components include transcription factors, kinases, and vesicle fusion machinery [53–56]. The apical actin cytoskeleton forms a band around the circumference of the cell that can tune barrier properties and dynamics through increased tension [57]. This entire structure, as well as the structure mirrored on the adjoined cell, is termed the "tight junction". This should be contrasted with the term "strand", which refers collectively to the transmembrane protein components within the tight junction. Excellent reviews of the protein constituents of the tight junction are available [30,34,58–60].

Several studies confirm the position of claudins at the top of the tight junction hierarchy with respect to tight junction structural assembly. For example, claudin 1 expression is sufficient to form strands in claudin-free in vitro cell systems [61,62]. More recently, tight junctions were found to be absent in quintuple claudin-knockout Madin–Darby canine kidney (MDCK) cells, whereas rescue experiments with claudin 3 could restore strand formation [63,64]. Remarkably, rescue occurred even in the absence of the claudin 3 PDZ binding motif. Futhermore, both cis interactions and trans interactions between claudins determine strand inclusion [40,64]. For example, Gonschoir et al. show claudin segregation of either pore-forming or sealing claudins in restricted regions of the strand [65]. These findings are consistent with previous data and models of stand formation where claudins compete by self-assembly processes for space in the strand [66,67].

4. Claudins Exhibit Dynamic Self-Assembly

Claudins within the junction strands are believed to undergo dynamic remodeling under physiological conditions, with altered claudin mobility after exposure to proinflammatory cytokines or growth factors [66,68]. Claudin mobility within the membrane exhibits isoform-specific dynamics when expressed in junction-deficient SF9 insect cells [69]. The nature of these dynamics is not entirely clear; however, data suggest that only static, immobile claudins participate in tight junction barrier function [66]. The tight junction structure as a whole also undergoes dynamic remodeling, with ZO-1 and actin moving constitutively into and out of the junctional region [70]. Recent studies show that there is likely intermittent association between claudins, ZO proteins, and actin. Furthermore, newly synthesized claudins integrate into the strand at strand break sites, which notably are increased in IBD [20,71]. Recent studies show that extrajunctional claudins serve as reservoirs of material to repair broken strands [72]. Additionally, Van Itallie et al. speculate that the intermittent actin association through ZO proteins allow for barrier functions during alterations in cell shape or movement [71]. Reduced ZO-1/ZO-2 expression by knockdown results in the mislocalization of some but not all claudins, indicating preferential ZO-1 binding for particular claudins. For example, claudins 1 and 2 are reduced in these double ZO-1/ZO-2 knockdown cells, whereas claudins 3 and 4 remain at normal levels [73]. Indeed, in vitro studies demonstrate claudin-isoform-specific ZO protein interactions [74].

For example, the first PDZ domain of ZO-1 preferentially binds claudin isoforms that contain a tyrosine residue at the negative 6 position [75]. Importantly, Claudins 2 and 4 are antagonistic at the protein level, as shown by overexpression and fluorescence recovery after photobleaching studies, and compete for occupancy within the junction [66]. These findings have been confirmed in more detail by recent investigations, which also identified competition between claudin 4 and claudins 7, 15, and 19 [45].

The studies discussed thus far provide important clues as to the steps of claudin strand assembly and dynamics, but what can we learn from these studies that might improve our understanding of IBD pathogenesis? Firstly, these studies show that cells lacking claudins 1, 2, 3, 4, and 7 fail to make strands. Importantly, the ablated claudins are among the most abundant transcripts out of the dozen isoforms found at the RNA level in MDCK II cells [46]. Therefore, it is likely that there must be sufficient claudin expression to support strand formation and that a reduction in claudin levels below a certain threshold is likely to produce strand defects and a non-functional tight junction. In addition, there appears to be a hierarchy to strand assembly, where some claudins can nucleate strand formation and others cannot. Thirdly, claudins compete for inclusion in stands, providing a molecular mechanism for claudin switching and dynamic strand reconstitution. Indicative of claudin switching processes, strand breakage occurs with increased frequency in IBD, coincident with changes in claudin gene expression [20]. Lastly, claudin isoform expression levels can dictate barrier properties; this is supported by studies showing claudin 2 density increases sodium flux through the paracellular space [47,48]. Given these observations, claudin stoichiometries are likely to be of great functional significance, as these studies demonstrate that pore-forming claudin function comes at the expense of sealing claudins. Alterations in claudin expression are expected to be highly impactful with respect to tight junction function, as the strands are assembled from available claudins.

In combination, it appears that claudin expression dictates the availability and character of paracellular pores, the density of pores in the strand, the architecture of the strands themselves, and, likely, the identity and volume of plaque/signaling proteins associated with the junction. Therefore, claudin expression changes during IBD are likely to have a variety of downstream effects that impact both barrier function and tissue homeostasis.

5. Claudins Regulate Cell Proliferation and Cell Migration

The above molecular studies demonstrate the central role of claudins in the tight junction structure. Therefore, changes in the complement of claudins during IBD could have far reaching effects on tight junction function. Most IBD studies have focused on claudins as regulators of pericellular antigen flux. However, understanding the role of claudin changes in IBD may require a broadening of our perspective to include non-canonical functions. Indeed, claudins have been discovered in some unexpected places, performing roles that are considered non-canonical, such as promoting cell migration and proliferation. Importantly, enhancement of non-canonical processes has the potential to compromise barrier properties.

Proliferation and cell migration occur during colonic tissue homeostasis as the gut replenishes shed and lost cells through stem cell replication in the colonic crypt base. These new cells migrate up the crypt towards the lumen-facing mucosal surface where they are ultimately shed. During migration, cells acquire differentiated states, producing sensory, secretory, or barrier cells [49]. Claudin isoforms are exchanged coincident with migration, following spatial and temporal patterns irrespective of cell fate (see above and Figure 2), and crypt regions are rich in claudins 2, 5, 10, and 15. Most of these claudins are believed to play a role in cell proliferation, given that claudin changes correlate with carcinogenesis (reviewed here [10]). In laboratory models, a direct role has been uncovered for claudins in enhancing proliferation, with the strongest evidence presented for claudin 2 in the colon epithelia. In claudin-2-overexpressing transgenic animals, a doubling of actively dividing crypt cells was determined relative to wild-type animals [12]. Although proliferation regulation could occur secondary to a number of tissue-specific factors, it is important to note that enhanced proliferative effects were found in in vitro overexpression systems, with Caco-2, SW480, and HCT116 cells exhibiting enhanced growth through claudin 2 functions [50]. In addition, claudin 2 interacts with ZO-1 and the transcription factor ZONAB/DbpA in colon cancer cells [51]. ZONAB/DpbA has been shown to regulate cell growth [52]. Claudin 15 provides another dramatic example, were ablation in knockout mice led to a megaintestine phenotype [53]. However, there are no studies that confirm direct claudin 15 participation, such as the in vitro studies performed for claudin 2, which further highlights the continuing utility of in vitro systems [54]. Other examples of claudin's role in cell growth exist in the literature. For example, claudin 3 is a tumor suppressor, as demonstrated by tumor growth in intestinal-claudin-3-knockout mice [55]. Conversely, claudin 3 was found to enhance proliferation when overexpressed in HT-29 cancer cells [56]. Claudin-7-overexpressing colon cancer cells show enhanced proliferation [76]. These counter examples lead to the proposition that these claudins act in a context-dependent manner [22,58]. Yet together, these studies show that claudins are active participants in the proliferative process, regulating signaling and transcription factor components.

Claudins have recently been given attention as regulators of cell migration, initially as indicators of epithelial-to-mesenchymal transition given that claudins are present in differentiated/polarized cells. However, an active role for claudins in cell migration has become apparent (reviewed here [22]). Indeed, claudin 1 overexpression reduces cell migration in breast epithelial cancer cells [59]. Notably, forced expression of claudin 1 in these cells increased the protein expression of ZO-1 and occludin. Conversely, knockdown of claudin 1 in colon cancer cells increased migration in PKM2-stimulated cells [60]. Claudin 2 overexpression in colon cancer cells also increases migration and invasiveness [50,77]. Claudin 7 expression has been found to increase proliferation in lung cancer cells, yet these cells were deficient in migratory behaviors [78]. Knockdown of claudin 3 promotes cell migration in endothelial cells as well [79]. Studies in intestine-specific knockout mice also show that claudins influence migration. These examples demonstrate direct participation of claudins in cell migration.

Cell proliferation in the crypts and cell shedding at the lumen surface increase during IBD. Both cell division and migration are cellular processes; however, for the mucosal tissue to remain intact, cell-cell junctions and barrier function must be maintained at the multicell/tissue level. These data support a model of intestinal barrier disruption where, for example, claudin 2 promotes cell proliferative and migratory behavior, yet creates additional paracellular antigen flux. This insight may resolve conflicting data on the role of claudin 2 in colitis: is this claudin beneficial or harmful? This topic remains an active debate, and the answer may be that it is both and that wound restitution may require a delicate balance of claudin expression.

6. Claudins Participate in Mechanotransduction

The increased cell proliferation and migration seen in IBD would be expected to add additional physical strain on cellular barriers [80]. Given that the tight junction and actin cytoskeleton are mechanically linked, it has been long understood that intercellular forces on the actin ring reduces barrier function [57]. This sets up the potential conflict that increased physical forces during cell proliferation and migration increase antigen penetration into the gut. The role of claudins in these processes is not well understood; however, recent studies suggest that diverse claudin expression may play a role in these processes.

Collective cell migration is a highly integrated processes with ECM–cell tension and cell-cell friction (termed tissue fluidity) both coming into play [81]. Of these forces, tissue fluidity is the least understood, although studies that manipulate ZO-1 provide clues as to the role of tight junctions in collective migration. By manipulating ZO-1/actin associations, it has been shown that weak actin–tight junction linkages are associated with "tight" barrier function, whereas strong actin associations produce a leakier monolayer [82]. Second, in Xenopus embryos is was shown that the collective cell migration can be simulated by strengthening cell-to-cell tension in the migrating sheet [83]. In mice, disruption of claudins

3 and 4 arrests neural tube closure by preventing proper actin contractility through pMLC (phospho-myosin light chain) and Rho/ROCK [84]. In ZO-1/ZO-2-double-knockdown MDCK cells, loss of these scaffolds dramatically reduced cell migration and enhanced actin/myosin networks at adhesive junctions [85]. It appears that without ZO-1/ZO-2, leader cells at the wound edge fail to transduce mechanical force to follower cells behind the wound. Therefore, it appears that cells must balance migratory efficiency and barrier function and that efficient cell migration and antigen exclusion may be at odds biophysically.

Increased shear strain at the tight junction is expected as cells jostle and migrate along the crypt axis towards the surface. Remarkably, recent studies show that tight junction proteins function in a mechanotransduction role that is nonredundant to adherens junctions [86]. Changes in junction morphology take place when associations between ZO-1 and claudins are altered. The degree of claudin/ZO-1/actin integration can lead to differing morphologies at the cell junction. For example, non-linear tight junctions, or ruffles, correlate with high claudin 2, high ZO-1 expression at the junctions, and decreased barrier function [87,88]. Additionally, forces at the junction have been shown to stretch ZO-1, thereby exposing a binding site for ZONAB/DbpA and stimulating actin polymerization at junction sites in mammary epithelia Eph4 cells. In this model, DbpA sequestration at the junction by ZO-1 during tension inhibits cell growth [89]. Importantly, reduced ZO-1 at the membrane would not be expected to transfer these forces, leading to dysregulation of ZONAB/DbpA, a regulator of cell proliferation [90]. It is plausible that claudins play a role in this process by providing binding sites to ZO-1; however, this has not been tested.

Lastly, claudin-based tight junctions are challenged to maintain barrier function during cytokinesis [91]. In Xenopus embryos, Higashi et al. showed a remarkable stability for claudin 6 and ZO-1 during cytokinesis, supporting a membrane pinching model of cell division that does not require new tight junction material at the cleavage site. The exception here is the appearance of tricellulin at the final stages of cleavage. Importantly, tricellulin expression is known to increase transepithelial antigen leak [92,93]. Remarkably, barrier function is retained during this process, with the caveat that immunofluorescence-based assessments of the barrier likely measure the unrestricted pathway and not leak or ion pore pathways [8,91]. It would be interesting to determine if this remarkable tight junction stability persists during inflammation, when the tissue experiences increased division and migration. This is of particular interest given the known role of proinflammatory cytokines as stimulators of claudin gene expression, tight junction dynamics, and actin contractility [13,57,94].

7. Concluding Remarks

Chronic barrier disfunction presents a persistent challenge to host peripheral immune tolerance systems by exposing host tissues to antigens or opportunistic pathogens. Antigens present a constant stimulus to mucosal innate immune systems and risk aberrant immune activation. Our discussions thus far concern the potential ramifications of claudin gene family changes in IBD, and a core question remains: are these changes adaptive or pathological? This review argues for a maladaptive claudin response in IBD patients based on key observations: (1) Claudins are keystone tight junction proteins that regulate the paracellular space and sequester the scaffolding, signaling, and actin structures responsible for non-canonical functions such as cell growth and migration. (2) Claudin strand self-assembly is deterministic, with a given claudin isoform pool competitively restricting potential tight junction structure and barrier function. (3) Claudin changes in IBD induce claudin switching, thereby changing junction dynamics. (4) Claudin isoforms differentially support antigen exclusion, cell division, and/or migration. (5) Cell division and migration challenge junctions to tune cell monolayer fluidity and manage shear stress with barrier function (Figure 3A). (6) Inflammation-induced actin contractility at the junction regulates barrier function.

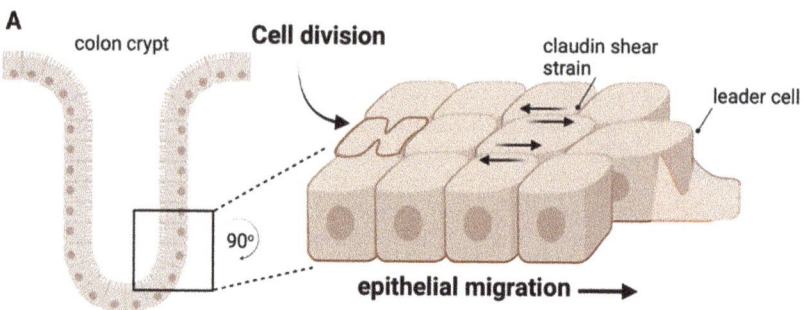

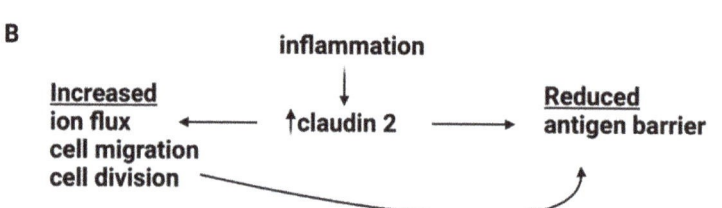

Figure 3. (**A**) A postulated increases in shear strain at claudin junctions from IBD-induced cell division and collective cell migration. (**B**) Proposed conflicting roles of claudin 2 in IBD pathogenesis. Increased antigen flux directly or secondarily produced by increased claudin 2.

The above studies largely support a model where the altered claudin expression seen in IBD drives tight junction remodeling towards structures that are more conducive to cell migration and division than antigen exclusion (Figure 3). Cell division requires extensive actin contractility and strong tight junction associations support cell migration but not robust barriers. It appears these cellular phenomena are likely working in opposition to a restrictive leak pathway, which is a tissue-wide phenomena. The best supporting data for this model are provided by studies of claudin 2, which supports cell proliferation and migration at the cellular level yet exposes tissue-wide vulnerabilities through increased antigen flux (Figure 3B). This may be due to claudin 2 expression directly or secondarily through claudin-2-mediated cell migration/division. With this in mind, the conflicting data for claudin 2 in mouse models of colitis may be resolved when considering the methods of colitis induction. If an insult/antigen is acute (DSS, pathogen), high claudin 2 levels are likely beneficial as this claudin supports wound repair; however, for chronic insults (immune dysfunction), high claudin 2 is likely detrimental as antigen exposure would increase (Figure 3B).

This conclusion follows from viewing claudin changes in IBD broadly, taking into account canonical barrier and non-canonical roles in relation to both cellular and tissue functions. This review is by no means exhaustive, and a similar analysis may fruitfully take into consideration that claudins participate in processes not discussed here, such as ion balance, cell shedding, and immune cell regulation [95]. However, limited data exist on these topics that are linked to IBD pathogenesis.

Ideally, sufficient claudin complexity exists to serve as a failsafe, preventing excessive antigen leak regardless of tissue requirements. However, this does not appear to be the case for IBD patients. Moving forward, new IBD therapies that focus on improving the intestinal barrier should consider the potential tradeoffs between barrier function and speedy wound restitution based on the underlying causes of disease.

Funding: This research was funded by grants from the National Institutes of Health (NIH), National Institute of General Medical Sciences (NIGMS), IDeA Networks of Biomedical Research Excellence (INBRE), Award number: P20GM103466, and NIH NIDDK grant # 1R15DK127369-01A1.

Acknowledgments: The author would like to thank Andrei Ivanov and Michael Koval for helpful comments. The content is solely the responsibility of the author and does not necessarily represent the official views of the National Institutes of Health. Graphics Created with BioRender.com.

Conflicts of Interest: The author declares no conflict of interest.

References

1. Kobayashi, T.; Siegmund, B.; Le Berre, C.; Wei, S.C.; Ferrante, M.; Shen, B.; Bernstein, C.N.; Danese, S.; Peyrin-Biroulet, L.; Hibi, T. Ulcerative colitis. *Nat. Rev. Dis. Primers* **2020**, *6*, 74. [CrossRef] [PubMed]
2. Roda, G.; Chien Ng, S.; Kotze, P.G.; Argollo, M.; Panaccione, R.; Spinelli, A.; Kaser, A.; Peyrin-Biroulet, L.; Danese, S. Crohn's disease. *Nat. Rev. Dis. Primers* **2020**, *6*, 22. [CrossRef] [PubMed]
3. Leung, G.; Muise, A.M. Monogenic Intestinal Epithelium Defects and the Development of Inflammatory Bowel Disease. *Physiology* **2018**, *33*, 360–369. [CrossRef] [PubMed]
4. Villablanca, E.J.; Selin, K.; Hedin, C.R.H. Mechanisms of mucosal healing: Treating inflammatory bowel disease without immunosuppression? *Nat. Rev. Gastroenterol. Hepatol.* **2022**, *19*, 493–507. [CrossRef]
5. Odenwald, M.A.; Turner, J.R. Intestinal permeability defects: Is it time to treat? *Clin. Gastroenterol. Hepatol.* **2013**, *11*, 1075–1083. [CrossRef]
6. Weidinger, C.; Krug, S.M.; Voskens, C.; Moschen, A.R.; Atreya, I. Editorial: Loss of Epithelial Barrier Integrity in Inflammatory Diseases: Cellular Mediators and Therapeutic Targets. *Front. Med.* **2021**, *8*, 813153. [CrossRef]
7. Williams, J.M.; Duckworth, C.A.; Watson, A.J.; Frey, M.R.; Miguel, J.C.; Burkitt, M.D.; Sutton, R.; Hughes, K.R.; Hall, L.J.; Caamano, J.H.; et al. A mouse model of pathological small intestinal epithelial cell apoptosis and shedding induced by systemic administration of lipopolysaccharide. *Dis. Model. Mech.* **2013**, *6*, 1388–1399. [CrossRef]
8. Chanez-Paredes, S.D.; Abtahi, S.; Kuo, W.T.; Turner, J.R. Differentiating Between Tight Junction-Dependent and Tight Junction-Independent Intestinal Barrier Loss In Vivo. *Methods Mol. Biol.* **2021**, *2367*, 249–271. [CrossRef]
9. Van Itallie, C.M.; Anderson, J.M. Architecture of tight junctions and principles of molecular composition. *Semin. Cell. Dev. Biol.* **2014**, *36*, 157–165. [CrossRef]
10. Zhu, L.; Han, J.; Li, L.; Wang, Y.; Li, Y.; Zhang, S. Claudin Family Participates in the Pathogenesis of Inflammatory Bowel Diseases and Colitis-Associated Colorectal Cancer. *Front. Immunol.* **2019**, *10*, 1441. [CrossRef]
11. Barkas, F.; Liberopoulos, E.; Kei, A.; Elisaf, M. Electrolyte and acid-base disorders in inflammatory bowel disease. *Ann. Gastroenterol.* **2013**, *26*, 23–28.
12. Ahmad, R.; Chaturvedi, R.; Olivares-Villagomez, D.; Habib, T.; Asim, M.; Shivesh, P.; Polk, D.B.; Wilson, K.T.; Washington, M.K.; Van Kaer, L.; et al. Targeted colonic claudin-2 expression renders resistance to epithelial injury, induces immune suppression, and protects from colitis. *Mucosal Immunol.* **2014**, *7*, 1340–1353. [CrossRef]
13. Capaldo, C.T.; Nusrat, A. Claudin switching: Physiological plasticity of the Tight Junction. *Semin. Cell. Dev. Biol.* **2015**, *42*, 22–29. [CrossRef]
14. Garcia-Hernandez, V.; Quiros, M.; Nusrat, A. Intestinal epithelial claudins: Expression and regulation in homeostasis and inflammation. *Ann. N. Y. Acad. Sci.* **2017**, *1397*, 66–79. [CrossRef]
15. Serigado, J.M.; Foulke-Abel, J.; Hines, W.C.; Hanson, J.A.; In, J.; Kovbasnjuk, O. Ulcerative Colitis: Novel Epithelial Insights Provided by Single Cell RNA Sequencing. *Front. Med.* **2022**, *9*, 868508. [CrossRef]
16. Ahmad, R.; Sorrell, M.F.; Batra, S.K.; Dhawan, P.; Singh, A.B. Gut permeability and mucosal inflammation: Bad, good or context dependent. *Mucosal Immunol.* **2017**, *10*, 307–317. [CrossRef]
17. Barrett, K.E. Claudin-2 pore causes leak that breaches the dam in intestinal inflammation. *J. Clin. Invest.* **2020**, *130*, 5100–5101. [CrossRef]
18. Capaldo, C.T.; Nusrat, A. Cytokine regulation of tight junctions. *Biochim. Biophys. Acta* **2009**, *1788*, 864–871. [CrossRef]
19. Schmitz, H.; Barmeyer, C.; Fromm, M.; Runkel, N.; Foss, H.D.; Bentzel, C.J.; Riecken, E.O.; Schulzke, J.D. Altered tight junction structure contributes to the impaired epithelial barrier function in ulcerative colitis. *Gastroenterology* **1999**, *116*, 301–309. [CrossRef]
20. Zeissig, S.; Burgel, N.; Gunzel, D.; Richter, J.; Mankertz, J.; Wahnschaffe, U.; Kroesen, A.J.; Zeitz, M.; Fromm, M.; Schulzke, J.D. Changes in expression and distribution of claudin 2, 5 and 8 lead to discontinuous tight junctions and barrier dysfunction in active Crohn's disease. *Gut* **2007**, *56*, 61–72. [CrossRef]
21. Rodriguez, P.; Heyman, M.; Candalh, C.; Blaton, M.A.; Bouchaud, C. Tumour necrosis factor-alpha induces morphological and functional alterations of intestinal HT29 cl.19A cell monolayers. *Cytokine* **1995**, *7*, 441–448. [CrossRef] [PubMed]
22. Li, J. Context-Dependent Roles of Claudins in Tumorigenesis. *Front. Oncol.* **2021**, *11*, 676781. [CrossRef] [PubMed]
23. Seker, M.; Fernandez-Rodriguez, C.; Martinez-Cruz, L.A.; Muller, D. Mouse Models of Human Claudin-Associated Disorders: Benefits and Limitations. *Int. J. Mol. Sci.* **2019**, *20*, 5504. [CrossRef] [PubMed]
24. Ding, L.; Lu, Z.; Foreman, O.; Tatum, R.; Lu, Q.; Renegar, R.; Cao, J.; Chen, Y.H. Inflammation and disruption of the mucosal architecture in claudin-7-deficient mice. *Gastroenterology* **2012**, *142*, 305–315. [CrossRef] [PubMed]

25. Shen, L.; Weber, C.R.; Raleigh, D.R.; Yu, D.; Turner, J.R. Tight junction pore and leak pathways: A dynamic duo. *Annu. Rev. Physiol.* **2011**, *73*, 283–309. [CrossRef]
26. Hempel, C.; Rosenthal, R.; Fromm, A.; Krug, S.M.; Fromm, M.; Gunzel, D.; Piontek, J. Tight junction channels claudin-10b and claudin-15: Functional mapping of pore-lining residues. *Ann. N. Y. Acad. Sci.* **2022**, *1515*, 129–142. [CrossRef]
27. Gunzel, D.; Yu, A.S. Claudins and the modulation of tight junction permeability. *Physiol. Rev.* **2013**, *93*, 525–569. [CrossRef]
28. Mitchell, L.A.; Overgaard, C.E.; Ward, C.; Margulies, S.S.; Koval, M. Differential effects of claudin-3 and claudin-4 on alveolar epithelial barrier function. *Am. J. Physiol. Lung Cell. Mol. Physiol.* **2011**, *301*, L40–L49. [CrossRef]
29. Liu, X.; Yang, G.; Geng, X.R.; Cao, Y.; Li, N.; Ma, L.; Chen, S.; Yang, P.C.; Liu, Z. Microbial products induce claudin-2 to compromise gut epithelial barrier function. *PLoS ONE* **2013**, *8*, e68547. [CrossRef]
30. Tanaka, H.; Takechi, M.; Kiyonari, H.; Shioi, G.; Tamura, A.; Tsukita, S. Intestinal deletion of Claudin-7 enhances paracellular organic solute flux and initiates colonic inflammation in mice. *Gut* **2015**, *64*, 1529–1538. [CrossRef]
31. Tsai, P.Y.; Zhang, B.; He, W.Q.; Zha, J.M.; Odenwald, M.A.; Singh, G.; Tamura, A.; Shen, L.; Sailer, A.; Yeruva, S.; et al. IL-22 Upregulates Epithelial Claudin-2 to Drive Diarrhea and Enteric Pathogen Clearance. *Cell. Host Microbe* **2017**, *21*, 671–681.e674. [CrossRef]
32. Raju, P.; Shashikanth, N.; Tsai, P.Y.; Pongkorpsakol, P.; Chanez-Paredes, S.; Steinhagen, P.R.; Kuo, W.T.; Singh, G.; Tsukita, S.; Turner, J.R. Inactivation of paracellular cation-selective claudin-2 channels attenuates immune-mediated experimental colitis in mice. *J. Clin. Invest.* **2020**, *130*, 5197–5208. [CrossRef]
33. Furuse, M.; Fujita, K.; Hiiragi, T.; Fujimoto, K.; Tsukita, S. Claudin-1 and -2: Novel integral membrane proteins localizing at tight junctions with no sequence similarity to occludin. *J. Cell. Biol.* **1998**, *141*, 1539–1550. [CrossRef]
34. Gunzel, D.; Fromm, M. Claudins and other tight junction proteins. *Compr. Physiol.* **2012**, *2*, 1819–1852. [CrossRef]
35. Morita, K.; Furuse, M.; Fujimoto, K.; Tsukita, S. Claudin multigene family encoding four-transmembrane domain protein components of tight junction strands. *Proc. Natl. Acad. Sci. USA* **1999**, *96*, 511–516. [CrossRef]
36. Daugherty, B.L.; Ward, C.; Smith, T.; Ritzenthaler, J.D.; Koval, M. Regulation of heterotypic claudin compatibility. *J. Biol. Chem.* **2007**, *282*, 30005–30013. [CrossRef]
37. Colegio, O.R.; Van Itallie, C.; Rahner, C.; Anderson, J.M. Claudin extracellular domains determine paracellular charge selectivity and resistance but not tight junction fibril architecture. *Am. J. Physiol. Cell. Physiol.* **2003**, *284*, C1346–C1354. [CrossRef]
38. Rosenthal, R.; Gunzel, D.; Krug, S.M.; Schulzke, J.D.; Fromm, M.; Yu, A.S. Claudin-2-mediated cation and water transport share a common pore. *Acta Physiol.* **2017**, *219*, 521–536. [CrossRef]
39. Milatz, S.; Krug, S.M.; Rosenthal, R.; Gunzel, D.; Muller, D.; Schulzke, J.D.; Amasheh, S.; Fromm, M. Claudin-3 acts as a sealing component of the tight junction for ions of either charge and uncharged solutes. *Biochim. Biophys. Acta* **2010**, *1798*, 2048–2057. [CrossRef]
40. Zhao, J.; Krystofiak, E.S.; Ballesteros, A.; Cui, R.; Van Itallie, C.M.; Anderson, J.M.; Fenollar-Ferrer, C.; Kachar, B. Multiple claudin-claudin cis interfaces are required for tight junction strand formation and inherent flexibility. *Commun. Biol.* **2018**, *1*, 50. [CrossRef]
41. Suzuki, H.; Tani, K.; Tamura, A.; Tsukita, S.; Fujiyoshi, Y. Model for the architecture of claudin-based paracellular ion channels through tight junctions. *J. Mol. Biol.* **2015**, *427*, 291–297. [CrossRef] [PubMed]
42. Itoh, M.; Furuse, M.; Morita, K.; Kubota, K.; Saitou, M.; Tsukita, S. Direct binding of three tight junction-associated MAGUKs, ZO-1, ZO-2, and ZO-3, with the COOH termini of claudins. *J. Cell. Biol.* **1999**, *147*, 1351–1363. [CrossRef] [PubMed]
43. Lee, H.J.; Zheng, J.J. PDZ domains and their binding partners: Structure, specificity, and modification. *Cell. Commun. Signal.* **2010**, *8*, 8. [CrossRef] [PubMed]
44. Tang, V.W. Proteomic and bioinformatic analysis of epithelial tight junction reveals an unexpected cluster of synaptic molecules. *Biol. Direct* **2006**, *1*, 37. [CrossRef]
45. Shashikanth, N.; France, M.M.; Xiao, R.; Haest, X.; Rizzo, H.E.; Yeste, J.; Reiner, J.; Turner, J.R. Tight junction channel regulation by interclaudin interference. *Nat. Commun.* **2022**, *13*, 3780. [CrossRef]
46. Ye, Q.; Phan, T.; Hu, W.S.; Liu, X.; Fan, L.; Tan, W.S.; Zhao, L. Transcriptomic Characterization Reveals Attributes of High Influenza Virus Productivity in MDCK Cells. *Viruses* **2021**, *13*, 2200. [CrossRef]
47. Amasheh, S.; Meiri, N.; Gitter, A.H.; Schoneberg, T.; Mankertz, J.; Schulzke, J.D.; Fromm, M. Claudin-2 expression induces cation-selective channels in tight junctions of epithelial cells. *J. Cell. Sci.* **2002**, *115*, 4969–4976. [CrossRef]
48. Van Itallie, C.M.; Holmes, J.; Bridges, A.; Gookin, J.L.; Coccaro, M.R.; Proctor, W.; Colegio, O.R.; Anderson, J.M. The density of small tight junction pores varies among cell types and is increased by expression of claudin-2. *J. Cell. Sci.* **2008**, *121*, 298–305. [CrossRef]
49. Beumer, J.; Clevers, H. Cell fate specification and differentiation in the adult mammalian intestine. *Nat. Rev. Mol. Cell. Biol.* **2021**, *22*, 39–53. [CrossRef]
50. Dhawan, P.; Ahmad, R.; Chaturvedi, R.; Smith, J.J.; Midha, R.; Mittal, M.K.; Krishnan, M.; Chen, X.; Eschrich, S.; Yeatman, T.J.; et al. Claudin-2 expression increases tumorigenicity of colon cancer cells: Role of epidermal growth factor receptor activation. *Oncogene* **2011**, *30*, 3234–3247. [CrossRef]
51. Buchert, M.; Papin, M.; Bonnans, C.; Darido, C.; Raye, W.S.; Garambois, V.; Pelegrin, A.; Bourgaux, J.F.; Pannequin, J.; Joubert, D.; et al. Symplekin promotes tumorigenicity by up-regulating claudin-2 expression. *Proc. Natl. Acad. Sci. USA* **2010**, *107*, 2628–2633. [CrossRef]

52. Lima, W.R.; Parreira, K.S.; Devuyst, O.; Caplanusi, A.; N'Kuli, F.; Marien, B.; Van Der Smissen, P.; Alves, P.M.; Verroust, P.; Christensen, E.I.; et al. ZONAB promotes proliferation and represses differentiation of proximal tubule epithelial cells. *J. Am. Soc. Nephrol.* **2010**, *21*, 478–488. [CrossRef]
53. Tamura, A.; Hayashi, H.; Imasato, M.; Yamazaki, Y.; Hagiwara, A.; Wada, M.; Noda, T.; Watanabe, M.; Suzuki, Y.; Tsukita, S. Loss of claudin-15, but not claudin-2, causes Na+ deficiency and glucose malabsorption in mouse small intestine. *Gastroenterology* **2011**, *140*, 913–923. [CrossRef]
54. Lechuga, S.; Braga-Neto, M.B.; Naydenov, N.G.; Rieder, F.; Ivanov, A.I. Understanding disruption of the gut barrier during inflammation: Should we abandon traditional epithelial cell lines and switch to intestinal organoids? *Front. Immunol.* **2023**, *14*, 1108289. [CrossRef]
55. Ahmad, R.; Kumar, B.; Chen, Z.; Chen, X.; Muller, D.; Lele, S.M.; Washington, M.K.; Batra, S.K.; Dhawan, P.; Singh, A.B. Loss of claudin-3 expression induces IL6/gp130/Stat3 signaling to promote colon cancer malignancy by hyperactivating Wnt/beta-catenin signaling. *Oncogene* **2017**, *36*, 6592–6604. [CrossRef]
56. de Souza, W.F.; Fortunato-Miranda, N.; Robbs, B.K.; de Araujo, W.M.; de-Freitas-Junior, J.C.; Bastos, L.G.; Viola, J.P.; Morgado-Diaz, J.A. Claudin-3 overexpression increases the malignant potential of colorectal cancer cells: Roles of ERK1/2 and PI3K-Akt as modulators of EGFR signaling. *PLoS ONE* **2013**, *8*, e74994. [CrossRef]
57. Lechuga, S.; Ivanov, A.I. Disruption of the epithelial barrier during intestinal inflammation: Quest for new molecules and mechanisms. *Biochim. Biophys. Acta Mol. Cell. Res.* **2017**, *1864*, 1183–1194. [CrossRef]
58. Venugopal, S.; Anwer, S.; Szaszi, K. Claudin-2: Roles beyond Permeability Functions. *Int. J. Mol. Sci.* **2019**, *20*, 5655. [CrossRef]
59. Geoffroy, M.; Kleinclauss, A.; Kuntz, S.; Grillier-Vuissoz, I. Claudin 1 inhibits cell migration and increases intercellular adhesion in triple-negative breast cancer cell line. *Mol. Biol. Rep.* **2020**, *47*, 7643–7653. [CrossRef]
60. Kim, H.; Kim, S.H.; Hwang, D.; An, J.; Chung, H.S.; Yang, E.G.; Kim, S.Y. Extracellular pyruvate kinase M2 facilitates cell migration by upregulating claudin-1 expression in colon cancer cells. *Biochem. Cell. Biol.* **2020**, *98*, 219–226. [CrossRef]
61. Sasaki, H.; Matsui, C.; Furuse, K.; Mimori-Kiyosue, Y.; Furuse, M.; Tsukita, S. Dynamic behavior of paired claudin strands within apposing plasma membranes. *Proc. Natl. Acad. Sci. USA* **2003**, *100*, 3971–3976. [CrossRef] [PubMed]
62. Furuse, M.; Sasaki, H.; Fujimoto, K.; Tsukita, S. A single gene product, claudin-1 or -2, reconstitutes tight junction strands and recruits occludin in fibroblasts. *J. Cell. Biol.* **1998**, *143*, 391–401. [CrossRef] [PubMed]
63. Otani, T.; Nguyen, T.P.; Tokuda, S.; Sugihara, K.; Sugawara, T.; Furuse, K.; Miura, T.; Ebnet, K.; Furuse, M. Claudins and JAM-A coordinately regulate tight junction formation and epithelial polarity. *J. Cell. Biol.* **2019**, *218*, 3372–3396. [CrossRef] [PubMed]
64. Fujiwara, S.; Nguyen, T.P.; Furuse, K.; Fukazawa, Y.; Otani, T.; Furuse, M. Tight junction formation by a claudin mutant lacking the COOH-terminal PDZ domain-binding motif. *Ann. N. Y. Acad. Sci.* **2022**, *1516*, 85–94. [CrossRef]
65. Gonschior, H.; Schmied, C.; Van der Veen, R.E.; Eichhorst, J.; Himmerkus, N.; Piontek, J.; Gunzel, D.; Bleich, M.; Furuse, M.; Haucke, V.; et al. Nanoscale segregation of channel and barrier claudins enables paracellular ion flux. *Nat. Commun.* **2022**, *13*, 4985. [CrossRef]
66. Capaldo, C.T.; Farkas, A.E.; Hilgarth, R.S.; Krug, S.M.; Wolf, M.F.; Benedik, J.K.; Fromm, M.; Koval, M.; Parkos, C.; Nusrat, A. Proinflammatory cytokine-induced tight junction remodeling through dynamic self-assembly of claudins. *Mol. Biol. Cell.* **2014**, *25*, 2710–2719. [CrossRef]
67. Kirschner, M.; Gerhart, J.; Mitchison, T. Molecular "vitalism". *Cell* **2000**, *100*, 79–88. [CrossRef]
68. Twiss, F.; Oldenkamp, M.; Hiemstra, A.; Zhou, H.; Matheron, L.; Mohammed, S.; de Rooij, J. HGF signaling regulates Claudin-3 dynamics through its C-terminal tyrosine residues. *Tissue Barriers* **2013**, *1*, e27425. [CrossRef]
69. Yamazaki, Y.; Tokumasu, R.; Kimura, H.; Tsukita, S. Role of claudin species-specific dynamics in reconstitution and remodeling of the zonula occludens. *Mol. Biol. Cell.* **2011**, *22*, 1495–1504. [CrossRef]
70. Shen, L.; Weber, C.R.; Turner, J.R. The tight junction protein complex undergoes rapid and continuous molecular remodeling at steady state. *J. Cell. Biol.* **2008**, *181*, 683–695. [CrossRef]
71. Van Itallie, C.M.; Tietgens, A.J.; Anderson, J.M. Visualizing the dynamic coupling of claudin strands to the actin cytoskeleton through ZO-1. *Mol. Biol. Cell.* **2017**, *28*, 524–534. [CrossRef]
72. Higashi, T.; Saito, A.C.; Fukazawa, Y.; Furuse, M.; Higashi, A.Y.; Ono, M.; Chiba, H. EpCAM proteolysis and release of complexed claudin-7 repair and maintain the tight junction barrier. *J. Cell. Biol.* **2023**, *222*, e202204079. [CrossRef]
73. Fanning, A.S.; Van Itallie, C.M.; Anderson, J.M. Zonula occludens-1 and -2 regulate apical cell structure and the zonula adherens cytoskeleton in polarized epithelia. *Mol. Biol. Cell.* **2012**, *23*, 577–590. [CrossRef]
74. Kalyoncu, S.; Keskin, O.; Gursoy, A. Interaction prediction and classification of PDZ domains. *BMC Bioinform.* **2010**, *11*, 357. [CrossRef]
75. Nomme, J.; Antanasijevic, A.; Caffrey, M.; Van Itallie, C.M.; Anderson, J.M.; Fanning, A.S.; Lavie, A. Structural Basis of a Key Factor Regulating the Affinity between the Zonula Occludens First PDZ Domain and Claudins. *J. Biol. Chem.* **2015**, *290*, 16595–16606. [CrossRef]
76. Darido, C.; Buchert, M.; Pannequin, J.; Bastide, P.; Zalzali, H.; Mantamadiotis, T.; Bourgaux, J.F.; Garambois, V.; Jay, P.; Blache, P.; et al. Defective claudin-7 regulation by Tcf-4 and Sox-9 disrupts the polarity and increases the tumorigenicity of colorectal cancer cells. *Cancer Res.* **2008**, *68*, 4258–4268. [CrossRef]
77. Takehara, M.; Nishimura, T.; Mima, S.; Hoshino, T.; Mizushima, T. Effect of claudin expression on paracellular permeability, migration and invasion of colonic cancer cells. *Biol. Pharm. Bull.* **2009**, *32*, 825–831. [CrossRef]

78. Kim, D.H.; Lu, Q.; Chen, Y.H. Claudin-7 modulates cell-matrix adhesion that controls cell migration, invasion and attachment of human HCC827 lung cancer cells. *Oncol. Lett.* **2019**, *17*, 2890–2896. [CrossRef]
79. Lei, N.; Cheng, Y.; Wan, J.; Blasig, R.; Li, A.; Bai, Y.; Haseloff, R.F.; Blasig, I.E.; Zhu, L.; Qin, Z. Claudin-3 inhibits tumor-induced lymphangiogenesis via regulating the PI3K signaling pathway in lymphatic endothelial cells. *Sci. Rep.* **2022**, *12*, 17440. [CrossRef]
80. Krndija, D.; El Marjou, F.; Guirao, B.; Richon, S.; Leroy, O.; Bellaiche, Y.; Hannezo, E.; Matic Vignjevic, D. Active cell migration is critical for steady-state epithelial turnover in the gut. *Science* **2019**, *365*, 705–710. [CrossRef]
81. Mayor, R.; Etienne-Manneville, S. The front and rear of collective cell migration. *Nat. Rev. Mol. Cell. Biol.* **2016**, *17*, 97–109. [CrossRef] [PubMed]
82. Belardi, B.; Hamkins-Indik, T.; Harris, A.R.; Kim, J.; Xu, K.; Fletcher, D.A. A Weak Link with Actin Organizes Tight Junctions to Control Epithelial Permeability. *Dev. Cell.* **2020**, *54*, 792–804.e797. [CrossRef] [PubMed]
83. Marchant, C.L.; Malmi-Kakkada, A.N.; Espina, J.A.; Barriga, E.H. Cell clusters softening triggers collective cell migration in vivo. *Nat. Mater.* **2022**, *21*, 1314–1323. [CrossRef]
84. Baumholtz, A.I.; Simard, A.; Nikolopoulou, E.; Oosenbrug, M.; Collins, M.M.; Piontek, A.; Krause, G.; Piontek, J.; Greene, N.D.E.; Ryan, A.K. Claudins are essential for cell shape changes and convergent extension movements during neural tube closure. *Dev. Biol.* **2017**, *428*, 25–38. [CrossRef] [PubMed]
85. Skamrahl, M.; Pang, H.; Ferle, M.; Gottwald, J.; Rubeling, A.; Maraspini, R.; Honigmann, A.; Oswald, T.A.; Janshoff, A. Tight Junction ZO Proteins Maintain Tissue Fluidity, Ensuring Efficient Collective Cell Migration. *Adv. Sci.* **2021**, *8*, e2100478. [CrossRef]
86. Angulo-Urarte, A.; van der Wal, T.; Huveneers, S. Cell-cell junctions as sensors and transducers of mechanical forces. *Biochim. Biophys. Acta Biomembr.* **2020**, *1862*, 183316. [CrossRef]
87. Lynn, K.S.; Peterson, R.J.; Koval, M. Ruffles and spikes: Control of tight junction morphology and permeability by claudins. *Biochim. Biophys. Acta Biomembr.* **2020**, *1862*, 183339. [CrossRef]
88. Tokuda, S.; Higashi, T.; Furuse, M. ZO-1 knockout by TALEN-mediated gene targeting in MDCK cells: Involvement of ZO-1 in the regulation of cytoskeleton and cell shape. *PLoS ONE* **2014**, *9*, e104994. [CrossRef]
89. Spadaro, D.; Le, S.; Laroche, T.; Mean, I.; Jond, L.; Yan, J.; Citi, S. Tension-Dependent Stretching Activates ZO-1 to Control the Junctional Localization of Its Interactors. *Curr. Biol.* **2017**, *27*, 3783–3795.e3788. [CrossRef]
90. Spadaro, D.; Tapia, R.; Jond, L.; Sudol, M.; Fanning, A.S.; Citi, S. ZO proteins redundantly regulate the transcription factor DbpA/ZONAB. *J. Biol. Chem.* **2014**, *289*, 22500–22511. [CrossRef]
91. Higashi, T.; Arnold, T.R.; Stephenson, R.E.; Dinshaw, K.M.; Miller, A.L. Maintenance of the Epithelial Barrier and Remodeling of Cell-Cell Junctions during Cytokinesis. *Curr. Biol.* **2016**, *26*, 1829–1842. [CrossRef]
92. Monaco, A.; Ovryn, B.; Axis, J.; Amsler, K. The Epithelial Cell Leak Pathway. *Int. J. Mol. Sci.* **2021**, *22*, 7677. [CrossRef]
93. Krug, S.M. Contribution of the tricellular tight junction to paracellular permeability in leaky and tight epithelia. *Ann. N. Y. Acad. Sci.* **2017**, *1397*, 219–230. [CrossRef]
94. Lechuga, S.; Ivanov, A.I. Actin cytoskeleton dynamics during mucosal inflammation: A view from broken epithelial barriers. *Curr. Opin. Physiol.* **2021**, *19*, 10–16. [CrossRef]
95. Kawai, Y.; Hamazaki, Y.; Fujita, H.; Fujita, A.; Sato, T.; Furuse, M.; Fujimoto, T.; Jetten, A.M.; Agata, Y.; Minato, N. Claudin-4 induction by E-protein activity in later stages of CD4/8 double-positive thymocytes to increase positive selection efficiency. *Proc. Natl. Acad. Sci. USA* **2011**, *108*, 4075–4080. [CrossRef]

Disclaimer/Publisher's Note: The statements, opinions and data contained in all publications are solely those of the individual author(s) and contributor(s) and not of MDPI and/or the editor(s). MDPI and/or the editor(s) disclaim responsibility for any injury to people or property resulting from any ideas, methods, instructions or products referred to in the content.

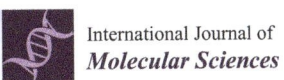

Review

Intestinal Behcet's Disease: A Review of the Immune Mechanism and Present and Potential Biological Agents

Kun He [1,†], Xiaxiao Yan [2,†] and Dong Wu [1,3,*]

1. Department of Gastroenterology, Peking Union Medical College Hospital, Chinese Academy of Medical Sciences and Peking Union Medical College, Beijing 100730, China
2. Eight-year Medical Doctor Program, Chinese Academy of Medical Sciences and Peking Union Medical College, Beijing 100730, China
3. Clinical Epidemiology Unit, Peking Union Medical College Hospital, Chinese Academy of Medical Sciences and Peking Union Medical College, Beijing 100730, China
* Correspondence: wudong@pumch.cn
† These authors contributed equally to this work.

Abstract: Behcet's disease (BD) is a chronic and recurrent systemic vasculitis involving almost all organs and tissues. Intestinal BD is defined as BD with predominant gastrointestinal involvement, presenting severe complications such as massive gastrointestinal hemorrhage, perforation, and obstruction in some cases. To some extent, intestinal BD is classified as a member of inflammatory bowel disease (IBD), as it has a lot in common with classical IBD including Crohn's disease (CD) and ulcerative colitis (UC). Certainly, the underlying pathogenesis is not the same and dysregulation of immune function is believed to be one of the main pathogeneses in intestinal BD, although the etiology has not been clear up to now. Biological agents are an emerging category of pharmaceuticals for various diseases, including inflammatory diseases and cancers, in recent decades. Based on the deep understanding of the immune mechanism of intestinal BD, biological agents targeting potential pathogenic cells, cytokines and pathways are optimized options. Recently, the adoption of biological agents such as anti-tumor necrosis factor agents has allowed for the effective treatment of patients with refractory intestinal BD who show poor response to conventional medications and are faced with the risk of surgical treatment. In this review, we have tried to summarize the immune mechanism and present potential biological agents of intestinal BD.

Keywords: intestinal Behcet's disease; inflammatory bowel disease; immune mechanism; biological agents

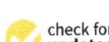

1. Introduction

Behcet's disease (BD) is a chronic and recurrent systemic variant vasculitis that mainly involves the skin, mucosa, joints, eyes, arteries and veins, nervous system and gastrointestinal organs [1,2]. Guan et al. in 2022 suggested that BD should be classified into eight subtypes: mucocutaneous BD, ocular BD, intestinal BD, cardiac BD, vascular BD, nervous BD, blood BD and articular BD [3]. Different subtypes present various disease courses, treatment responses and prognoses, suggesting a clinical heterogeneity and potential diversity of pathogenesis [4,5]. BD with gastrointestinal involvement is termed intestinal Behcet's disease (intestinal BD). Intestinal BD can involve the entire gastrointestinal tract, most commonly the ileocecal region. Clinical manifestations include abdominal pain, diarrhea, nausea, vomiting, gastrointestinal bleeding, and perforation. A colonoscopy reveals ulcers and histopathology shows neutrophil infiltration in the vessel wall, perivascular and intravascular areas [6]. Intestinal BD can cause serious complications and has high rates of disability and mortality, showing poor outcomes and calling for active treatment [7]. The incidence of gastrointestinal BD is about 3–60% and it shows regional differences, with approximately 2.8–4.0% in Turkey, India and Saudi Arabia, 10% in China, 38–53% in Japan,

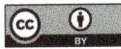

and 50–60% in British [7]. According to a 30-year retrospective analysis in Japan, the clinical cluster of gastrointestinal involvement shows an increasing trend [8]. The diagnosis of intestinal BD mainly depends on clinical and endoscopic manifestations. It is worth noting that the relationship between intestinal BD and classical inflammatory bowel disease (IBD) including Crohn's disease (CD) and ulcerative colitis (UC) is still disputed up to now [6]. Considering the similarity of genetic backgrounds, clinical manifestations, and therapeutic strategies between intestinal BD and classical IBD (especially CD), some experts place these two diseases in the same category or different spectrums of the same disease [9]. Certainly, there are still independent characteristics between intestinal BD and CD by careful clinical evaluation (Table 1), suggesting different underlying pathogenesis [10].

Table 1. The clinical characteristics of intestinal BD and CD.

	Intestinal Behcet's Disease	Crohn's Disease
Lesion distribution	Common in ileocecal region, rare in rectum and anus, short segment lesions	Common in ileocecal region, long segment lesions, jumping distribution
Bowel morphology	Not prone to stenosis	Thickening and stenosis
Gastrointestinal manifestations	Abdominal pain, diarrhea, hematochezia, with or without abdominal mass sometimes	Abdominal pain, diarrhea, hematochezia, abdominal mass, with or without perianal lesion
Extra-gastrointestinal manifestations	Oral and vulval ulcers, folliculitis or acne-like skin lesions, systemic manifestations (for example, ocular, vascular, neurological and articular symptoms)	Oral ulcers, nodular erythema, pyoderma, arthritis and so on
Laboratory tests	Positive in acupuncture test, HLA-B5 and ASCA	Positive in ASCA
Endoscopic findings	Round or oval ulcers, volcano-like ulcers, single or multiple ulcers ≤ 5, with definite boundary and smooth mucosa around the ulcer	Discontinuous distribution of longitudinal ulcers, paving stone-like pattern, aphthous ulcers
Pathologic findings	Signs of vasculitis.	Transmural inflammation, fissure-like ulcers, non-caseous granuloma

BD: Behcet's disease; CD: Crohn's disease; HLA-B5: human leukocyte antigen-B5; ASCA: anti-saccharomyces cerevisiae antibody.

However, the pathogenesis of BD, including intestinal BD, is not clear. The well-known hypothesis reveals that the intricate interplay between environmental factors and genetic susceptibility causes immune dysfunction, which is thought to be an inflammatory disorder between autoimmune and autoinflammatory conditions [11]. The main conventional medications for intestinal BD include 5-aminosalicylic acids (5-ASAs), corticosteroids, and immunomodulators, although there are still several patients who are refractory to conventional treatment. For intestinal BD, mucosal healing is associated with a decreased risk of recurrence and surgery, and should be considered the outcome of monitoring disease activity and targets of management [12]. In the past decade, the adoption of biological agents in BD allowed for effective treatment of these refractory patients [5,13,14]. As 2018 European League Against Rheumatism (EULAR) recommendations suggested, for severe and/or refractory intestinal BD patients, monoclonal anti-tumor necrosis factor (TNF) antibodies should be considered [5]. A recent study reported that earlier and more aggressive treatment may be beneficial to patients with BD who had the highest risk for a severe disease course [15]. Based on the deep understanding of the immune mechanism of intestinal BD, biological agents targeting potential pathogenic cells, cytokines and pathways are optimized options [14,16]. In this review, we summarize the immune mechanism and present and potential biological agents of intestinal BD, aiming to improve clinicians' understanding.

2. Immunity Mechanism

Both innate immunity and adaptive immunity show abnormalities in the pathogenesis of BD, which is activated by environmental factors in genetically predisposed patients [17–19]. For intestinal BD, abnormal activation of innate and adaptive immunity contributes to recurrent intestinal inflammatory reactions and destruction of intestinal vessels, the intestinal barrier and a series of injuries by inducing changes in the complex cytokine network and pathways [20].

2.1. Immunogens

Immune reactions are significantly important in the pathogenesis of BD, and infections, as one of various environmental factors, have been proven to be an important triggering factor. Bacterial infections, such as *Streptococcus sanguis* and *Helicobacter pylori*, and viral infections, including herpes simplex virus 1, Epstein–Barr virus, cytomegalovirus, and so on, have been reported to be related to the etiology of BD [21]. Molecular mimicry between microbes and autoantigens due to sequence homology rather than direct infection in the development of BD is considered a possible mechanism [17,22]. For example, the sequence homology between microbial and human heat-shock proteins, streptococcal cell wall M proteins and tropomyosin was reported to be associated with autoimmune reactions in BD [23–25].

In addition, as for intestinal BD, the location of lesions has direct contact with intestinal flora, and there may be a close relationship between gastrointestinal involvement of BD and the intestinal microbiome in theory. Several previous studies reported changes in the intestinal flora in patients with BD. By comparing the fecal microflora of BD patients with healthy controls, it was found that patients had significantly lower flora diversity and decreased short-chain fatty acid content in the intestine, which could cause intestinal epithelial barrier damage and imbalance in T-cell differentiation [26–28]. A Japanese study found that the relatively high abundance of *Bifidobacteria* in the intestinal flora of BD patients may trigger immune disorders by affecting intestinal pH [28]. A recent study has found deviations in microbiota composition between BD patients with skin mucosa, ocular and vascular involvement [29]. However, these studies did not separately analysis intestinal BD patients; some even excluded intestinal BD patients. There has been a lack of studies on the interaction between the development of intestinal BD and the imbalance of the intestinal microbiome thus far, which is a gap needed to be filled urgently.

2.2. Cellular Immunity in Adaptive Immunity

In the adaptive immunity of BD, cellular immunity is considered to play an important role, and T cells are the main lymphocytes, mainly Th1 cells, regulatory T cells (Tregs), and Th17 cells [30,31]. Studies have found mixed Th1 and Th2 cytokines in BD patients with different organ involvement [32–34]. Imamura et al. found that intestinal BD lesions expressed interferon (IFN)-γ, TNF-α, and interleukin (IL)-12, which were signature Th1 cytokines. Th1-related CCR5 was detected in intestinal samples from BD, while Th2-related CCR3 and CCR4 were mainly in inactive patients. This evidence of Th1 polarization indicated that Th1-dominant immune response has a close association with the pathogenesis of intestinal BD [35]. In addition, accumulating evidence has revealed that the expression levels of Th17 cells and related cytokines such as IL-17, IL-21, IL-22, and IL-23 are significantly higher in active BD than in inactive BD and BD at the remission stage [36–38]. In intestinal BD, the role of Th17 cells in the development of gastrointestinal involvement in BD is controversial. Ferrante et al. reported that the expression levels of Th1-related cytokines, such as TNF-α, IFN-γ, IL-12, and IL-27, were upregulated at the mRNA level in 11 patients with intestinal BD compared with healthy controls, which could inhibit the differentiation of Th0 cells into Th17 cells [30]. However, another study showed that partial CD4 clones isolated from the intestinal mucosa of eight patients at the early stage of intestinal BD produced IFN-γ and IL-17 (Th1/Th17 profile), suggesting that both Th1 and Th17 cells drive inflammation leading to mucosal damage in the early stage of intestinal BD [31]. Considering the small number of included patients, studies with a large sample size are required to explore the roles of Th1 and Th17 cells in intestinal BD. Tregs are considered a sublineage of CD4+ T cells and have a critical role in the regulation of immune tolerance and homeostasis by expressing immunosuppressive cytokines such as IL-10, IL-35, and transforming growth factor (TGF)-β as well as other functional proteins such as transcription factor forkhead box protein 3 (Foxp3) [39,40]. However, the expression levels of Tregs in BD are also inconsistent based on previous studies [41,42]. In addition, other T cells, such as Th22 cells and related cytokines, are also involved in the pathogenesis of BD. Th22 cells are CD4+ effector T cells and mainly secrete IL-22 and TNF-α, with expression of chemokine receptors as CCR4, CCR6, and CCR10. For example, the overexpression of Th22-related cytokines such as IL-22, TNF-α and chemokine receptor CCR10 was detected in the ocular samples of patients with active BD [43]. As well, the increased level of IL-22 also seemed to be associated with active uveitis and the recurrence of ulcers in patients with BD [44].

2.3. Humoral Immunity in Adaptive Immunity

Although cellular immunity plays a critical role in the pathogenesis of BD, humoral immunity also contributes to the immune reactions in the development of BD, as it takes effect in other autoimmune diseases [45]. For example, Suzuki et al. reported that patients with active BD had an increase in B cells spontaneously secreting immunoglobulin (IgG+IgA+IgM) and a decreased B-cell response to the T-cell-independent B-cell mitogen, such as *Staphylococcus aureus* Cowan 1. T-cell-dependent polyclonal activator, pokeweed mitogen. No response to the T-cell-dependent polyclonal activator as a pokeweed mitogen was also found in these patients, suggesting that B-cell abnormalities may be involved in the pathogenesis of BD [46]. Moreover, Eksioglu-Demiralp et al. found that compared with healthy controls, there was a remarkable increase in subsets of B cells marked as CD13, CD33, CD80, and CD45RO in patients with BD, although the total number of B cells marked as CD19+ was normal [47].

2.4. Innate Immunity

Innate immune cells are mainly composed of neutrophils, mononuclear phagocytes, dendritic cells, natural killer (NK) cells, γδ T cells, mast cells, and so on, of which abnormal activation plays an important role in the pathogenesis of BD [48].

Neutrophils, which act as the first line of defense against pathogens, can cause bodily injury and further the immune response, especially in patients with autoinflammatory and autoimmune disorders [49]. Previous studies reported that hyperactive neutrophils were associated with perivascular infiltration in lesion sites of patients with BD. Moreover, by increasing chemotaxis, phagocytosis, and superoxide production, neutrophils could contribute to high levels of proinflammatory cytokines such as IL-8, IL-12, TNF-α, INF-γ, and vascular endothelial dysfunction [50–52]. It is noteworthy that neutrophils act as a key factor in mediating thrombosis in BD [22,53].

NK cells are another important component of innate immunity, which regulates other immune cells, such as T cells and dendritic cells, and defends against infected cells and tumor cells by cytotoxicity and cytokine secretion, with IFN-γ as the hallmark cytokine [54–56]. Accumulating evidence has reported that the number of NK cells in the peripheral blood of patients with BD is less than that in healthy controls, suggesting that NK cells play a protective role in BD [54,57].

γδ T cells are also involved in the regulation of the autoimmune response, of which the number could increase from minority to majority of all circulating T cells in a short time once infected [58]. Sutton et al. reported that γδ T cells activated by IL-1β and IL-23 could produce IL-17, IL-21 and IL-22 without T-cell receptor engagement and mediate autoimmune inflammation in autoimmune diseases [59]. In patients with active BD, Parlakgul et al. found functional changes in γδ T cells and decreased related cytokine responses, although there was no increase in the number of γδ T cells [60].

For intestinal BD, Ahn et al. revealed that extracellular high-mobility group Box 1 (HMGB1) expression, which could activate the release of cytokines and mediate inflammation in innate immunity, was significantly increased in BD patients with gastrointestinal involvement compared to BD patients without gastrointestinal involvement and healthy controls [61]. Kirino et al. reported that Toll-like receptor 4 (TLR4), which mediates activation of the innate immune system, was upregulated with a reduction in the anti-inflammatory enzyme heme oxygenase (HO)-1 in peripheral blood mononuclear cells in patients with BD, suggesting the involvement of innate immunity in the pathogenesis of BD [62].

3. Present and Potential Biological Agents

The key points of intestinal BD treatment focus on the suppression of inflammatory exacerbations and the prevention of recurrences. As for intestinal BD, mucosal healing tends to have a better prognosis after the remission of clinical symptoms and normalization of C-reactive protein (CRP) [63]. Biological agents are an emerging category of pharmaceuticals for various diseases, including inflammatory diseases and cancers, in recent decades. They are defined by their derivation from biological sources, including monoclonal antibodies, fusion receptor proteins, hormones, and cytokines [64,65]. Table 2 lists the immune-targeted biological agents and possible applicable subtypes in BD according to current studies. And based on the immune mechanism of BD, including intestinal BD, biological agents are promising choices for the achievement of intestinal BD treatment targets. We list present and potential biological agents in intestinal BD as well as related targets, including pathogenic cells, cytokines, and pathways.

Table 2. Immune-targeted biological agents and possible applicable subtypes in BD.

Biological Agents	Immune-Related Targets	Structure	Possible Applicable Subtypes in BD
Infliximab, adalimumab	TNF-α	Monoclonal antibodies against TNF-α	All subtypes of BD * [5]
Golimumab			Intestinal BD [66]; BD with ocular and neurological involvement [67–70]
Etanercept		Soluble receptors against TNF-α	Intestinal BD [71]; BD with mucocutaneous and articular involvement * [5]
IFN-α	Not clear	Recombinant human IFN-α-2a	Intestinal BD [72–74]; BD with mucocutaneous, articular, ocular, and vascular involvement * [5]
Anakinra	IL-1	Recombinant human IL-1 receptor antagonist	Intestinal BD [75,76]; BD with mucocutaneous * and ocular involvement [77–79]
Canakinumab		Anti-IL-1β humanized monoclonal antibodies	Controversial in intestinal BD [80,81]; BD with ocular involvement [80,82]
Gevokizumab			
Tocilizumab	IL-6	Human IL-6 receptor monoclonal antibody	Controversial in intestinal BD; BD with ocular, neurological, and vascular involvement [83–85]
Secukinumab	IL-17	Human IL-17A monoclonal antibody	Unclear in intestinal BD; BD with mucocutaneous and articular involvement [86–88]
Ustekinumab	IL-12/IL-23	Human IL-12/IL-23p40 monoclonal antibody	Unclear in intestinal BD but effective in CD [89,90]; BD with mucocutaneous and ocular involvement [91–93]
Baricitinib	JAK1/JAK2	JAK1/JAK2 inhibitor; small molecule drug	Intestinal BD [94]
Apremilast	Phosphodiesterase 4	Phosphodiesterase 4 inhibitor; small molecule drug	Intestinal BD [95]; BD with mucocutaneous [95,96]
Rituximab	CD20	Chimeric mouse/human monoclonal antibody against CD20 antigen on the B lymphocyte	Unclear in intestinal BD; BD with mucocutaneous, articular, neurological, and ocular involvement [97,98]
Abatacept	B7	Selective T-cell costimulation modulator and a protein drug	Unclear in intestinal BD; BD with mucocutaneous and ocular involvement [99]
Alemtuzumab	CD52	Humanized monoclonal antibody against CD52	Unclear in intestinal BD; BD with ocular, vascular, and neurological involvement [100,101]
Vedolizumab	α4β7 integrin	Humanized anti-α4β7 integrin monoclonal antibody	Intestinal BD [102]

BD: Behcet's disease; *: Recommendation from international guidelines; IL: interleukin; CD: Crohn's disease; JAK: Janus kinase.

3.1. Anti-TNF-α Agents

TNF-α is an important proinflammatory cytokine in both innate immunity and adaptive immunity in BD patients with significantly elevated serum concentrations and mediating mucosal damage [103]. TNF-α antagonists can be classified into two groups based on different mechanisms of action: a. monoclonal antibodies such as infliximab, adalimumab, and golimumab. b. soluble receptors such as etanercept. Anti-TNF-α agents such as infliximab and adalimumab have been proven to be rapidly effective in inducing and maintaining remission of intestinal BD and are recommended by various international guidelines of intestinal BD as the only definitely effective biological agent [16,104,105]. Tanida et al. conducted a study at 12 sites in Japan in patients with intestinal BD ($n = 20$) who were refractory to corticosteroid and/or immunomodulator therapies. The results showed that most patients achieved improvement in global gastrointestinal symptoms and endoscopic scores at weeks 24 and 52, with complete remission in 20% of patients at weeks 24 and 52. No new safety signals were observed and no death occurred. Four of six patients experienced an infection after the dose escalated [106]. Another prospective study conducted by Zou et al. in patients with moderate-to-severe active intestinal BD ($n = 27$) revealed that 84.6%, 70%, and 70% of patients achieved clinical responses at weeks 14, 30, and 52 after infliximab treatment, respectively, with proportions of clinical remission of 69.2%, 40%, and 55%. Infliximab therapy was generally well tolerated in all patients, and five patients (18.5%) developed infectious adverse events [107]. Recently, Zhang et al. performed a systemic and meta-analysis including 13 studies on the application of anti-TNF-α agents in patients ($n = 739$) with intestinal BD, suggesting that anti-TNF agents, including infliximab and adalimumab, were an efficient therapy for intestinal BD. The pooled clinical remission rate at Months 3, 6, 12, and 24 were 0.61 (95%CI 0.48–0.78), 0.51 (95%CI 0.40–0.66), 0.57 (95%CI 0.48–0.67), and 0.38 (95%CI 0.16–0.88), respectively. The pooled mucosal healing rate at Months 3, 6, 12, and 24 were 0.66 (95%CI 0.50–0.86), 0.82 (95%CI 0.48–0.98), 0.65 (95%CI 0.51–0.81), and 0.69 (95%CI 0.39–1.00), respectively. The pooled estimate of the proportion of overall adverse reactions for infliximab was 0.22 (95%CI 7–69%). The majority was acute or delayed infusion reaction or infection. The pooled proportions of infusion reactions and infection were respectively 12% (95%CI 5–29%) and 21% (95%CI 6–80%) related to infliximab [108].

3.2. IFN-α

IFN-α has antiviral and antitumor functions as well as involvement in the regulation of the cytokine network and innate and adaptive immunity [109]. Because of the hypothesis of viral pathogenesis, treatment with IFNs has been suggested [73]. Data reporting the efficacy of IFN-α in BD patients can be traced back to 1986 [110]. Accumulating evidence has proven its positive role in BD, especially with ocular involvement [111–120]. IFNα may prompt the reperfusion of occluded vessels, resulting in complete remission of ocular vasculitis [121]. The EULAR updated the recommendations for BD in 2018 and recommended the application of IFN-α in BD patients with mucocutaneous, articular, ocular, and vascular involvement [5]. However, there is a lack of data about the efficacy of IFN-α in intestinal BD, except for a few case reports. Monastirli et al. reported a 40-year-old woman with BD under severe conditions with acute myelitis and intestinal involvement who achieved a nearly complete remission at week 10 after treatment with IFN-α and conventional medications. In this case report, complete remission of intestinal ulcers was observed after a 9-day combined application of IFN-α with corticosteroids followed by a 4-week IFN-α monotherapy [72]. Another two case reports showed that patients with ocular and gastrointestinal involvement at the same time experienced the disappearance of peptic ulcers after treatment with IFN-α-targeting ophthalmitis [73,74]. Based on these limited experiences, potential side effects mainly include flu-like syndrome (such as fever and arthralgia) and transient leukopenia. Further large-sample studies are required to validate the efficacy and safety of IFN-α treatment in intestinal BD.

3.3. IL-1 Antagonist

Previous studies have revealed that IL-1 acts as an important proinflammatory cytokine in the development of inflammatory diseases by inducing an acute phase response, activating endothelial cells, and expressing cell adhesion molecules and coagulation factors [122]. Elevated IL-1 levels have been found in BD since 1990 and have been confirmed in subsequent studies, laying a theoretical foundation for the use of an IL-1 antagonist as a therapeutic agent in BD [123,124]. IL-1 antagonists inhibit local inflammatory effects of IL-1, mainly including IL-1 receptor antagonists such as anakinra (ANA) and anti-IL-1β humanized monoclonal antibodies such as canakinumab (CAN) and gevokizumab (GEV). The efficacy of ANA and CAN in patients with BD was mainly reported in retrospective case series, which were not specific to intestinal BD [77–79]. Cantarini et al. conducted a study in BD patients ($n = 9$) with multiorgan involvement who were refractory to anti-TNF-α agents and standardized therapies. A total of 33.3% of patients had gastrointestinal involvement. Within 1 or 2 weeks after treatment with ANA, eight out of nine patients received a prompt response, while most patients experienced a relapse over time for an unknown reason. With regard to anakinra safety, three of nine BD patients suffered a mild itchy skin rash at the sites of anakinra injection. No serious adverse events occurred in all nine patients [75]. Another study conducted by Vitale et al. found that three adult patients with BD who were refractory to conventional medications all achieved prompt and sustained clinical remission after treatment with CAN, of whom two had gastrointestinal involvement [76]. GEV did not obtain a significantly positive result in a phase 3 trial, although a rapid clinical response and inflammation control were observed in BD patients refractory to conventional treatments in a phase 2 trial [80,81]. Certainly, future large-sample studies are needed.

3.4. IL-6 Antagonist

IL-6 is another important proinflammatory cytokine in the innate immunity of BD that is usually produced by NK cells and γδ T cells [125,126]. IL-6 usually increases TH2 differentiation and inhibits TH1 differentiation. Under inflammatory conditions, IL-6, accompanied by IL-1β and IL-21, plays a key role in the relationship between Treg and Th17 cells by inducing the differentiation of naive T cells into Th17 cells and promoting the expansion of differentiated Th17 cells [126–128]. Both Th1/Th2 and Th1/Th17 profiles have been discussed in the pathogenesis of BD, providing support for the use of IL-6 antagonists. Tocilizumab is a humanized monoclonal antibody that can block IL-6-mediated proinflammatory reactions by specific binding of the IL-6 receptor [129]. Accumulating evidence based on small-scale studies revealed that tocilizumab was effective for refractory ocular, neurological and vascular BD, while it did not play a positive role in BD patients with gastrointestinal, mucocutaneous, and articular involvement [83,84,130]. In contrast, there is one case report presenting a positive effect of tocilizumab on intestinal BD. Chen et al. reported in 2016 that a young female patient with intestinal BD was refractory to multiple conventional medications with limited application of anti-TNF-α agents due to side effects. Therefore, tocilizumab was considered a therapeutic option. Symptoms and endoscopic images of this patient improved during nine months of administration and no adverse events were reported [85]. Undoubtedly, further studies are required for a definite conclusion.

3.5. IL-17 Antagonist

As mentioned in the Immunity mechanism section in our review, IL-17 also plays a proinflammatory role in the pathogenesis of BD. Previous studies revealed that serum IL-17 concentration and TH17 cells and the number of Th17 cells were higher in active BD than in inactive BD, which also showed a positive relationship with other inflammatory markers, such as erythrocyte sedimentation rate (ESR) and CRP [38,131]. Secukinumab, which has been approved for the treatment of psoriatic arthritis and ankylosing spondylitis, is a human IL-17A-binding monoclonal antibody [132]. However, its role in intestinal BD is controversial and needs further investigation. Di Scala G et al. conducted a study in five BD patients with mucocutaneous and joint involvement who were refractory to at least one anti-TNF-α agent. The results revealed that all patients could achieve complete response after treatment with secukinumab at a dose of 300 mg/month. The treatment was well tolerated and no significant drug reaction was observed. Only mild infections of the urinary tract were recorded in two patients [86]. Fagni et al. conducted a multicenter retrospective study of BD patients ($n = 15$) with mucosal and articular subphenotypes who were refractory to conventional medications and at least one anti-TNF-α agent. After treatment with secukinumab, the proportion of patients achieving a response (complete or partial) increased with follow-up time: 66.7% at 3 months, 86.7% at 6 months, 76.9% at 12 months, 90.0% at 18 months and 100.0% after 24 months. No serious or dose-related adverse effects were observed [87]. In contrast, in a randomized, controlled clinical trial of 118 patients with Behçet's uveitis, there were no statistically significant differences in the primary outcome of uveitis recurrence between the secukinumab treatment groups and placebo groups, although treatment with secukinumab may reduce the use of concomitant immunosuppressive medication based on the secondary outcome of the randomized controlled trial (RCT). Greater percentages of patients in the secukinumab treatment groups experienced ocular or nonocular adverse events compared with the placebo group [88]. Barrado-Solís et al. also reported that BD developed in two patients with psoriasis a few weeks after receiving secukinumab treatment [133]. Although no related studies have been conducted in intestinal BD thus far, it is worth noting that in a high-quality RCT of 59 patients with moderate to severe CD, treatment with secukinumab has been proven to be ineffective and to have higher rates of adverse events than placebo. Drug-related serious adverse events, including worsening of CD, pilonidal cyst, and ileostomy, occurred in six patients receiving secukinumab. Twenty infections were seen on secukinumab while none on placebo [134]. Considering that intestinal BD is similar to CD in its clinical symptoms, imaging findings and endoscopic characteristics, exploration of secukinumab treatment in intestinal BD should be more rigorous and careful.

3.6. IL-12/IL-23 Antagonist

IL-12 and IL-23, which both belong to the IL-12 cytokine family, share the same p40 subunit [135,136]. The former has a significant role in differentiating naive T cells into Th1 cells, and the latter is indispensable for the differentiation of Th17 cells [137]. Previous studies have shown that IL-12 and IL-23 are involved in the immune mechanism of BD [138,139]. Genome Wide Association Studies (GWAS) have reported that IL12R-IL23RB2 region is associated with BD, suggesting the role of IL12 and IL23 receptors in the disease onset [140]. Ustekinumab, a fully humanized monoclonal antibody targeting the p40 subunit of IL-12 and IL-23, has been reported to be effective in BD, although there are no related studies in intestinal BD [91–93]. In addition, ustekinumab has been proven to be effective in treating active CD. The rates of adverse events were similar in ustekinumab and placebo group, mainly including infections, arthralgia, headache, and nausea [89,90]. In summary, considering the similarity between CD and intestinal BD, ustekinumab may be a potential biological agent in intestinal BD.

3.7. Small Molecule Targeted Agents

Small molecule targeted agents are chemically synthesized but have high selectivity and efficacy similar to those of typical biological agents, which were considered special biological agents in a broad sense. Among them, baricitinib as an oral Janus kinase (JAK)-inhibitors (JAKi) and apremilast as an oral phosphodiesterase 4 inhibitor, were reported in case series to be potential drugs in the treatment of intestinal BD [94,95]. Baricitinib, a new class of targeted synthetic DMARDs (tsDMARDs), interferes with signal transduction pathways of a variety of cytokines. It can suppress the differentiation of plasmablasts, Th1 and Th17 cells, as well as innate immunity, showing potential in immune-related diseases [141]. Thirteen intestinal BD patients received baricitinib 2–4 mg daily, with background glucocorticoids and immunosuppressants. 76.92% (10/13) patients achieved complete remission of global gastrointestinal symptom scores, and 66.7% (6/9) had mucosal healing on endoscopy. The disease activity index for intestinal Behçet's disease (DAIBD) and CRP level decreased significantly [94]. Certainly, future large-sample studies are required to confirm the potential of these biological agents.

3.8. Other Biological Agents

In addition to the drugs mentioned above, there are other biological agents with potential applications in intestinal BD as well. Considering the lack of related studies in intestinal BD, our review plan is to perform a preliminary overview of these drugs: a. Rituximab, a chimeric mouse/human monoclonal antibody, could cause B-cell lysis by specifically binding CD20 antigen on the B lymphocyte. Previous studies have shown that it may have positive effects on BD with mucocutaneous, articular, neurological, and ocular subphenotypes. According to the pilot RCT study, in the rituximab group, two of ten patients had conjunctivitis during the first infusion, one patient had pneumonia 4 months after the infusion and one patient had herpes zoster 4 months after the infusion. The remaining side effects were infusion-related, all during the first infusion [97,98]. b. Abatacept, a soluble fusion protein consisting of the extracellular domain of human cytotoxic T-lymphocyte-associated protein 4 (CTLA4), is a selective T-cell costimulation modulator and a protein drug for autoimmune diseases [142]. A case report published by Maciel suggested that abatacept may be effective for refractory ocular and mucocutaneous BD [99]. c. Alemtuzumab, a humanized monoclonal antibody against CD52, is a glycoprotein expressed on the surface of most lymphocytes and in myeloid cells to a lesser extent. Therefore, it could induce deep depletion of lymphocytes and then restore T cells and B cells with a regulatory phenotype [143]. Previous studies revealed that alemtuzumab may provide an alternative treatment strategy for refractory BD with ocular, vascular, and neurological involvement [100,101,144]. d. Vedolizumab, a humanized anti-$\alpha 4 \beta 7$ integrin monoclonal antibody, can modulate gut lymphocyte trafficking. It has been approved for both induction and maintenance treatment of inflammatory bowel diseases (IBD) such as CD and ulcerative colitis. Its gastrointestinal-specific interaction reduces the side effects associated with systemic immunosuppression [90]. Up to now, there has been only one case report of a patient with intestinal BD suggesting its efficacy as a valid option for treatment. This 49-year-old female was unsuccessfully treated with conventional immunosuppressive and several biological agents and received vedolizumab at 0, 2, and 6 weeks and then every 4 weeks. After the second dose of vedolizumab, a marked improvement of intestinal BD was achieved and clinical remission was achieved at 6 months without side effects [102].

4. Conclusions

Intestinal BD has been classified into IBD to some extent, of which typical members are UC and CD, considering the similarity of genetic backgrounds, clinical manifestations, and therapeutic strategies. As well, there is no doubt that progress in our understanding of the pathogenesis of intestinal BD as well as the other members of IBD will pave the way for seeking effective approaches. Based on the immunological perspective, we have come to know that immune cells, related cytokines, and specific autoantibodies play important roles in the pathogenesis of intestinal BD, although the etiology remains unclear. Biological agents targeting potential pathogenic cells, cytokines, and pathways are optimized options in the treatment of intestinal BD. Some of them have been considered to be definitely effective in intestinal BD and are widely used in clinical practice, such as anti-TNF-α agents, while others require further well-designed multi-center RCT or other study designs that would provide high-quality evidence to confirm their efficacy. Detailed issues accompanied by the wide use of biological agents in the near future, such as adjustment of dosage form or dosage for an invalid biological agent, transition to other biological agents, combination of different kinds of drugs and prevention of adverse effects, call for in-depth thinking and further extensive studies. Certainly, drugs related to immune mechanisms in preclinical stages also deserve attention. Furthermore, considering that intestinal BD is a specific and less common phenotype of BD, separate studies focused on intestinal involvement and comparisons of different phenotypes will become the trend of future research, especially from the perspective of pathogenesis. These will provide more precise explanations of mechanisms and more individualized treatment strategies for different organ involvement.

Author Contributions: Conceptualization, K.H., X.Y. and D.W.; methodology, K.H.; validation, K.H., X.Y. and D.W.; formal analysis, K.H. and X.Y.; investigation, K.H. and X.Y.; resources, D.W.; writing—original draft preparation, K.H. and X.Y.; writing—review and editing, D.W.; visualization, K.H. and X.Y.; supervision, D.W.; project administration, D.W. All authors have read and agreed to the published version of the manuscript.

Funding: This research received financial support from National Key Clinical Specialty Construction Project (ZK108000).

Institutional Review Board Statement: Not applicable.

Informed Consent Statement: Not applicable.

Data Availability Statement: The data underlying this article are available in the article.

Acknowledgments: The authors would like to thank Yabing Wang and Tao Wang for their comments to the manuscript.

Conflicts of Interest: The authors declare no conflict of interest.

References

1. Hatemi, G.; Seyahi, E.; Fresko, I.; Talarico, R.; Ucar, D.; Hamuryudan, V. Behcet's syndrome: One year in review 2022. *Clin. Exp. Rheumatol.* **2022**, *40*, 1461–1471. [CrossRef] [PubMed]
2. Yazici, H.; Seyahi, E.; Hatemi, G.; Yazici, Y. Behcet syndrome: A contemporary view. *Nat. Rev. Rheumatol.* **2018**, *14*, 107–119. [CrossRef] [PubMed]
3. Guan, J. *New Concept of Behcet's Disease*; Fudan University Press: Shanghai, China, 2021; pp. 55–91.
4. Bettiol, A.; Hatemi, G.; Vannozzi, L.; Barilaro, A.; Prisco, D.; Emmi, G. Treating the Different Phenotypes of Behcet's Syndrome. *Front. Immunol.* **2019**, *10*, 2830. [CrossRef] [PubMed]
5. Hatemi, G.; Christensen, R.; Bang, D.; Bodaghi, B.; Celik, A.F.; Fortune, F.; Gaudric, J.; Gul, A.; Kotter, I.; Leccese, P.; et al. 2018 update of the EULAR recommendations for the management of Behcet's syndrome. *Ann. Rheum. Dis.* **2018**, *77*, 808–818. [CrossRef] [PubMed]
6. Hatemi, I.; Hatemi, G.; Celik, A.F. Gastrointestinal Involvement in Behcet Disease. *Rheum. Dis. Clin. N. Am.* **2018**, *44*, 45–64. [CrossRef] [PubMed]
7. Skef, W.; Hamilton, M.J.; Arayssi, T. Gastrointestinal Behcet's disease: A review. *World J. Gastroenterol.* **2015**, *21*, 3801–3812. [CrossRef]
8. Soejima, Y.; Kirino, Y.; Takeno, M.; Kurosawa, M.; Takeuchi, M.; Yoshimi, R.; Sugiyama, Y.; Ohno, S.; Asami, Y.; Sekiguchi, A.; et al. Changes in the proportion of clinical clusters contribute to the phenotypic evolution of Behçet's disease in Japan. *Arthritis Res. Ther.* **2021**, *23*, 49. [CrossRef]
9. Kim, D.H.; Cheon, J.H. Intestinal Behcet's Disease: A True Inflammatory Bowel Disease or Merely an Intestinal Complication of Systemic Vasculitis? *Yonsei Med. J.* **2016**, *57*, 22–32. [CrossRef]
10. He, K.; Wu, D. Clinical characteristics, diagnosis and evaluation of intestinal Behcet's disease. *Chin. J. Gen. Pract.* **2022**, *21*, 1101–1106. [CrossRef]
11. Salmaninejad, A.; Zamani, M.R.; Shabgah, A.G.; Hosseini, S.; Mollaei, F.; Hosseini, N.; Sahebkar, A. Behcet's disease: An immunogenetic perspective. *J. Cell. Physiol.* **2019**, *234*, 8055–8074. [CrossRef]
12. Gong, L.; Zhang, Y.L.; Sun, L.X.; Chen, G.R.; Wu, D. Mucosal healing in intestinal Behcet's disease: A systematic review and meta-analysis. *J. Dig. Dis.* **2021**, *22*, 83–90. [CrossRef] [PubMed]
13. Nguyen, A.; Upadhyay, S.; Javaid, M.A.; Qureshi, A.M.; Haseeb, S.; Javed, N.; Cormier, C.; Farooq, A.; Sheikh, A.B. Behcet's Disease: An In-Depth Review about Pathogenesis, Gastrointestinal Manifestations, and Management. *Inflamm. Intest. Dis.* **2021**, *6*, 175–185. [CrossRef] [PubMed]
14. Alibaz-Oner, F.; Direskeneli, H. Biologic treatments in Behcet's disease. *Eur. J. Rheumatol.* **2021**, *8*, 217–222. [CrossRef]
15. Bozkurt, T.; Karabacak, M.; Karatas, H.; KutlugAgackiran, S.; Ergun, T.; Direskeneli, H.; Alibaz-Oner, F. Earlier and more aggressive treatment with biologics may prevent relapses and further new organ involvement in Behcet's disease. *Clin. Immunol.* **2023**, *248*, 109263. [CrossRef]
16. Watanabe, K.; Tanida, S.; Inoue, N.; Kunisaki, R.; Kobayashi, K.; Nagahori, M.; Arai, K.; Uchino, M.; Koganei, K.; Kobayashi, T.; et al. Evidence-based diagnosis and clinical practice guidelines for intestinal Behcet's disease 2020 edited by Intractable Diseases, the Health and Labour Sciences Research Grants. *J. Gastroenterol.* **2020**, *55*, 679–700. [CrossRef]

17. Tong, B.; Liu, X.; Xiao, J.; Su, G. Immunopathogenesis of Behcet's Disease. *Front. Immunol.* **2019**, *10*, 665. [CrossRef] [PubMed]
18. Iris, M.; Ozcikmak, E.; Aksoy, A.; Alibaz-Oner, F.; Inanc, N.; Ergun, T.; Direskeneli, H.; Mumcu, G. The assessment of contributing factors to oral ulcer presence in Behcet's disease: Dietary and non-dietary factors. *Eur. J. Rheumatol.* **2018**, *5*, 240–243. [CrossRef]
19. Mumcu, G.; Direskeneli, H. Triggering agents and microbiome as environmental factors on Behcet's syndrome. *Intern. Emerg. Med.* **2019**, *14*, 653–660. [CrossRef]
20. Yan, X.; Wu, D. Research progress on the pathogenesis of intestinal Behcet's syndrome. *Chin. J. Alergy Clin. Immunol.* **2022**, *16*, 501–505. (In Chinese) [CrossRef]
21. Park, U.C.; Kim, T.W.; Yu, H.G. Immunopathogenesis of ocular Behcet's disease. *J. Immunol. Res.* **2014**, *2014*, 653539. [CrossRef]
22. Pineton de Chambrun, M.; Wechsler, B.; Geri, G.; Cacoub, P.; Saadoun, D. New insights into the pathogenesis of Behçet's disease. *Autoimmun. Rev.* **2012**, *11*, 687–698. [CrossRef] [PubMed]
23. Direskeneli, H.; Saruhan-Direskeneli, G. The role of heat shock proteins in Behet's disease. *Clin. Exp. Rheumatol.* **2003**, *21* (Suppl. S30), S44–S48. [PubMed]
24. Birtas-Atesoglu, E.; Inanc, N.; Yavuz, S.; Ergun, T.; Direskeneli, H. Serum levels of free heat shock protein 70 and anti-HSP70 are elevated in Behçet's disease. *Clin. Exp. Rheumatol.* **2008**, *26* (Suppl. S50), S96–S98. [PubMed]
25. Mahesh, S.P.; Li, Z.; Buggage, R.; Mor, F.; Cohen, I.R.; Chew, E.Y.; Nussenblatt, R.B. Alpha tropomyosin as a self-antigen in patients with Behcet's disease. *Clin. Exp. Immunol.* **2005**, *140*, 368–375. [CrossRef]
26. Consolandi, C.; Turroni, S.; Emmi, G.; Severgnini, M.; Fiori, J.; Peano, C.; Biagi, E.; Grassi, A.; Rampelli, S.; Silvestri, E.; et al. Behçet's syndrome patients exhibit specific microbiome signature. *Autoimmun. Rev.* **2015**, *14*, 269–276. [CrossRef]
27. Shimizu, J.; Kubota, T.; Takada, E.; Takai, K.; Fujiwara, N.; Arimitsu, N.; Ueda, Y.; Wakisaka, S.; Suzuki, T.; Suzuki, N. Relative abundance of Megamonas hypermegale and Butyrivibrio species decreased in the intestine and its possible association with the T cell aberration by metabolite alteration in patients with Behcet's disease (210 characters). *Clin. Rheumatol.* **2019**, *38*, 1437–1445. [CrossRef]
28. Shimizu, J.; Kubota, T.; Takada, E.; Takai, K.; Fujiwara, N.; Arimitsu, N.; Ueda, Y.; Wakisaka, S.; Suzuki, T.; Suzuki, N. Bifidobacteria Abundance-Featured Gut Microbiota Compositional Change in Patients with Behcet's Disease. *PLoS ONE* **2016**, *11*, e0153746. [CrossRef]
29. Yasar Bilge, N.S.; Perez Brocal, V.; Kasifoglu, T.; Bilge, U.; Kasifoglu, N.; Moya, A.; Dinleyici, E.C. Intestinal microbiota composition of patients with Behcet's disease: Differences between eye, mucocutaneous and vascular involvement. The Rheuma-BIOTA study. *Clin. Exp. Rheumatol.* **2020**, *38* (Suppl. S127), 60–68.
30. Ferrante, A.; Ciccia, F.; Principato, A.; Giardina, A.R.; Impastato, R.; Peralta, S.; Triolo, G. A Th1 but not a Th17 response is present in the gastrointestinal involvement of Behcet's disease. *Clin. Exp. Rheumatol.* **2010**, *28* (Suppl. S60), S27–S30.
31. Emmi, G.; Silvestri, E.; Bella, C.D.; Grassi, A.; Benagiano, M.; Cianchi, F.; Squatrito, D.; Cantarini, L.; Emmi, L.; Selmi, C.; et al. Cytotoxic Th1 and Th17 cells infiltrate the intestinal mucosa of Behcet patients and exhibit high levels of TNF-alpha in early phases of the disease. *Medicine* **2016**, *95*, e5516. [CrossRef]
32. Aridogan, B.C.; Yildirim, M.; Baysal, V.; Inaloz, H.S.; Baz, K.; Kaya, S. Serum Levels of IL-4, IL-10, IL-12, IL-13 and IFN-gamma in Behcet's disease. *J. Dermatol.* **2003**, *30*, 602–607. [CrossRef] [PubMed]
33. Ahn, J.K.; Yu, H.G.; Chung, H.; Park, Y.G. Intraocular cytokine environment in active Behcet uveitis. *Am. J. Ophthalmol.* **2006**, *142*, 429–434. [CrossRef] [PubMed]
34. Horai, R.; Caspi, R.R. Cytokines in autoimmune uveitis. *J. Interferon Cytokine Res.* **2011**, *31*, 733–744. [CrossRef] [PubMed]
35. Imamura, Y.; Kurokawa, M.S.; Yoshikawa, H.; Nara, K.; Takada, E.; Masuda, C.; Tsukikawa, S.; Ozaki, S.; Matsuda, T.; Suzuki, N. Involvement of Th1 cells and heat shock protein 60 in the pathogenesis of intestinal Behcet's disease. *Clin. Exp. Immunol.* **2005**, *139*, 371–378. [CrossRef]
36. Chi, W.; Zhu, X.; Yang, P.; Liu, X.; Lin, X.; Zhou, H.; Huang, X.; Kijlstra, A. Upregulated IL-23 and IL-17 in Behcet patients with active uveitis. *Invest. Ophthalmol. Vis. Sci.* **2008**, *49*, 3058–3064. [CrossRef] [PubMed]
37. Nanke, Y.; Yago, T.; Kotake, S. The Role of Th17 Cells in the Pathogenesis of Behcet's Disease. *J. Clin. Med.* **2017**, *6*, 74. [CrossRef] [PubMed]
38. Hamzaoui, K.; Bouali, E.; Ghorbel, I.; Khanfir, M.; Houman, H.; Hamzaoui, A. Expression of Th-17 and RORgammat mRNA in Behcet's Disease. *Med. Sci. Monit.* **2011**, *17*, CR227–CR234. [CrossRef]
39. Campbell, D.J.; Koch, M.A. Phenotypical and functional specialization of FOXP3+ regulatory T cells. *Nat. Rev. Immunol.* **2011**, *11*, 119–130. [CrossRef]
40. Sakaguchi, S.; Miyara, M.; Costantino, C.M.; Hafler, D.A. FOXP3+ regulatory T cells in the human immune system. *Nat. Rev. Immunol.* **2010**, *10*, 490–500. [CrossRef]
41. Geri, G.; Terrier, B.; Rosenzwajg, M.; Wechsler, B.; Touzot, M.; Seilhean, D.; Tran, T.A.; Bodaghi, B.; Musset, L.; Soumelis, V.; et al. Critical role of IL-21 in modulating TH17 and regulatory T cells in Behcet disease. *J. Allergy Clin. Immunol.* **2011**, *128*, 655–664. [CrossRef]
42. Hamzaoui, K.; Borhani Haghighi, A.; Ghorbel, I.B.; Houman, H. RORC and Foxp3 axis in cerebrospinal fluid of patients with neuro-Behcet's disease. *J. Neuroimmunol.* **2011**, *233*, 249–253. [CrossRef]
43. Duhen, T.; Geiger, R.; Jarrossay, D.; Lanzavecchia, A.; Sallusto, F. Production of interleukin 22 but not interleukin 17 by a subset of human skin-homing memory T cells. *Nat. Immunol.* **2009**, *10*, 857–863. [CrossRef]

44. Aktas Cetin, E.; Cosan, F.; Cefle, A.; Deniz, G. IL-22-secreting Th22 and IFN-γ-secreting Th17 cells in Behçet's disease. *Mod. Rheumatol.* **2014**, *24*, 802–807. [CrossRef] [PubMed]
45. Yanaba, K.; Bouaziz, J.D.; Matsushita, T.; Magro, C.M.; St Clair, E.W.; Tedder, T.F. B-lymphocyte contributions to human autoimmune disease. *Immunol. Rev.* **2008**, *223*, 284–299. [CrossRef] [PubMed]
46. Suzuki, N.; Sakane, T.; Ueda, Y.; Tsunematsu, T. Abnormal B cell function in patients with Behcet's disease. *Arthritis Rheum.* **1986**, *29*, 212–219. [CrossRef] [PubMed]
47. Eksioglu-Demiralp, E.; Kibaroglu, A.; Direskeneli, H.; Yavuz, S.; Karsli, F.; Yurdakul, S.; Yazici, H.; Akoglu, T. Phenotypic characteristics of B cells in Behcet's disease: Increased activity in B cell subsets. *J. Rheumatol.* **1999**, *26*, 826–832.
48. Beutler, B. Innate immunity: An overview. *Mol. Immunol.* **2004**, *40*, 845–859. [CrossRef]
49. Nathan, C. Neutrophils and immunity: Challenges and opportunities. *Nat. Rev. Immunol.* **2006**, *6*, 173–182. [CrossRef]
50. Neves, F.S.; Spiller, F. Possible mechanisms of neutrophil activation in Behcet's disease. *Int. Immunopharmacol.* **2013**, *17*, 1206–1210. [CrossRef]
51. Keller, M.; Spanou, Z.; Schaerli, P.; Britschgi, M.; Yawalkar, N.; Seitz, M.; Villiger, P.M.; Pichler, W.J. T cell-regulated neutrophilic inflammation in autoinflammatory diseases. *J. Immunol.* **2005**, *175*, 7678–7686. [CrossRef]
52. Kobayashi, M.; Ito, M.; Nakagawa, A.; Matsushita, M.; Nishikimi, N.; Sakurai, T.; Nimura, Y. Neutrophil and endothelial cell activation in the vasa vasorum in vasculo-Behcet disease. *Histopathology* **2000**, *36*, 362–371. [CrossRef]
53. Becatti, M.; Emmi, G.; Silvestri, E.; Bruschi, G.; Ciuccarelli, L.; Squatrito, D.; Vaglio, A.; Taddei, N.; Abbate, R.; Emmi, L.; et al. Neutrophil Activation Promotes Fibrinogen Oxidation and Thrombus Formation in Behcet Disease. *Circulation* **2016**, *133*, 302–311. [CrossRef]
54. Kucuksezer, U.C.; Aktas Cetin, E.; Esen, F.; Tahrali, I.; Akdeniz, N.; Gelmez, M.Y.; Deniz, G. The Role of Natural Killer Cells in Autoimmune Diseases. *Front. Immunol.* **2021**, *12*, 622306. [CrossRef]
55. Cooper, M.A.; Fehniger, T.A.; Turner, S.C.; Chen, K.S.; Ghaheri, B.A.; Ghayur, T.; Carson, W.E.; Caligiuri, M.A. Human natural killer cells: A unique innate immunoregulatory role for the CD56(bright) subset. *Blood* **2001**, *97*, 3146–3151. [CrossRef] [PubMed]
56. Moretta, A.; Marcenaro, E.; Parolini, S.; Ferlazzo, G.; Moretta, L. NK cells at the interface between innate and adaptive immunity. *Cell. Death Differ.* **2008**, *15*, 226–233. [CrossRef] [PubMed]
57. Hasan, M.S.; Ryan, P.L.; Bergmeier, L.A.; Fortune, F. Circulating NK cells and their subsets in Behcet's disease. *Clin. Exp. Immunol.* **2017**, *188*, 311–322. [CrossRef] [PubMed]
58. Eberl, M.; Moser, B. Monocytes and gammadelta T cells: Close encounters in microbial infection. *Trends Immunol.* **2009**, *30*, 562–568. [CrossRef]
59. Sutton, C.E.; Lalor, S.J.; Sweeney, C.M.; Brereton, C.F.; Lavelle, E.C.; Mills, K.H. Interleukin-1 and IL-23 induce innate IL-17 production from gammadelta T cells, amplifying Th17 responses and autoimmunity. *Immunity* **2009**, *31*, 331–341. [CrossRef] [PubMed]
60. Parlakgul, G.; Guney, E.; Erer, B.; Kilicaslan, Z.; Direskeneli, H.; Gul, A.; Saruhan-Direskeneli, G. Expression of regulatory receptors on gammadelta T cells and their cytokine production in Behcet's disease. *Arthritis Res. Ther.* **2013**, *15*, R15. [CrossRef]
61. Ahn, J.K.; Cha, H.S.; Bae, E.K.; Lee, J.; Koh, E.M. Extracellular high-mobility group box 1 is increased in patients with Behcet's disease with intestinal involvement. *J. Korean Med. Sci.* **2011**, *26*, 697–700. [CrossRef]
62. Kirino, Y.; Takeno, M.; Watanabe, R.; Murakami, S.; Kobayashi, M.; Ideguchi, H.; Ihata, A.; Ohno, S.; Ueda, A.; Mizuki, N.; et al. Association of reduced heme oxygenase-1 with excessive Toll-like receptor 4 expression in peripheral blood mononuclear cells in Behcet's disease. *Arthritis Res. Ther.* **2008**, *10*, R16. [CrossRef] [PubMed]
63. He, K.; Wu, D. The treatment principles and targets for intestinal Behcet's disease. *Therap. Adv. Gastroenterol.* **2023**, *16*, 17562848231167283. [CrossRef] [PubMed]
64. Corominas, M.; Gastaminza, G.; Lobera, T. Hypersensitivity reactions to biological drugs. *J. Investig. Allergol. Clin. Immunol.* **2014**, *24*, 212–225.
65. Purcell, R.T.; Lockey, R.F. Immunologic responses to therapeutic biologic agents. *J. Investig. Allergol. Clin. Immunol.* **2008**, *18*, 335–342.
66. Vitale, A.; Emmi, G.; Lopalco, G.; Fabiani, C.; Gentileschi, S.; Silvestri, E.; Gerardo, D.S.; Iannone, F.; Frediani, B.; Galeazzi, M.; et al. Long-term efficacy and safety of golimumab in the treatment of multirefractory Behcet's disease. *Clin. Rheumatol.* **2017**, *36*, 2063–2069. [CrossRef] [PubMed]
67. Fabiani, C.; Sota, J.; Rigante, D.; Vitale, A.; Emmi, G.; Vannozzi, L.; Franceschini, R.; Bacherini, D.; Frediani, B.; Galeazzi, M.; et al. Rapid and Sustained Efficacy of Golimumab in the Treatment of Multirefractory Uveitis Associated with Behcet's Disease. *Ocul. Immunol. Inflamm.* **2019**, *27*, 58–63. [CrossRef] [PubMed]
68. Mesquida, M.; Victoria Hernandez, M.; Llorenc, V.; Pelegrin, L.; Espinosa, G.; Dick, A.D.; Adan, A. Behcet disease-associated uveitis successfully treated with golimumab. *Ocul. Immunol. Inflamm.* **2013**, *21*, 160–162. [CrossRef]
69. Yao, M.; Gao, C.; Zhang, C.; Di, X.; Liang, W.; Sun, W.; Wang, Q.; Zheng, Z. Behcet's disease with peripheral nervous system involvement successfully treated with golimumab: A case report and review of the literature. *Rheumatol. Int.* **2021**, *41*, 197–203. [CrossRef]
70. Kon, T.; Hasui, K.; Suzuki, C.; Nishijima, H.; Tomiyama, M. Isolated myelitis in a patient with Behcet's disease during golimumab therapy. *J. Neuroimmunol.* **2021**, *354*, 577533. [CrossRef]

71. Melikoglu, M.; Fresko, I.; Mat, C.; Ozyazgan, Y.; Gogus, F.; Yurdakul, S.; Hamuryudan, V.; Yazici, H. Short-term trial of etanercept in Behcet's disease: A double blind, placebo controlled study. *J. Rheumatol.* **2005**, *32*, 98–105.
72. Monastirli, A.; Chroni, E.; Georgiou, S.; Ellul, J.; Pasmatzi, E.; Papathanasopoulos, P.; Tsambaos, D. Interferon-alpha treatment for acute myelitis and intestinal involvement in severe Behcet's disease. *QJM* **2010**, *103*, 787–790. [CrossRef] [PubMed]
73. Grimbacher, B.; Wenger, B.; Deibert, P.; Ness, T.; Koetter, I.; Peter, H.H. Loss of vision and diarrhoea. *Lancet* **1997**, *350*, 1818. [CrossRef] [PubMed]
74. Kotter, I.; Vonthein, R.; Zierhut, M.; Eckstein, A.K.; Ness, T.; Gunaydin, I.; Grimbacher, B.; Blaschke, S.; Peter, H.H.; Stubiger, N. Differential efficacy of human recombinant interferon-alpha2a on ocular and extraocular manifestations of Behcet disease: Results of an open 4-center trial. *Semin. Arthritis Rheum.* **2004**, *33*, 311–319. [CrossRef] [PubMed]
75. Cantarini, L.; Vitale, A.; Scalini, P.; Dinarello, C.A.; Rigante, D.; Franceschini, R.; Simonini, G.; Borsari, G.; Caso, F.; Lucherini, O.M.; et al. Anakinra treatment in drug-resistant Behcet's disease: A case series. *Clin. Rheumatol.* **2015**, *34*, 1293–1301. [CrossRef]
76. Vitale, A.; Rigante, D.; Caso, F.; Brizi, M.G.; Galeazzi, M.; Costa, L.; Franceschini, R.; Lucherini, O.M.; Cantarini, L. Inhibition of interleukin-1 by canakinumab as a successful mono-drug strategy for the treatment of refractory Behcet's disease: A case series. *Dermatology* **2014**, *228*, 211–214. [CrossRef]
77. Ugurlu, S.; Ucar, D.; Seyahi, E.; Hatemi, G.; Yurdakul, S. Canakinumab in a patient with juvenile Behcet's syndrome with refractory eye disease. *Ann. Rheum. Dis.* **2012**, *71*, 1589–1591. [CrossRef]
78. Cantarini, L.; Vitale, A.; Borri, M.; Galeazzi, M.; Franceschini, R. Successful use of canakinumab in a patient with resistant Behcet's disease. *Clin. Exp. Rheumatol.* **2012**, *30* (Suppl. S72), S115.
79. Botsios, C.; Sfriso, P.; Furlan, A.; Punzi, L.; Dinarello, C.A. Resistant Behcet disease responsive to anakinra. *Ann. Intern. Med.* **2008**, *149*, 284–286. [CrossRef]
80. Tugal-Tutkun, I.M.; Kadayifcilar, S.M.; Khairallah, M.M.; Lee, S.C.M.P.; Ozdal, P.; Ozyazgan, Y.; Song, J.H.M.; Yu, H.G.M.P.; Lehner, V.P.; de Cordoue, A.M.; et al. Safety and Efficacy of Gevokizumab in Patients with Behcet's Disease Uveitis: Results of an Exploratory Phase 2 Study. *Ocul. Immunol. Inflamm.* **2017**, *25*, 62–70. [CrossRef]
81. Tugal-Tutkun, I.; Pavesio, C.; De Cordoue, A.; Bernard-Poenaru, O.; Gul, A. Use of Gevokizumab in Patients with Behcet's Disease Uveitis: An International, Randomized, Double-Masked, Placebo-Controlled Study and Open-Label Extension Study. *Ocul. Immunol. Inflamm.* **2018**, *26*, 1023–1033. [CrossRef]
82. Gul, A.; Tugal-Tutkun, I.; Dinarello, C.A.; Reznikov, L.; Esen, B.A.; Mirza, A.; Scannon, P.; Solinger, A. Interleukin-1beta-regulating antibody XOMA 052 (gevokizumab) in the treatment of acute exacerbations of resistant uveitis of Behcet's disease: An open-label pilot study. *Ann. Rheum. Dis.* **2012**, *71*, 563–566. [CrossRef] [PubMed]
83. Atienza-Mateo, B.; Calvo-Río, V.; Beltrán, E.; Martínez-Costa, L.; Valls-Pascual, E.; Hernández-Garfella, M.; Atanes, A.; Cordero-Coma, M.; Miquel Nolla, J.; Carrasco-Cubero, C.; et al. Anti-interleukin 6 receptor tocilizumab in refractory uveitis associated with Behçet's disease: Multicentre retrospective study. *Rheumatology* **2018**, *57*, 856–864. [CrossRef] [PubMed]
84. Deroux, A.; Chiquet, C.; Bouillet, L. Tocilizumab in severe and refractory Behcet's disease: Four cases and literature review. *Semin. Arthritis Rheum.* **2016**, *45*, 733–737. [CrossRef] [PubMed]
85. Chen, J.; Chen, S.; He, J. A case of refractory intestinal Behçet's disease treated with tocilizumab, a humanised anti-interleukin-6 receptor antibody. *Clin. Exp. Rheumatol.* **2017**, *35*, 116–118.
86. Di Scala, G.; Bettiol, A.; Cojan, R.D.; Finocchi, M.; Silvestri, E.; Emmi, G. Efficacy of the anti-IL 17 secukinumab in refractory Behçet's syndrome: A preliminary study. *J. Autoimmun.* **2019**, *97*, 108–113. [CrossRef]
87. Fagni, F.; Bettiol, A.; Talarico, R.; Lopalco, G.; Silvestri, E.; Urban, M.L.; Russo, P.A.J.; Di Scala, G.; Emmi, G.; Prisco, D. Long-term effectiveness and safety of secukinumab for treatment of refractory mucosal and articular Behçet's phenotype: A multicentre study. *Ann. Rheum. Dis.* **2020**, *79*, 1098–1104. [CrossRef]
88. Dick, A.D.; Tugal-Tutkun, I.; Foster, S.; Zierhut, M.; Melissa Liew, S.H.; Bezlyak, V.; Androudi, S. Secukinumab in the treatment of noninfectious uveitis: Results of three randomized, controlled clinical trials. *Ophthalmology* **2013**, *120*, 777–787. [CrossRef]
89. Singh, S.; Murad, M.H.; Fumery, M.; Sedano, R.; Jairath, V.; Panaccione, R.; Sandborn, W.J.; Ma, C. Comparative efficacy and safety of biologic therapies for moderate-to-severe Crohn's disease: A systematic review and network meta-analysis. *Lancet Gastroenterol. Hepatol.* **2021**, *6*, 1002–1014. [CrossRef]
90. Feagan, B.G.; Sandborn, W.J.; Gasink, C.; Jacobstein, D.; Lang, Y.; Friedman, J.R.; Blank, M.A.; Johanns, J.; Gao, L.L.; Miao, Y.; et al. Ustekinumab as Induction and Maintenance Therapy for Crohn's Disease. *N. Engl. J. Med.* **2016**, *375*, 1946–1960. [CrossRef]
91. Lopalco, G.; Fabiani, C.; Venerito, V.; Lapadula, G.; Iannone, F.; Cantarini, L. Ustekinumab efficacy and safety in mucocutaneous multi-refractory Behçet's disease. *Clin. Exp. Rheumatol.* **2017**, *35*, 130–131.
92. Baerveldt, E.M.; Kappen, J.H.; Thio, H.B.; van Laar, J.A.; van Hagen, P.M.; Prens, E.P. Successful long-term triple disease control by ustekinumab in a patient with Behcet's disease, psoriasis and hidradenitis suppurativa. *Ann. Rheum. Dis.* **2013**, *72*, 626–627. [CrossRef] [PubMed]
93. Mirouse, A.; Barete, S.; Desbois, A.C.; Comarmond, C.; Sène, D.; Domont, F.; Bodaghi, B.; Ferfar, Y.; Cacoub, P.; Saadoun, D. Long-Term Outcome of Ustekinumab Therapy for Behçet's Disease. *Arthritis Rheumatol.* **2019**, *71*, 1727–1732. [CrossRef] [PubMed]
94. Liu, J.; Yu, X.; Wang, Z.; Liu, W.; Liu, X.; Wang, X.; Zhang, M.; Zhao, Y.; Zhang, F.; Yang, H.; et al. Baricitinib for the treatment of intestinal Behcet's disease: A pilot study. *Clin. Immunol.* **2023**, *247*, 109241. [CrossRef] [PubMed]

95. Atienza-Mateo, B.; Martín-Varillas, J.L.; Graña, J.; Espinosa, G.; Moriano, C.; Pérez-Sandoval, T.; García-Armario, M.D.; Castellví, I.; Román-Ivorra, J.A.; Olivé, A.; et al. Apremilast in refractory orogenital ulcers and other manifestations of Behçet's disease. A national multicentre study of 51 cases in clinical practice. *Clin. Exp. Rheumatol.* **2020**, *38* (Suppl. S127), 69–75.
96. Hatemi, G.; Mahr, A.; Ishigatsubo, Y.; Song, Y.W.; Takeno, M.; Kim, D.; Melikoglu, M.; Cheng, S.; McCue, S.; Paris, M.; et al. Trial of Apremilast for Oral Ulcers in Behcet's Syndrome. *N. Engl. J. Med.* **2019**, *381*, 1918–1928. [CrossRef]
97. Garcia-Estrada, C.; Casallas-Vanegas, A.; Zabala-Angeles, I.; Gomez-Figueroa, E.; Rivas-Alonso, V.; Flores-Rivera, J. Rituximab as an effective therapeutic option in refractory Neuro-Behçet syndrome. *J. Neuroimmunol.* **2020**, *346*, 577308. [CrossRef]
98. Davatchi, F.; Shams, H.; Rezaipoor, M.; Sadeghi-Abdollahi, B.; Shahram, F.; Nadji, A.; Chams-Davatchi, C.; Akhlaghi, M.; Faezi, T.; Naderi, N. Rituximab in intractable ocular lesions of Behcet's disease; randomized single-blind control study (pilot study). *Int. J. Rheum. Dis.* **2010**, *13*, 246–252. [CrossRef]
99. Maciel, M.L.; Novello, M.; Neves, F.S. Short-term efficacy of abatacept in the treatment of refractory ocular and cutaneous Behçet's disease. *Rheumatol. Adv. Pract.* **2017**, *1*, rkx004. [CrossRef]
100. Mohammad, A.J.; Smith, R.M.; Chow, Y.W.; Chaudhry, A.N.; Jayne, D.R. Alemtuzumab as Remission Induction Therapy in Behçet Disease: A 20-year Experience. *J. Rheumatol.* **2015**, *42*, 1906–1913. [CrossRef]
101. Perez-Pampin, E.; Campos-Franco, J.; Blanco, J.; Mera, A. Remission induction in a case of refractory Behçet disease with alemtuzumab. *J. Clin. Rheumatol.* **2013**, *19*, 101–103. [CrossRef]
102. Arbrile, M.; Radin, M.; Rossi, D.; Menegatti, E.; Baldovino, S.; Sciascia, S.; Roccatello, D. Vedolizumab for the Management of Refractory Behçet's Disease: From a Case Report to New Pieces of Mosaic in a Complex Disease. *Front. Immunol.* **2021**, *12*, 769785. [CrossRef] [PubMed]
103. Oztas, M.O.; Onder, M.; Gurer, M.A.; Bukan, N.; Sancak, B. Serum interleukin 18 and tumour necrosis factor-alpha levels are increased in Behçet's disease. *Clin. Exp. Dermatol.* **2005**, *30*, 61–63. [CrossRef] [PubMed]
104. Kone-Paut, I.; Barete, S.; Bodaghi, B.; Deiva, K.; Desbois, A.C.; Galeotti, C.; Gaudric, J.; Kaplanski, G.; Mahr, A.; Noel, N.; et al. French recommendations for the management of Behçet's disease. *Orphanet. J. Rare. Dis.* **2021**, *16*, 352. [CrossRef] [PubMed]
105. Inflammatory Enteropathy Group, Gastroenterology Branch, Chinese Medical Association. Chinese consensus on diagnosis and treatment of intestinal Behcet's disease. *Chin. J. Dig.* **2022**, *42*, 649–658. (In Chinese) [CrossRef]
106. Tanida, S.; Inoue, N.; Kobayashi, K.; Naganuma, M.; Hirai, F.; Iizuka, B.; Watanabe, K.; Mitsuyama, K.; Inoue, T.; Ishigatsubo, Y.; et al. Adalimumab for the treatment of Japanese patients with intestinal Behcet's disease. *Clin. Gastroenterol. Hepatol.* **2015**, *13*, 940–948.e943. [CrossRef]
107. Zou, J.; Ji, D.N.; Cai, J.F.; Guan, J.L.; Bao, Z.J. Long-Term Outcomes and Predictors of Sustained Response in Patients with Intestinal Behcet's Disease Treated with Infliximab. *Dig. Dis. Sci.* **2017**, *62*, 441–447. [CrossRef]
108. Zhang, M.; Liu, J.; Liu, T.; Han, W.; Bai, X.; Ruan, G.; Lv, H.; Shu, H.; Li, Y.; Li, J.; et al. The efficacy and safety of anti-tumor necrosis factor agents in the treatment of intestinal Behcet's disease, a systematic review and meta-analysis. *J. Gastroenterol. Hepatol.* **2022**, *37*, 608–619. [CrossRef]
109. Theofilopoulos, A.N.; Baccala, R.; Beutler, B.; Kono, D.H. Type I interferons (alpha/beta) in immunity and autoimmunity. *Annu. Rev. Immunol.* **2005**, *23*, 307–336. [CrossRef]
110. Tsambaos, D.; Eichelberg, D.; Goos, M. Behçet's syndrome: Treatment with recombinant leukocyte alpha-interferon. *Arch. Dermatol. Res.* **1986**, *278*, 335–336. [CrossRef]
111. Krause, L.; Altenburg, A.; Pleyer, U.; Kohler, A.K.; Zouboulis, C.C.; Foerster, M.H. Longterm visual prognosis of patients with ocular Adamantiades-Behcet's disease treated with interferon-alpha-2a. *J. Rheumatol.* **2008**, *35*, 896–903.
112. Gueudry, J.; Wechsler, B.; Terrada, C.; Gendron, G.; Cassoux, N.; Fardeau, C.; Lehoang, P.; Piette, J.C.; Bodaghi, B. Long-term efficacy and safety of low-dose interferon alpha2a therapy in severe uveitis associated with Behcet disease. *Am. J. Ophthalmol.* **2008**, *146*, 837–844.e831. [CrossRef] [PubMed]
113. Yang, P.; Huang, G.; Du, L.; Ye, Z.; Hu, Y.; Wang, C.; Qi, J.; Liang, L.; Wu, L.; Cao, Q.; et al. Long-Term Efficacy and Safety of Interferon Alpha-2a in the Treatment of Chinese Patients with Behcet's Uveitis Not Responding to Conventional Therapy. *Ocul. Immunol. Inflamm.* **2019**, *27*, 7–14. [CrossRef] [PubMed]
114. Celiker, H.; Kazokoglu, H.; Direskeneli, H. Factors Affecting Relapse and Remission in Behcet's Uveitis Treated with Interferon Alpha2a. *J. Ocul. Pharmacol. Ther.* **2019**, *35*, 58–65. [CrossRef] [PubMed]
115. Alpsoy, E.; Durusoy, C.; Yilmaz, E.; Ozgurel, Y.; Ermis, O.; Yazar, S.; Basaran, E. Interferon alfa-2a in the treatment of Behcet disease: A randomized placebo-controlled and double-blind study. *Arch. Dermatol.* **2002**, *138*, 467–471. [CrossRef] [PubMed]
116. Calguneri, M.; Onat, A.M.; Ozturk, M.A.; Ozcakar, L.; Ureten, K.; Akdogan, A.; Ertenli, I.; Kiraz, S. Transverse myelitis in a patient with Behcet's disease: Favorable outcome with a combination of interferon-alpha. *Clin. Rheumatol.* **2005**, *24*, 64–66. [CrossRef]
117. Nichols, J.C.; Ince, A.; Akduman, L.; Mann, E.S. Interferon-alpha 2a treatment of neuro-Behcet disease. *J. Neuroophthalmol.* **2001**, *21*, 109–111. [CrossRef]
118. Feron, E.J.; Rothova, A.; van Hagen, P.M.; Baarsma, G.S.; Suttorp-Schulten, M.S. Interferon-alpha 2b for refractory ocular Behcet's disease. *Lancet* **1994**, *343*, 1428. [CrossRef]
119. Lightman, S.; Taylor, S.R.; Bunce, C.; Longhurst, H.; Lynn, W.; Moots, R.; Stanford, M.; Tomkins-Netzer, O.; Yang, D.; Calder, V.L.; et al. Pegylated interferon-alpha-2b reduces corticosteroid requirement in patients with Behcet's disease with upregulation of circulating regulatory T cells and reduction of Th17. *Ann. Rheum. Dis.* **2015**, *74*, 1138–1144. [CrossRef]

120. Calguneri, M.; Ozturk, M.A.; Ertenli, I.; Kiraz, S.; Apras, S.; Ozbalkan, Z. Effects of interferon alpha treatment on the clinical course of refractory Behcet's disease: An open study. *Ann. Rheum. Dis.* **2003**, *62*, 492–493. [CrossRef]
121. Kötter, I.; Eckstein, A.K.; Stübiger, N.; Zierhut, M. Treatment of ocular symptoms of Behçet's disease with interferon alpha 2a: A pilot study. *Br. J. Ophthalmol.* **1998**, *82*, 488–494. [CrossRef]
122. Dinarello, C.A. Biologic basis for interleukin-1 in disease. *Blood.* **1996**, *87*, 2095–2147. [CrossRef] [PubMed]
123. Pay, S.; Erdem, H.; Pekel, A.; Simsek, I.; Musabak, U.; Sengul, A.; Dinc, A. Synovial proinflammatory cytokines and their correlation with matrix metalloproteinase-3 expression in Behçet's disease. Does interleukin-1beta play a major role in Behçet's synovitis? *Rheumatol. Int.* **2006**, *26*, 608–613. [CrossRef] [PubMed]
124. Karasneh, J.; Hajeer, A.H.; Barrett, J.; Ollier, W.E.; Thornhill, M.; Gul, A. Association of specific interleukin 1 gene cluster polymorphisms with increased susceptibility for Behcet's disease. *Rheumatology* **2003**, *42*, 860–864. [CrossRef] [PubMed]
125. Korn, T.; Bettelli, E.; Oukka, M.; Kuchroo, V.K. IL-17 and Th17 Cells. *Annu. Rev. Immunol.* **2009**, *27*, 485–517. [CrossRef] [PubMed]
126. Ho, L.J.; Luo, S.F.; Lai, J.H. Biological effects of interleukin-6: Clinical applications in autoimmune diseases and cancers. *Biochem. Pharmacol.* **2015**, *97*, 16–26. [CrossRef] [PubMed]
127. Zhou, L.; Lopes, J.E.; Chong, M.M.; Ivanov, I.I.; Min, R.; Victora, G.D.; Shen, Y.; Du, J.; Rubtsov, Y.P.; Rudensky, A.Y.; et al. TGF-beta-induced Foxp3 inhibits T(H)17 cell differentiation by antagonizing RORgammat function. *Nature* **2008**, *453*, 236–240. [CrossRef]
128. Yang, L.; Anderson, D.E.; Baecher-Allan, C.; Hastings, W.D.; Bettelli, E.; Oukka, M.; Kuchroo, V.K.; Hafler, D.A. IL-21 and TGF-beta are required for differentiation of human T(H)17 cells. *Nature* **2008**, *454*, 350–352. [CrossRef]
129. Khanna, D.; Denton, C.P.; Jahreis, A.; van Laar, J.M.; Frech, T.M.; Anderson, M.E.; Baron, M.; Chung, L.; Fierlbeck, G.; Lakshminarayanan, S.; et al. Safety and efficacy of subcutaneous tocilizumab in adults with systemic sclerosis (faSScinate): A phase 2, randomised, controlled trial. *Lancet* **2016**, *387*, 2630–2640. [CrossRef]
130. Akiyama, M.; Kaneko, Y.; Takeuchi, T. Effectiveness of tocilizumab in Behcet's disease: A systematic literature review. *Semin. Arthritis Rheum.* **2020**, *50*, 797–804. [CrossRef] [PubMed]
131. Moseley, T.A.; Haudenschild, D.R.; Rose, L.; Reddi, A.H. Interleukin-17 family and IL-17 receptors. *Cytokine Growth Factor Rev.* **2003**, *14*, 155–174. [CrossRef]
132. McGonagle, D.G.; McInnes, I.B.; Kirkham, B.W.; Sherlock, J.; Moots, R. The role of IL-17A in axial spondyloarthritis and psoriatic arthritis: Recent advances and controversies. *Ann. Rheum. Dis.* **2019**, *78*, 1167–1178. [CrossRef] [PubMed]
133. Barrado-Solís, N.; Rodrigo-Nicolás, B.; De la Morena-Barrio, I.; Pérez-Pastor, G.; Sanchis-Sánchez, C.; Tomás-Cabedo, G.; Valcuende-Cavero, F. Report of two cases of Behçet's disease developed during treatment with secukinumab. *J. Eur. Acad. Dermatol. Venereol.* **2020**, *34*, e587–e589. [CrossRef] [PubMed]
134. Hueber, W.; Sands, B.E.; Lewitzky, S.; Vandemeulebroecke, M.; Reinisch, W.; Higgins, P.D.; Wehkamp, J.; Feagan, B.G.; Yao, M.D.; Karczewski, M.; et al. Secukinumab, a human anti-IL-17A monoclonal antibody, for moderate to severe Crohn's disease: Unexpected results of a randomised, double-blind placebo-controlled trial. *Gut* **2012**, *61*, 1693–1700. [CrossRef] [PubMed]
135. Chyuan, I.T.; Lai, J.H. New insights into the IL-12 and IL-23: From a molecular basis to clinical application in immune-mediated inflammation and cancers. *Biochem. Pharmacol.* **2020**, *175*, 113928. [CrossRef]
136. Benson, J.M.; Sachs, C.W.; Treacy, G.; Zhou, H.; Pendley, C.E.; Brodmerkel, C.M.; Shankar, G.; Mascelli, M.A. Therapeutic targeting of the IL-12/23 pathways: Generation and characterization of ustekinumab. *Nat. Biotechnol.* **2011**, *29*, 615–624. [CrossRef]
137. Trinchieri, G. Interleukin-12 and its role in the generation of TH1 cells. *Immunol. Today* **1993**, *14*, 335–338. [CrossRef]
138. Zhou, Z.Y.; Chen, S.L.; Shen, N.; Lu, Y. Cytokines and Behcet's disease. *Autoimmun. Rev.* **2012**, *11*, 699–704. [CrossRef]
139. Sadeghi, A.; Davatchi, F.; Shahram, F.; Karimimoghadam, A.; Alikhani, M.; Pezeshgi, A.; Mazloomzadeh, S.; Sadeghi-Abdollahi, B.; Asadi-Khiavi, M. Serum Profiles of Cytokines in Behcet's Disease. *J. Clin. Med.* **2017**, *6*, 49. [CrossRef]
140. Mizuki, N.; Meguro, A.; Ota, M.; Ohno, S.; Shiota, T.; Kawagoe, T.; Ito, N.; Kera, J.; Okada, E.; Yatsu, K.; et al. Genome-wide association studies identify IL23R-IL12RB2 and IL10 as Behçet's disease susceptibility loci. *Nat. Genet.* **2010**, *42*, 703–706. [CrossRef]
141. Kubo, S.; Nakayamada, S.; Sakata, K.; Kitanaga, Y.; Ma, X.; Lee, S.; Ishii, A.; Yamagata, K.; Nakano, K.; Tanaka, Y. Janus Kinase Inhibitor Baricitinib Modulates Human Innate and Adaptive Immune System. *Front. Immunol.* **2018**, *9*, 1510. [CrossRef]
142. Lon, H.K.; Liu, D.; DuBois, D.C.; Almon, R.R.; Jusko, W.J. Modeling pharmacokinetics/pharmacodynamics of abatacept and disease progression in collagen-induced arthritic rats: A population approach. *J. Pharmacokinet. Pharmacodyn.* **2013**, *40*, 701–712. [CrossRef] [PubMed]
143. Ruck, T.; Barman, S.; Schulte-Mecklenbeck, A.; Pfeuffer, S.; Steffen, F.; Nelke, C.; Schroeter, C.B.; Willison, A.; Heming, M.; Müntefering, T.; et al. Alemtuzumab-induced immune phenotype and repertoire changes: Implications for secondary autoimmunity. *Brain* **2022**, *145*, 1711–1725. [CrossRef] [PubMed]
144. Vitale, A.; Rigante, D.; Lopalco, G.; Emmi, G.; Bianco, M.T.; Galeazzi, M.; Iannone, F.; Cantarini, L. New therapeutic solutions for Behçet's syndrome. *Expert Opin. Investig. Drugs* **2016**, *25*, 827–840. [CrossRef] [PubMed]

Disclaimer/Publisher's Note: The statements, opinions and data contained in all publications are solely those of the individual author(s) and contributor(s) and not of MDPI and/or the editor(s). MDPI and/or the editor(s) disclaim responsibility for any injury to people or property resulting from any ideas, methods, instructions or products referred to in the content.

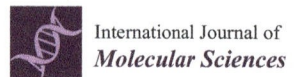

International Journal of *Molecular Sciences*

Article

Bacterial Lysate from the Multi-Strain Probiotic SLAB51 Triggers Adaptative Responses to Hypoxia in Human Caco-2 Intestinal Epithelial Cells under Normoxic Conditions and Attenuates LPS-Induced Inflammatory Response

Francesca Lombardi [1,*], Francesca Rosaria Augello [1], Paola Palumbo [1], Laura Bonfili [2], Serena Artone [1], Serena Altamura [1], Jenna Marie Sheldon [3], Giovanni Latella [1], Maria Grazia Cifone [1], Anna Maria Eleuteri [2] and Benedetta Cinque [1]

[1] Department of Life, Health & Environmental Sciences, University of L'Aquila, 67100 L'Aquila, Italy
[2] School of Biosciences and Veterinary Medicine, University of Camerino, 62032 Camerino, Italy
[3] Dr. Kiran C Patel College of Osteopathic Medicine, Nova Southeastern University, Fort Lauderdale, FL 33314-7796, USA
* Correspondence: francesca.lombardi@univaq.it; Tel.: +39-0862-433-555

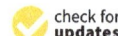

Citation: Lombardi, F.; Augello, F.R.; Palumbo, P.; Bonfili, L.; Artone, S.; Altamura, S.; Sheldon, J.M.; Latella, G.; Cifone, M.G.; Eleuteri, A.M.; et al. Bacterial Lysate from the Multi-Strain Probiotic SLAB51 Triggers Adaptative Responses to Hypoxia in Human Caco-2 Intestinal Epithelial Cells under Normoxic Conditions and Attenuates LPS-Induced Inflammatory Response. *Int. J. Mol. Sci.* **2023**, *24*, 8134. https://doi.org/10.3390/ijms24098134

Academic Editors: Baltasar Mayo and Carmine Stolfi

Received: 13 January 2023
Revised: 28 April 2023
Accepted: 1 May 2023
Published: 2 May 2023

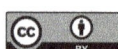

Copyright: © 2023 by the authors. Licensee MDPI, Basel, Switzerland. This article is an open access article distributed under the terms and conditions of the Creative Commons Attribution (CC BY) license (https://creativecommons.org/licenses/by/4.0/).

Abstract: Hypoxia-inducible factor-1α (HIF-1α), a central player in maintaining gut-microbiota homeostasis, plays a pivotal role in inducing adaptive mechanisms to hypoxia and is negatively regulated by prolyl hydroxylase 2 (PHD2). HIF-1α is stabilized through PI3K/AKT signaling regardless of oxygen levels. Considering the crucial role of the HIF pathway in intestinal mucosal physiology and its relationships with gut microbiota, this study aimed to evaluate the ability of the lysate from the multi-strain probiotic formulation SLAB51 to affect the HIF pathway in a model of in vitro human intestinal epithelium (intestinal epithelial cells, IECs) and to protect from lipopolysaccharide (LPS) challenge. The exposure of IECs to SLAB51 lysate under normoxic conditions led to a dose-dependent increase in HIF-1α protein levels, which was associated with higher glycolytic metabolism and L-lactate production. Probiotic lysate significantly reduced PHD2 levels and HIF-1α hydroxylation, thus leading to HIF-1α stabilization. The ability of SLAB51 lysate to increase HIF-1α levels was also associated with the activation of the PI3K/AKT pathway and with the inhibition of NF-κB, nitric oxide synthase 2 (NOS2), and IL-1β increase elicited by LPS treatment. Our results suggest that the probiotic treatment, by stabilizing HIF-1α, can protect from an LPS-induced inflammatory response through a mechanism involving PI3K/AKT signaling.

Keywords: HIF-1α; PHD2; AKT; intestinal epithelial cells; probiotics; LPS

1. Introduction

The hypoxia-inducible factor (HIF) pathway is a central and ubiquitous cellular mechanism promoting and coordinating the transcriptional response to low-oxygen (O_2) environments [1]. In the intestine, several HIF target genes are involved in the maintenance of the mucosal barrier, including genes critical for microbial defense, xenobiotic clearance, mucin production, and cellular energetics [2]. HIFs are heterodimers consisting of a hypoxia-inducible α-subunit (HIF-1α, HIF-2α, and HIF-3α) and β-subunit (aryl hydrocarbon receptor nuclear translocator (ARNT)/HIF-1β and ARNT2) [3]. In normoxic conditions, HIF-α subunits are continuously synthesized while proteasomal pathways rapidly degrade them, limiting their circulating levels within cells [4]. Two prolyl residues in the O_2-dependent degradation domain of HIF-α subunits are hydroxylated by the HIF prolyl 4-hydroxylases family (PHDs), primarily by PHD2 contributing to ubiquitination mediated by the von Hippel–Lindau (VHL) ubiquitin ligase [5,6]. Under hypoxia, when the cellular demand for O_2 exceeds its supply, HIF-α subunits are stabilized following the loss of activity of PHDs due to the low availability of O_2, one of their substrates. The subsequent translocation of the HIF-α subunit into the nucleus, where it dimerizes with HIF-1β, permits it to function as a transcription factor by binding to hypoxia-response elements of its target genes and leading to their expression [5,7].

The stabilization of HIF-1α associated with low O_2 availability stimulates adaptive mechanisms to hypoxia, including enhancing anaerobic ATP generation through glycolysis [1]. Upregulated HIF-1α expression and increased glycolysis are dependent on the PI3K/AKT (protein kinase B) signaling, a pathway playing a central role in regulating energy metabolism. In particular, activated PI3K/AKT upregulates HIF-1α transcription and translation, stabilizing and trans-activating HIF-1α regardless of O_2 levels [8,9]. In animal models, both genetic and pharmacologic stabilization of HIFs is disease protective. At the same time, the loss of these factors could lead to detrimental effects such as an increased susceptibility to colitis associated with diminished levels of epithelial HIF-1α [10–14].

Hypoxia mimetic agents able to increase HIF-1α expression have been hypothesized as potentially able to exert a positive effect in pathological contexts [15,16], such as gut inflammation, whereby the HIF pathway is induced by pharmacologic PHD inhibitors (PHI) [5,17]. PHI such as dimethyloxalylglycine (DMOG), FG-4497, AKB-4924, TRC160334, or CG-598 have been reported to exert protective effects in experimental murine colitis [12,13,18–20]. Recently, the effect of PHI on improving colonic anastomotic healing in a mouse model has been described [21].

Lipopolysaccharide (LPS) plays an important pathogenic role in intestinal inflammation: through the interaction with Toll-like receptors 4 (TLR4) it can activate the NF-κB pathways [22] that represent master regulators of inflammatory gene expression [23]. The increase in intestinal permeability associated with intestinal inflammation leads to the translocation of LPS into the blood circulation, triggering the release of pro-inflammatory cytokines such as tumor necrosis factor-α (TNF-α), IL-1β, or IL-6 [23]. These cytokines contribute to amplifying the activation of NF-κB signaling pathways in epithelial cells, decreasing the expression of tight junction (TJ) proteins, such as ZO-1 and occludin, and further increasing intestinal permeability [24]. NF-κB activation has been shown to stabilize HIF-1α in hypoxia and in inflammation. On the other hand, HIF-1α has been shown to repress NF-κB in vivo and in vitro under inflammatory conditions. It seems, therefore, that HIF-1α acts through negative feedback to NF-κB to reduce the host inflammatory response by restricting NF-κB-dependent gene expression [25,26].

The activation of NF-κB is also known to induce the expression of nitric oxide synthase 2 (NOS2), which is responsible for the increased NO production at the site of inflammation [27]. In the intestinal epithelium, the upregulation of NOS2 and the consequent chronic release of NO at high concentrations have been associated with the pathogenesis of inflammatory bowel disease (IBD) [28], mainly through the generation of peroxynitrite [29]. Moreover, NO can regulate HIF-1α accumulation, HIF-1 activity, and HIF-1-dependent target gene expression. However, studies addressing the regulation of HIF-1 by NO revealed a complex and paradoxical picture. It appears that short-term exposure to NO stabilizes HIF-1α, while chronic exposure to NO destabilizes HIF-1α. Several mechanisms were found to contribute to this variable role of NO in regulating HIF-1. It has been shown that NO regulates HIF-1 by modulating the activity of the O_2-sensor enzymes, PHDs, and factor inhibiting HIF-1 (FIH-1) [30].

SLAB51 is a probiotic mixture consisting of *Streptococcus thermophilus* (DSM 32245), *B. lactis* (DSM 32246), *B. lactis* (DSM 32247), *L. acidophilus* (DSM 32241), *L. helveticus* (DSM 32242), *L. paracasei* (DSM 32243), *L. plantarum* (DSM 32244), and *L. brevis* (DSM 27961), previously studied both in vitro and in vivo, in animal models and patients, on hypoxia-related conditions [31–36]. Bacterial species present within this multi-strain probiotic formulation constitute common inhabitants of the human gut, mostly ingested with food, especially dairy products [37,38]. Consolidated knowledge shows that within the human gut, microorganisms are variably distributed with respect to quantity and types along the different gut districts. Environmental pH and available trophic sources represent the main factors driving such peculiar distribution, while age, geographical origin of the host, and lifestyle impact the global quantity of the different bacterial species in the gut microbiota [39,40]. Species of lactobacilli, streptococci, and bifidobacteria, present in the formulation used in our study, are mainly harbored in the most proximal parts of the gut such as the duodenum, jejunum, and ileum where a more limited bacterial load normally exists.

Several studies have registered beneficial effects of the multi-strain probiotic formulation, SLAB51, on humans and animal models; in particular, this probiotic proved to be protective in neurodegenerative disorders by promoting antioxidant and neuroprotective effects [31,41–43]. Moreover, it was able to keep the gut integrity, preserving its functionality in a mouse model of chemotherapy-induced peripheral neuropathy [44]. A recent study reported that SLAB51 alleviated the respiratory conditions in subjects with SARS-CoV-2 infections concluding that the probiotic was able to increase oxygen supply to other organs [33]. Of note, evaluating the neuroprotective effects of SLAB51 oral supplementation on neuroinflammation in Alzheimer's disease (AD), a recent study showed its ability to induce HIF-1α stabilization and to reduce the PHD2 expression, along with inhibition of NOS2 expression and activity in the brain of an AD animal model [31].

Considering the crucial role of the HIF pathway in intestinal mucosal pathophysiology, we aimed to evaluate the ability of the SLAB51 probiotic lysate to influence the HIF-1α pathway and counteract the inflammatory stimulus of LPS in a model of in vitro intestinal epithelium.

Our findings show evidence that probiotic exposure, by positively impacting the HIF pathway through a mechanism involving PI3K/AKT upregulation, could predispose cells for better survival and reactivity in a pathologically hypoxic and inflammatory environment.

2. Results

2.1. Effect of SLAB51 Lysate on HIF-1α Levels on Caco-2 Cells

We first investigated the ability of SLAB51 to modulate HIF-1α levels on Caco-2 cells treated for 6 or 24 h with increasing concentrations of the probiotic lysate (10, 50, and 100 μg/mL). The treatment induced a dose-dependent increase in HIF-1α levels as assayed by Western blotting, being statistically significant after 6 h at 100 μg/mL ($p < 0.01$) (Figure 1). After 24 h of treatment, HIF-1α levels were significantly higher than the control at 50 and 100 μg/mL ($p < 0.05$ and $p < 0.01$, respectively, vs. untreated cells). Based on the obtained results, the SLAB51 concentration of 100 μg/mL, being the most efficient in influencing HIF-1α levels, was chosen for the following experiments.

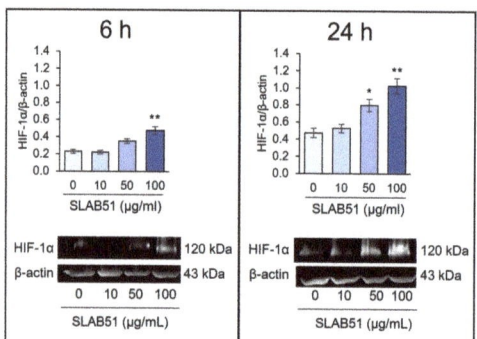

Figure 1. Effect of SLAB51 lysate on HIF-1α levels in Caco-2 cells. Cells were incubated with increasing concentrations of SLAB51 bacterial lysate for 6 and 24 h; HIF-1α levels were then evaluated by Western blotting. Following the densitometric analysis, the obtained values were normalized to β-actin. Values are expressed as means ± SEM of three independent experiments. Representative immunoblots are also shown. For the comparative analysis of the data, the one-way analysis of variance (ANOVA) followed by the Dunnett test was used. * $p < 0.05$, ** $p < 0.01$ vs. untreated cells.

2.2. Effect of SLAB51 Lysate on PHD2 Activity and Expression

To investigate whether SLAB51 lysate affected HIF-1α levels through regulation of PHD2 activity or expression under normoxia, the levels of HIF-1α and hydroxylated HIF-1α were first analyzed. HIF-1α proline hydroxylation was determined using an antibody specific for the proline-hydroxylation site (Pro564) following proteasomal degradation inhibition through MG132 incubation to allow the accumulation of HIF-1α hydroxylated form. Immunoblotting in Figure 2 shows HIF-1α and hydroxyl-HIF-1α (HIF-1α-OH) protein levels. The effect of MG132 on proteasomal degradation inhibition of hydroxylated HIF-1α was demonstrated by the accumulation of HIF-1α (Figure 2A) as well as its hydroxylated form (Figure 2B). Treatment with deferoxamine (DFO) was used as a positive control, being an iron chelator known to attenuate PHD activity and, in turn, stabilize HIF-1α; it increased HIF-1α and reduced the accumulation of (hydroxyproline) Hyp-564 under normoxia (Figure 2B). Likewise, SLAB51 treatment decreased Hyp-564 compared with the control under normoxia after 6 h of incubation, increasing HIF-1α levels. We next assessed the ability of SLAB51 lysate to influence PHD2 expression. The treatment with the probiotic lysate significantly reduced PHD2 expression at 6 h (Figure 2C) as evaluated through Western blot (% reduction vs. control ~17%).

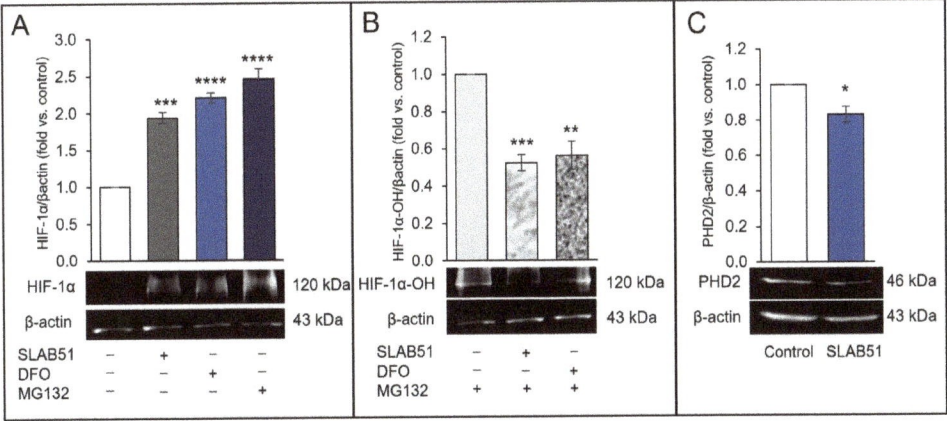

Figure 2. Effect of SLAB51 lysate on HIF-1α levels and PHD2 activity and expression. Cells were incubated in normoxia with SLAB51 lysate (100 μg/mL) or DFO (150 μM, positive control) with or without proteasome inhibitor MG132 (10 μM) for 6 h: (**A**) HIF-1α, (**B**) HIF-1α-OH, and (**C**) PHD2 levels were then evaluated by Western blotting. Following the densitometric analysis, the obtained values were normalized to β-actin. Values are expressed as means ± SEM of three independent experiments. Representative immunoblots are also shown. For the comparative analysis of the data, ANOVA followed by the Dunnett test or Student's unpaired *t*-test were used, for comparison of the mean values among the groups and for comparison between two means, respectively. * $p < 0.05$, ** $p < 0.01$, *** $p < 0.001$, **** $p < 0.0001$ vs. untreated cells.

2.3. Effect of SLAB51 Lysate on Cell Metabolism and AKT Pathway

Given the ability of HIF-1α to induce genes encoding glycolytic enzymes [45], the effect of SLAB51 on glycolytic metabolism was studied next. The levels of L-lactate, a key metabolite of the glycolysis pathway, were evaluated in culture media. The relative glycolysis rate was also analyzed as the ECAR/OCR ratio. ECAR stands for the extracellular acidification rate of the media, a parameter that reflects glycolysis, while OCR is the O_2 consumption rate used to determine oxidative phosphorylation [46]. Both levels of L-lactate (Figure 3A) and the ECAR/OCR ratio were significantly increased in Caco-2 cells after 24 h incubation with the probiotic lysate (Figure 3B). Upregulated HIF-1α expression and increased glycolysis are dependent on the activated PI3K/AKT pathway, which plays a central role in regulating the energy metabolism [8]. To verify the ability of SLAB51 lysate to modulate the AKT pathway, the analysis of AKT phosphorylation was performed. As shown in Figure 3C, phospho-AKT (pAKT, Ser473) protein levels were significantly upregulated after 6 h treatment with SLAB51 lysate compared with control cells.

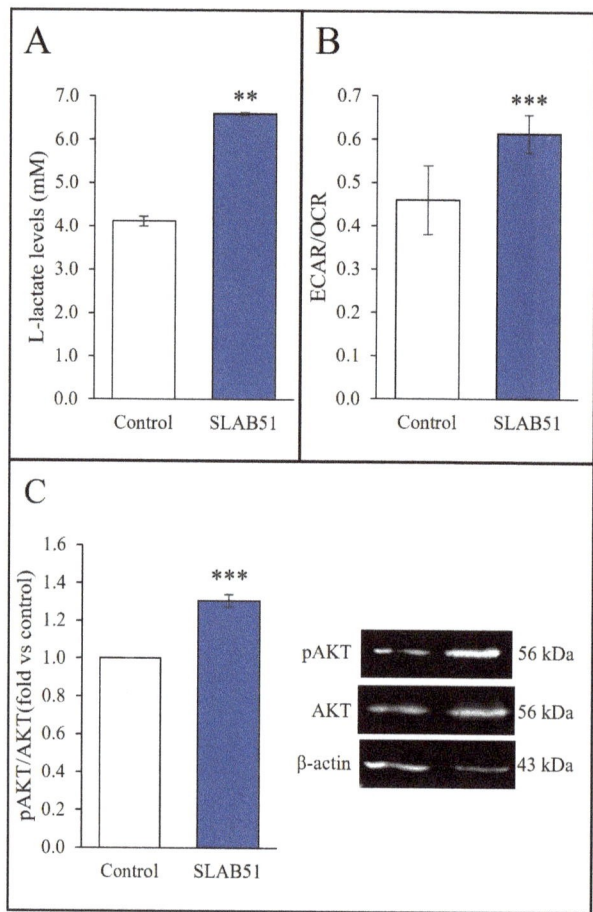

Figure 3. Effect of SLAB51 lysate on L-lactate production, glycolysis rate, and pAKT levels. Caco-2 cells were treated with or without SLAB51 lysate (100 µg/mL) for (**C**) 6 h or (**A,B**) 24 h. The levels of lactate were analyzed through a colorimetric assay on cell culture supernatants. Values are expressed as the means ± SEM of three independent experiments in triplicate (**A**). The relative glycolysis rate ECAR/OCR was assessed using the Seahorse XF Analyzer. Values are expressed as the means ± SD of a representative experiment (N = 9) out of three independent experiments (**B**). pAKT levels were evaluated by Western blotting. Following the densitometric analysis, the obtained values were normalized vs. AKT. Values are expressed as the means ± SEM of three independent experiments. Representative immunoblots of pAKT, AKT, and β-actin are also shown (**C**). For comparison between two means, the Student's unpaired *t*-test was used ** $p < 0.01$; *** $p < 0.001$.

2.4. Involvement of AKT Pathway in SLAB51's Ability to Increase HIF-1α Levels

The involvement of the PI3K/AKT pathway was further verified by analyzing the influence of perifosine and LY294002, i.e., AKT and PI3K inhibitors, respectively, on the effect of SLAB51 on HIF-1α levels of Caco-2 cells. The cells were pre-treated for 30 min with perifosine or LY294002 and then incubated with SLAB51 lysate for 6 h. Pretreatment with each inhibitor counteracting the pAKT increase induced by SLAB51 inhibited its ability to increase HIF-1α, lowering the protein expression to levels comparable to those of the control (Figure 4). These data suggest that the activation of the PI3K/AKT pathway is required for the HIF-1α increase induced by SLAB51 lysate treatment.

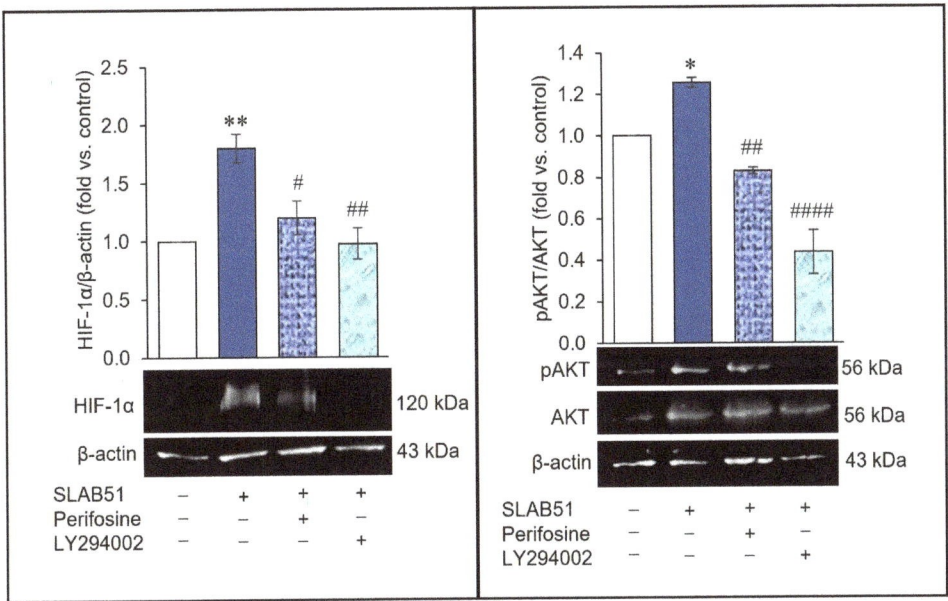

Figure 4. Effect of AKT and PI3K inhibition on SLAB51 lysate's ability to increase HIF-1α levels. Caco-2 cells were pre-treated with perifosine or LY294002 for 30 min and then incubated with SLAB51 lysate (100 µg/mL) for 6 h. HIF-1α and pAKT levels were evaluated by Western blotting. Following the densitometric analysis, the obtained values were normalized to β-actin or AKT. Representative immunoblots of HIF-1α, pAKT, AKT, and β-actin are also shown. Values are expressed as the means ± SEM of three independent experiments. The ANOVA followed by the Tukey test was used for the comparative analysis of the data. * $p < 0.05$, ** $p < 0.01$ vs. untreated cells; # $p < 0.05$, ## $p < 0.01$, #### $p < 0.0001$ vs. SLAB51.

2.5. Effect of SLAB51 Lysate on HIF-1α Levels on an In Vitro Model of Intestinal Inflammation

The effect of the SLAB51 lysate was then evaluated on Caco-2 cells exposed to LPS, 10 µg/mL. In our experimental conditions at 24 h, LPS treatment was unable to increase HIF-1α levels, which were not different compared to the control. On the other hand, the ability of the SLAB51 treatment to increase HIF-1α levels was not affected by the concomitant treatment with LPS (Figure 5A). The effect on AKT activation was also evaluated. LPS did not significantly influence the AKT pathway nor the ability of SLAB51 lysate to increase pAKT levels (Figure 5B).

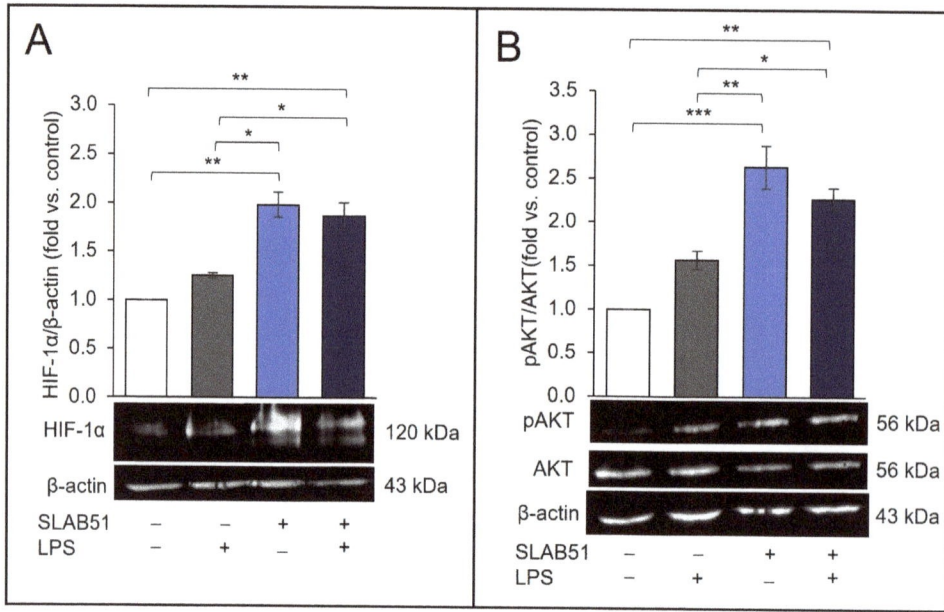

Figure 5. Effect of SLAB51 lysate on HIF-1α and pAKT levels in LPS-stimulated Caco-2 cells. Caco-2 cells were treated for 24 h with or without LPS (10 μg/mL) and SLAB51 lysate (100 μg/mL). (**A**) HIF-1α and (**B**) pAKT levels were evaluated by Western blotting. Following the densitometric analysis, the obtained values were normalized with respect to β-actin or AKT. Values are expressed as the means ± SEM of three independent experiments. Representative immunoblots are also shown. For the comparative analysis of the data, ANOVA was used followed by the Tukey test. * $p < 0.05$, ** $p < 0.01$, *** $p < 0.001$,.

2.6. Probiotic Prevention of LPS-Induced Pro-Inflammatory Stress in Caco-2 Cells

As known, LPS induces NF-κB signaling and upregulates the production of inflammatory cytokines at the intestinal level [23]. Moreover, in our experiments, LPS significantly enhanced the levels of phospho-NF-κB p65 in Caco-2 cells (Figure 6A) and the secretion of the pro-inflammatory cytokine IL-1β into the culture medium (Figure 6B). Of note, these effects were counteracted by the treatment with SLAB51 lysate.

The transcription factor NF-κB represents a key mediator of inflammatory responses as it is able to induce the expression of various pro-inflammatory genes, including NOS2 [47]. Thus, the effect of SLAB51 lysate was next assessed on the expression and activity of NOS2 induced by LPS. Nitrite levels in the culture medium at 24 h after LPS stimulation were increased with respect to control cells. The treatment with SLAB51 abrogated the ability of LPS to promote NOS2 activity, bringing the nitrite levels back to those of the control (Figure 7A); the specificity of the assay was verified using the NOS2 inhibitor, 1400W. In Figure 7B, the results of Western blot analysis of NOS2 protein are shown; as expected, LPS was able to induce the NOS2 expression. Of note, this effect was counteracted by the concomitant treatment with SLAB51 lysate, with the NOS2 expression not significantly different from untreated controls. As expected, no effect on NOS2 protein level was observed after treatment with the inhibitor of the NOS2 activity, 1400W.

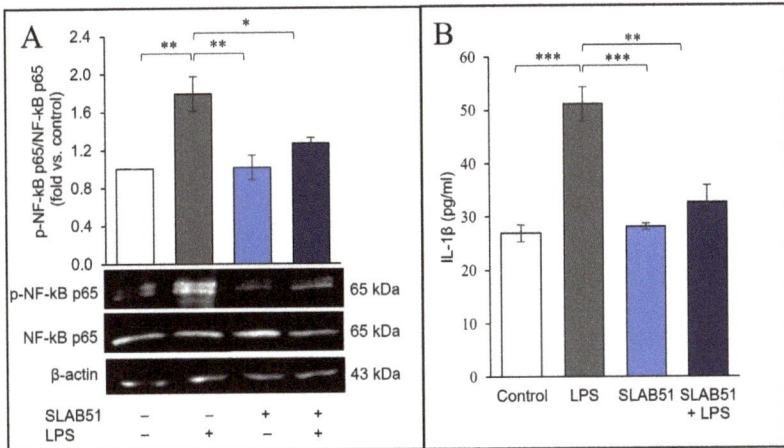

Figure 6. Effect of SLAB51 lysate treatment on inflammatory markers in LPS-stimulated Caco-2 cells. Caco-2 cells were treated for 24 h with or without LPS (10 μg/mL) and SLAB51 lysate (100 μg/mL). (**A**) p-NF-κB p65 and NF-κB p65 were analyzed by Western blotting. Following the densitometric analysis, the obtained values for p-NF-κB p65 were normalized with respect to NF-κB p65. Representative immunoblots of p-NF-κB p65, NF-κB p65, and β-actin are also shown. (**B**) IL-1β levels in the culture medium were assayed by ELISA kit. Data shown are expressed as mean ± SEM of three independent experiments. For the comparative analysis of the data, ANOVA was used followed by the Tukey test. * $p < 0.05$, ** $p < 0.01$, *** $p < 0.001$.

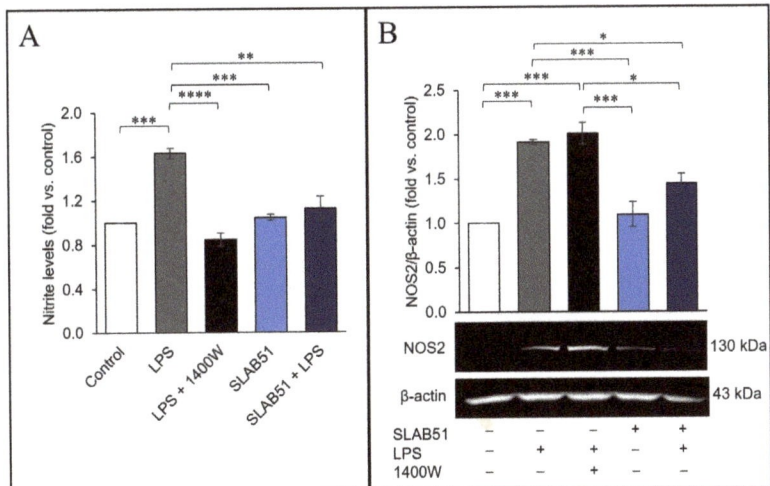

Figure 7. Effect of SLAB51 lysate on NOS2 expression and activity in LPS-stimulated Caco-2 cells. Caco-2 cells were treated for 24 h with or without LPS (10 μg/mL), NOS2 inhibitor 1400W (100 μM), SLAB51 lysate (100 μg/mL). (**A**) Nitrite levels in the culture medium were assayed by Griess reagent. Values are expressed as fold of nitrite levels vs. control. (**B**) Western blotting for NOS2 on cell lysates. Following the densitometric analysis, the obtained values were normalized with respect to β-actin. Representative immunoblots of NOS2 and β-actin are also shown. Data shown are expressed as means ± SEM of three independent experiments. For the comparative analysis of the data, ANOVA was used followed by the Tukey test. * $p < 0.05$, ** $p < 0.01$, *** $p < 0.001$, **** $p < 0.0001$.

Finally, we verified the hypothesis that the anti-inflammatory effect of SLAB51 observed in our model could be mediated by the ability of the probiotic to modulate the HIF-1α pathway. For this purpose, the cells were incubated with AKT and PI3K inhibitors 30 min prior to the treatment with SLAB51 lysate and LPS, and then the effect on NOS2 activity was evaluated after 24 h treatment. The results demonstrated that the two inhibitors were able to significantly interfere with the ability of SLAB51 lysate to reduce NOS2 activity (Figure 8). Indeed, nitrite levels in the culture medium after SLAB51 + LPS + perifosine or LY24002 were significantly higher than SLAB51 + LPS treatment ($p < 0.05$). However, both inhibitors were unable to totally abrogate the effect of SLAB51 since nitrite levels in the medium of the cells treated also with perifosine or LY24002 were still significantly lower than LPS treatment ($p < 0.05$).

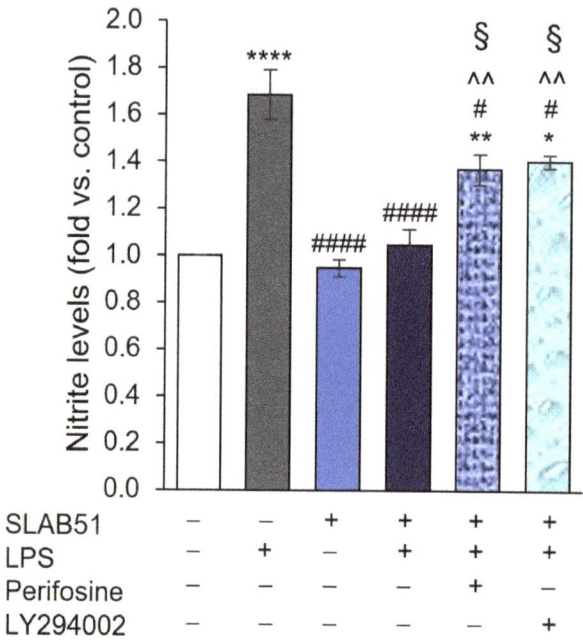

Figure 8. Effect of AKT and PI3K inhibition on SLAB51 lysate's ability to modulate NOS2 activity in LPS-stimulated Caco-2 cells. Caco-2 cells were incubated in the presence or absence of perifosine or LY294002 for 30 min and then treated for 24 h with or without LPS (10 µg/mL) and SLAB51 lysate (100 µg/mL). Nitrite levels in the culture medium were assayed by Griess reagent. Values are expressed as fold of nitrite levels vs. control. Data shown are expressed as means ± SEM of three independent experiments. For the comparative analysis of the data, ANOVA was used followed by the Tukey test. * $p < 0.05$, ** $p < 0.01$, **** $p < 0.0001$ vs. control; # $p < 0.05$, #### $p < 0.0001$ vs. LPS; ^^ $p < 0.01$ vs. SLAB51; § $p < 0.05$ vs. SLAB51 + LPS.

3. Discussion

The role of the HIF pathway in regulating gut homeostasis is an area of active interest, as demonstrated by the plethora of studies highlighting the therapeutic potential of targeting pathological hypoxia signaling pathways in IBD [16,48]. Among HIFs, the HIF-1α subunit is the most ubiquitously expressed. Recent studies emphasize the potential role of HIF-1α as the central hypoxia sensor in preserving gut homeostasis by improving the survival of gut microresidents [2,3,49]. In addition, HIF-1α plays a crucial role in maintaining the integrity of the intestinal epithelial mucosa by upregulating genes involved in gut barrier functions such as MUC2, ITF, CLDN1, and other tight junction proteins [2].

Despite the increasing attention on the role of HIFs in regulating mucosal barrier function, metabolism, inflammatory processes, and immune response in the gut, the ability of probiotics to influence the HIF pathway has not been thoroughly investigated. The existing studies evaluating probiotics' influence on HIF-1α stabilization in the intestinal environment are limited to investigating the effect of short-chain fatty acids, mainly butyrate, a product of microbial fermentation of dietary fibers in the lower intestinal tract able to directly and non-competitively inhibit PHD [50]. This effect has been linked to the colonization of the colon by probiotics while no evidence has been produced about activities directly exerted by probiotics in their transit through the upper intestine.

Ingested probiotics must pass the stomach, survive the gastric acid, bile salts, and pancreatic enzymes, and travel through the intestine until they reach the ileocecal valve. It is the common opinion that a substantial reduction in viable probiotic bacteria during transit in the gastrointestinal tract reduces the benefits of probiotics [51]. Even though the joint FAO/WHO working group specifically recommended that candidate bacteria for use as probiotics be resistant to gastric acidity and bile compounds, there is always a proportion of bacteria undergoing destruction before reaching the colon. The contents of these destroyed bacteria could have a biological effect at the small intestine level, where the bulk of nutrient and calorie absorption takes place. So, even though the number of bacteria in the proximal tract of the intestine is low, their biological relevance may play a pivotal role in influencing the host physiology as many of the systemic effects of the gut are generated in the small intestine [52]. Particularly, bacteria in the duodenum and the upper part of the intestine could influence hypoxia through the modulation of the HIF pathway. It has been recently reported that vertical sleeve gastrectomy (VSG) facilitated the richness of *Lactobacillus* spp. by reducing the amount of gastric acid reaching the duodenum and was associated with a consistent increase in HIF2α signaling [53].

Regarding the possibility of a direct action of the probiotic at the level of the duodenum and upper part of the intestine, we would like to mention a recent study by Ceccarelli et al., which has reported a significant and rapid improvement in the respiratory conditions of patients positive for SARS-CoV-2 infection if treated with SLAB51 [33]. After 24 h from the start of bacteriotherapy, the group treated with SLAB51 had an improved blood oxygenation compared to the group that received only routinely administered anti-COVID-19 treatment, as evidenced by the analysis of pO_2, O_2Hb, and SaO_2 values. The mechanism by which SLAB51 lysate leads to the improvement of lung functions are not yet identified. Furthermore, treatment with SLAB51 has recently been shown to induce HIF-1α stabilization, reduce PHD2 expression, and inhibit NOS2 expression in the brain of the AD mouse model [31]. These findings indicate that the probiotic formulation can exert positive effects not only in the gastrointestinal tract, but also in extraintestinal organs. In the small intestine, the modulation of the HIF pathways is more probably a consequence of direct, enzymatic action of the probiotic rather than the result of the bacterial fermentation process, as could be in the colon.

Driven by the need to deepen our understanding of the crucial role of the HIF in intestinal mucosal physiology, in this study, we have evaluated the effect of the SLAB51 lysate on the HIF pathway in Caco-2 IECs. The data obtained show that exposure of Caco-2 IECs to SLAB51 under normoxic conditions positively influenced the HIF pathway. Specifically, a dose-dependent upregulation in HIF-1α levels was associated with an increase in L-lactate levels and the relative glycolysis rate in the treated cells. SLAB51's ability to stabilize HIF-1α was associated with the inhibition of PHD2 activity and expression. The involvement of the PI3K/AKT pathway underlying the ability of the SLAB51 lysate to induce the increase in HIF-1α levels was also verified, per previous reports supporting that upregulated HIF-1α expression and increased glycolysis are dependent on the activation of this pathway, regardless of oxygen levels [8]. Moreover, PHD2 inhibition induced by SLAB51 lysate could also lead to AKT activation, thus indirectly contributing to the observed increase in HIF-1α levels [54,55]. PHD2 can directly hydroxylate AKT on two major proline residues, thus leading to its inactivation [54]. On the other hand, the deletion of PHD2 leads to AKT activation [55]. Of note, the activation of PI3K/AKT signaling in melanoma cells has been reported to induce PHD2 inhibition, thereby promoting HIF-1α stability [56].

Although preliminary, our results are supported by previously published clinical data [31–34]. In this context, our observations lead us to hypothesize that the multi-strain probiotic SLAB51 is capable of conditioning cells to make them more prone to survive and respond to stresses to which they are exposed in a hypoxic and inflamed environment.

Probiotics have been shown to suppress inflammation by inhibiting various signaling pathways, such as the NF-κB pathway [57]. NF-κB signaling for transcriptional activation can occur through the classical (canonical) or the alternative (non-canonical) pathway, with both pathways leading to nuclear translocation and activation of NF-κB and binding of DNA. Both the canonical and non-canonical NF-κB pathways were found to be activated in IECs by IL-1β [24]. Interestingly, it was reported that hydroxylase inhibition led to the suppression of IL-1β-induced NF-kB-dependent gene expression [58]. Moreover, HIF-1α has been shown to repress the activation of NF-κB under inflammatory conditions [2]. In our experiments, LPS failed to induce an increase in HIF-1α levels; consistently, it has been demonstrated in a murine macrophage cell line that LPS stimulation induced the HIF-1α downregulation to below the basal level after an initial increase leading to pyroptosis [59]. Here, we demonstrated that SLAB51 lysate was able to counteract the NF-κB activation and IL-1β secretion induced by LPS stimulation. The probiotic also counteracted NOS2 expression and activity induced by LPS treatment. Notably, it has been shown that while acute exposure to NO stabilizes HIF-1α, chronic exposure to NO destabilizes HIF-1α [30].

SLAB51 possesses high levels of arginine deiminase (ADI) [33]. This prokaryotic enzyme, using the same substrate as NOS, L-arginine, indirectly inhibits the generation of NO due to substrate depletion [60]. The exposure of Caco-2 to SLAB51 induced a reduction in NOS2 activity [33]. In our conditions, the inhibition of the PI3K/AKT pathway was able to counteract the effect of SLAB51 on NOS activity, demonstrating a link between the activation of the AKT/PHD2/HIF pathway and the anti-inflammatory effect of the probiotic. Moreover, the inability of AKT signaling inhibition to totally counteract the effects of SLAB51 on NOS activity could be due to the ADI present in the probiotic.

In summary, our results broaden the knowledge of the beneficial effects of the multi-strain probiotic SLAB51, showing its ability to trigger a hypoxic response in intestinal epithelial cells in vitro under normoxic conditions. The increased HIF-1α levels associated with higher glycolytic metabolism and L-lactate production could be attributed to decreased PHD2 levels and activity, as well as to induced PI3K/AKT signaling. The ability of the probiotic lysate to activate the AKT pathway could be related to the modulation of TLR-mediated signaling. In this context, some probiotics or their bioactive compounds have been reported to modulate TLR signaling and inhibit the TLR4-mediated activation of inflammatory response elicited by LPS under inflammatory conditions [61–63].

It will be interesting to investigate the influence of SLAB51 treatment on the HIF pathway of the gut immune components under normoxia, physiological hypoxia, and pathological or inflammatory hypoxia. Furthermore, considering the suggested and partly opposite effects of HIF-1α vs. HIF-2α in gut homeostasis [11,64,65], it will be crucial to verify whether treatment with SLAB51 modulates the two isoforms of HIF differently. Identifying the SLAB51 lysate active components will also increase our understanding of the observed effect and advance the knowledge of evidence-based bacteriotherapy strategies.

Overall, these results support our hypothesis that, by increasing HIF-1α levels through the upregulation of the AKT pathway, the SLAB51 lysate can inhibit the NF-κB activation and its downstream signaling in IECs, counteracting the LPS-induced inflammatory response. To the best of our knowledge, this is the first report showing that a probiotic formulation led to HIF pathway activation in human IECs, by influencing PI3K/AKT signaling. In order to verify this hypothesis, studies are underway on supplementary cell lines and intestinal organoids using other complementary techniques and analyses, such as gene expression and flow cytometry. In addition, the suggestive hypothesis of potential immunomodulatory and anti-inflammatory bioactive peptides derived from SLAB51 strains will also be investigated in our experimental conditions [66,67].

Even though further studies are warranted to investigate the observed effects in further inflammatory models in vitro and in vivo, we can hypothesize that the SLAB51 formulation could act as a hypoxia mimetic agent, thus contributing to the preservation of intestinal homeostasis and the protection of IECs from the detrimental effects of chronic inflammation and pathologic hypoxia. On the other hand, a growing body of evidence supports that HIF-1α signaling can trigger contrasting responses depending on cell and tissue type [68]. Of particular interest, higher HIF-1α levels in diagnostic tumor biopsies have been associated with increased mortality risk in several cancers; these results were supported by experimental studies, which revealed that genetic manipulations leading to HIF-1α overexpression resulted in tumor overgrowth [69]. Conversely, the loss of HIF-1α activity resulted in reduced tumor expansion. Accordingly, HIF-1α overexpression has been observed in a variety of human cancers, including colon [70,71], and can enhance chemoresistance through the inhibition of apoptosis and senescence and the activation of drug efflux proteins [72]. Thus, targeting HIF-1α is considered a promising strategy for inhibiting cancer cell proliferation and overcoming chemoresistance. Of note, our preliminary and encouraging results indicate that the SLAB51 lysate was able to counteract the stabilization of HIF-1α in different human colorectal cancer cell lines, i.e., HT29 and HCT116 (not shown).

In conclusion, our data can partially explain the beneficial effects recorded following treatment with SLAB51 in animal models and patients with hypoxia-related conditions [31–36]. Despite this, to furnish the multi-strain SLAB51 probiotic with an authorized health claim approved by a regulatory agency, such as the U.S. Food and Drug Administration (FDA) or the European Food Safety Authority (EFSA), evidence has to be provided through well-designed human trials.

4. Materials and Methods

4.1. Preparation of Bacterial Lysate for Cell Treatments

SLAB51 probiotic formulation (sold as Sivomixx, Ormendes SA, Jouxtens-Mézery, Switzerland) contains eight different live bacterial strains: *Streptococcus thermophilus* DSM 32245, *Bifidobacterium lactis* DSM 32246, *Bifidobacterium lactis* DSM 32247, *Lactobacillus acidophilus* DSM 32241, *Lactobacillus helveticus* DSM 32242, *Lactobacillus paracasei* DSM 32243, *Lactobacillus plantarum* DSM 32244, and *Lactobacillus brevis* DSM 27961. Bacterial lysate was prepared as previously described [73]. Briefly, SLAB51 formulation was suspended at the concentration of 133×10^9 CFU in 10 mL of phosphate buffered saline (PBS, Euro Clone, West York, UK), centrifuged at $8600 \times g$, washed twice, and sonicated (30 min, alternating 10 s of sonication and 10 s of pause) using a Vibracell sonicator (Sonic and Materials, Danbury, CT, USA). Bacterial cell disruption was verified by measuring the absorbance of the sample at 590 nm with a spectrophotometer (Eppendorf Hamburg, Germany) before and after every sonication step. The samples were then centrifuged at $17,949 \times g$, and the supernatants were filtered using a 0.22 μm-pore filter (Corning Incorporated, Corning, NY, USA) to remove any whole remaining bacteria. Total protein content was determined by a Bradford assay, using bovine serum albumin (BSA, Sigma Aldrich, St. Louis, MO, USA) as the standard.

4.2. Caco-2 IECs

The Caco-2 cell line purchased from Sigma-Aldrich (St. Louis, MO, USA) was grown in tissue culture flasks at 37 °C, 5% CO_2, and 90% relative humidity environment. The culture medium (Dulbecco's modified Eagle's medium, DMEM), supplemented with 10% fetal calf serum (FCS), 1% non-essential amino acids, 1 mM sodium pyruvate, 2 mM L-glutamine, 100 U/mL penicillin, and 100 μg/mL streptomycin (Euro Clone, West York, UK), was refreshed every other day. After reaching 80% confluence, cells were detached with trypsin solution from bovine pancreas (Euro Clone, West York, UK) and seeded into Dickinson

96-well plates (Seahorse XF96 Cell Culture Microplate, Agilent, Santa Clara, CA, USA) for metabolic studies, or into sterile tissue culture 6-well plates (Becton, San Jose, CA, USA) for the other experiments. In both the culture plates, the cells were seeded at 60,000 cells/cm^2 and cell growth was monitored by microscopy. Fourteen days post-confluence, cells were incubated with or without the SLAB51 lysate at the indicated concentrations and with or without 10 µg/mL lipopolysaccharide (LPS, Sigma-Aldrich). Where indicated, the cells were also pre-treated for 30 min with 100 µM NOS2 inhibitor N-(3-(aminomethyl) benzyl) acetamidine (1400W) (Sigma-Aldrich, St. Louis, MO, USA) prior to the treatment with LPS. To inhibit the PI3K/AKT pathway, the cells were pre-treated for 30 min with perifosine at 20 µM (AKT inhibitor, Cell Signaling Technology, Danvers, MA, USA) or LY294002 10 µM (PI3K inhibitor, Cell Signaling Technology). MG132 10 µM (Merck KGaA, Darmstadt, Germany) was used to inhibit proteasomal degradation of hydroxylated HIF-1α. The iron chelator deferoxamine (DFO, 150 µM) was used to inhibit PHD2 activity. To evaluate the effect of the several treatments on cell viability and proliferation, the cells were washed with PBS, centrifuged for 10 min at 400× g, and the pellets incubated with a 0.04% Trypan blue (Euro Clone, West York, UK) solution for 5 min to analyze cell number and viability. Untreated cells were also analyzed and served as controls. Cells were transferred to a Bürker counting chamber and counted by microscopy (Eclipse 50i, Nikon Corporation, Minato, Tokyo, Japan). All the experimental conditions and treatments did not significantly influence the cell viability (always >90%) or basal proliferation level compared to the untreated controls at all the incubation times.

4.3. Western Blot Analysis

Cells were washed with cold PBS and removed from plates by scraping in RIPA Lysis Buffer (Merck KGaA, Darmstadt, Germany) containing 100 mM protease inhibitor cocktail (Sigma-Aldrich, St. Louis, MO, USA). The process was carried out on ice because HIF-1α degrades rapidly in normoxia. After the lysis, the samples were centrifuged at 17,949× g to eliminate cell debris. The supernatants were collected and assayed for protein content with a Bradford assay/DC Protein Assay (Bio-Rad Laboratories, Hercules, CA, USA). Then, 25 µg total proteins were resolved on a 10% sodium dodecyl sulphate–polyacrylamide gel electrophoresis (SDS-PAGE), and electroblotted onto nitrocellulose membranes (Bio-Rad Laboratories). Membranes were blocked with 5% nonfat dry milk for 1 h at room temperature and then incubated overnight at 4 °C with rabbit monoclonal antibody anti-HIF-1α (Cell Signaling Technology, Danvers, MA, USA) 1:1000, rabbit monoclonal antibody anti-Hydroxy-HIF-1α (Pro564, Cell Signaling Technology) 1:1000, rabbit monoclonal antibody anti-PHD2 (Abcam, Cambridge, UK) 1:1000, rabbit monoclonal antibody anti-phospho-AKT (Ser473, Cell Signaling Technology) 1:1000, rabbit monoclonal antibody anti-AKT (Cell Signaling Technology) 1:1000, rabbit polyclonal anti-NOS2 antibody (Boster Biological Technology, Pleasanton, CA, USA) 1:500, rabbit monoclonal antibody anti-NF-kB (Cell Signaling Technology), or with mouse monoclonal antibody anti-β-actin 1:1000 (OriGene Technologies, Inc, Rockville, MD, USA). Horseradish peroxidase- (HRP-) conjugated goat anti-rabbit IgG secondary antibody (Millipore EMD, Darmstadt, Germany) 1:2000 or HRP-conjugated goat anti-mouse IgG secondary antibody (Bio-Rad Laboratories, Hercules, CA, USA) 1:2000 were used. Immunoreactive bands were visualized by enhanced chemiluminescence (ECL, Amersham Pharmacia Biotech) according to the manufacturer's instructions. Band relative densities were determined using a chemiluminescence documentation system Alliance (UVITEC, Cambridge, UK), and values were given as relative units (Supplementary Figures S1–S3).

4.4. L-Lactate Assay

L-lactate levels in cell culture supernatants were analyzed via the L-lactate assay kit (Abcam, Cambridge, UK) according to the manufacturer's instructions. Accordingly, the supernatants were deproteinized with a 10 kDa NMWCO Centrifugal Filter Unit (Amicon, Millipore, Burlington, MA, USA), and the filtrate was added to reaction wells.

The absorbance was measured by spectrophotometric reading at 570 nm using a microplate reader (Bio-Rad Laboratories, Hercules, CA, USA). The L-lactate levels were determined by comparison to a standard curve.

4.5. Metabolic Studies

Cells treated as described above were assessed for extracellular acidification rate (ECAR) and O_2 consumption rate (OCR) to calculate glycolysis rate (ECAR/OCR) using the Seahorse XFe96 Analyzer (Agilent, Santa Clara, CA, USA) following the manufacturer's instructions. Briefly, on the day of the assay, the medium was changed for Seahorse XF DMEM Medium pH 7.4 supplemented with glucose (10 mmol/L), pyruvate (1 mmol/L), and glutamine (2 mmol/L) (Agilent), and the cells were allowed to equilibrate in a non-CO_2 incubator for 1 h; OCR and ECAR were then measured. XFp Mito Stress Test Kit was used to test mitochondrial function. Injection of oligomycin (1 µM), carbonyl cyanide-4 (trifluoromethoxy) phenylhydrazone (FCCP, 1 µM), and the mixture of rotenone and antimycin A (1 µM) allows for the determination of the key bioenergetic parameters: basal respiration, ATP production-linked respiration (ATP production), maximal respiration, spare respiratory capacity, nonmitochondrial respiration, proton leak, and coupling efficiency.

4.6. IL-1β ELISA

The levels of released IL-1β were quantified in the cell supernatants using a human IL-1β enzyme-linked immunosorbent assay (ELISA) kit (Sigma Aldrich, Saint Louis, MO, USA), as described in the manufacturer's instructions. The collected media were cleared of cellular debris/dead cells by centrifugation at $1000\times g$ for 15 min. The absorbance was measured by spectrophotometric reading at 450 nm. The IL-1β concentration was determined by comparison to a standard curve. Results are expressed as pg/mL.

4.7. Nitrite Level Assay

The enzymatic activity of NOS2 was evaluated by measuring nitrite levels using nitrate reductase and Griess reaction through a colorimetric assay (Nitrite Assay kit-Sigma-Aldrich Co., Milan, Italy). Nitrite levels were assayed in the supernatants of Caco-2 cells, treated as above described, applied to a 96-well microtiter plate, according to the manufacturer's instructions. The absorbance was measured by spectrophotometric reading at 550 nm using a microplate reader (Bio-Rad Laboratories). The nitrite content of each sample was evaluated with a standard curve obtained by linear regression made with sodium nitrite and expressed as fold vs. control.

4.8. Statistical Analysis

Statistical analysis of data was performed using GraphPad Prism 6.0 (GraphPad Software, San Diego, CA, USA). For comparison between two means, Student's unpaired *t*-test was used. For comparison of the mean values among the groups, a one-way ANOVA, followed by Dunnett or Tukey post hoc test, was used. The results were expressed as mean ± SEM, as specified in figure legends. *p* values less than 0.05 were considered to be statistically significant.

Supplementary Materials: The following supporting information can be downloaded at: https://www.mdpi.com/article/10.3390/ijms24098134/s1.

Author Contributions: Conceptualization, F.L. and B.C.; formal analysis, F.L., P.P. and S.A. (Serena Altamura); investigation, F.L., F.R.A. and S.A. (Serena Artone); resources, F.L., F.R.A., P.P., S.A. (Serena Artone) and B.C.; data curation, F.L. and P.P.; writing—original draft preparation, F.L., P.P., S.A. (Serena Altamura) and B.C.; writing—review and editing, J.M.S., L.B., G.L., M.G.C. and B.C.; supervision, F.L., A.M.E., M.G.C. and B.C.; project administration, M.G.C. and B.C.; funding acquisition, F.L., P.P., G.L., M.G.C. and B.C. All authors have read and agreed to the published version of the manuscript.

Funding: This research and the APC were funded by Department of Life, Health and Environmental Sciences, University of L'Aquila, grants "FFO MeSVA 2021", "FFO MeSVA 2022", and grant "Bando PSD-MESVA 2022".

Data Availability Statement: The datasets generated and analyzed during the current study are available from the corresponding authors upon reasonable request.

Acknowledgments: The authors thank Gasperina De Nuntiis (Department of Life, Health and Environmental Sciences, University of L'Aquila, L'Aquila, Italy) for excellent technical assistance.

Conflicts of Interest: The authors declare no conflict of interest.

References

1. Semenza, G.L. Oxygen sensing, homeostasis, and disease. *N. Engl. J. Med.* **2011**, *365*, 537–547. [CrossRef] [PubMed]
2. Kumar, T.; Pandey, R.; Chauhan, N.S. Hypoxia Inducible Factor-1alpha: The Curator of Gut Homeostasis. *Front. Cell. Infect. Microbiol.* **2020**, *10*, 227. [CrossRef] [PubMed]
3. Singhal, R.; Shah, Y.M. Oxygen battle in the gut: Hypoxia and hypoxia-inducible factors in metabolic and inflammatory responses in the intestine. *J. Biol. Chem.* **2020**, *295*, 10493–10505. [CrossRef]
4. Kaelin, W.G., Jr.; Ratcliffe, P.J. Oxygen sensing by metazoans: The central role of the HIF hydroxylase pathway. *Mol. Cell* **2008**, *30*, 393–402. [CrossRef] [PubMed]
5. Strowitzki, M.J.; Cummins, E.P.; Taylor, C.T. Protein Hydroxylation by Hypoxia-Inducible Factor (HIF) Hydroxylases: Unique or Ubiquitous? *Cells* **2019**, *8*, 384. [CrossRef] [PubMed]
6. Wong, B.W.; Kuchnio, A.; Bruning, U.; Carmeliet, P. Emerging novel functions of the oxygen-sensing prolyl hydroxylase domain enzymes. *Trends Biochem. Sci.* **2013**, *38*, 3–11. [CrossRef] [PubMed]
7. Demidenko, Z.N.; Blagosklonny, M.V. The purpose of the HIF-1/PHD feedback loop: To limit mTOR-induced HIF-1alpha. *Cell Cycle* **2011**, *10*, 1557–1562. [CrossRef]
8. Dong, S.; Liang, S.; Cheng, Z.; Zhang, X.; Luo, L.; Li, L.; Zhang, W.; Li, S.; Xu, Q.; Zhong, M.; et al. ROS/PI3K/Akt and Wnt/beta-catenin signalings activate HIF-1alpha-induced metabolic reprogramming to impart 5-fluorouracil resistance in colorectal cancer. *J. Exp. Clin. Cancer Res.* **2022**, *41*, 15. [CrossRef]
9. Manning, B.D.; Cantley, L.C. AKT/PKB signaling: Navigating downstream. *Cell* **2007**, *129*, 1261–1274. [CrossRef]
10. Hindryckx, P.; De Vos, M.; Jacques, P.; Ferdinande, L.; Peeters, H.; Olievier, K.; Bogaert, S.; Brinkman, B.; Vandenabeele, P.; Elewaut, D.; et al. Hydroxylase inhibition abrogates TNF-alpha-induced intestinal epithelial damage by hypoxia-inducible factor-1-dependent repression of FADD. *J. Immunol.* **2010**, *185*, 6306–6316. [CrossRef]
11. Karhausen, J.; Furuta, G.T.; Tomaszewski, J.E.; Johnson, R.S.; Colgan, S.P.; Haase, V.H. Epithelial hypoxia-inducible factor-1 is protective in murine experimental colitis. *J. Clin. Investig.* **2004**, *114*, 1098–1106. [CrossRef] [PubMed]
12. Keely, S.; Campbell, E.L.; Baird, A.W.; Hansbro, P.M.; Shalwitz, R.A.; Kotsakis, A.; McNamee, E.N.; Eltzschig, H.K.; Kominsky, D.J.; Colgan, S.P. Contribution of epithelial innate immunity to systemic protection afforded by prolyl hydroxylase inhibition in murine colitis. *Mucosal Immunol.* **2014**, *7*, 114–123. [CrossRef] [PubMed]
13. Robinson, A.; Keely, S.; Karhausen, J.; Gerich, M.E.; Furuta, G.T.; Colgan, S.P. Mucosal protection by hypoxia-inducible factor prolyl hydroxylase inhibition. *Gastroenterology* **2008**, *134*, 145–155. [CrossRef]
14. Tambuwala, M.M.; Cummins, E.P.; Lenihan, C.R.; Kiss, J.; Stauch, M.; Scholz, C.C.; Fraisl, P.; Lasitschka, F.; Mollenhauer, M.; Saunders, S.P.; et al. Loss of prolyl hydroxylase-1 protects against colitis through reduced epithelial cell apoptosis and increased barrier function. *Gastroenterology* **2010**, *139*, 2093–2101. [CrossRef] [PubMed]
15. Glover, L.E.; Lee, J.S.; Colgan, S.P. Oxygen metabolism and barrier regulation in the intestinal mucosa. *J. Clin. Investig.* **2016**, *126*, 3680–3688. [CrossRef]
16. Manresa, M.C.; Taylor, C.T. Hypoxia Inducible Factor (HIF) Hydroxylases as Regulators of Intestinal Epithelial Barrier Function. *Cell. Mol. Gastroenterol. Hepatol.* **2017**, *3*, 303–315. [CrossRef]
17. Cummins, E.P.; Strowitzki, M.J.; Taylor, C.T. Mechanisms and Consequences of Oxygen and Carbon Dioxide Sensing in Mammals. *Physiol. Rev.* **2020**, *100*, 463–488. [CrossRef]
18. Cummins, E.P.; Seeballuck, F.; Keely, S.J.; Mangan, N.E.; Callanan, J.J.; Fallon, P.G.; Taylor, C.T. The hydroxylase inhibitor dimethyloxalylglycine is protective in a murine model of colitis. *Gastroenterology* **2008**, *134*, 156–165. [CrossRef]
19. Gupta, R.; Chaudhary, A.R.; Shah, B.N.; Jadhav, A.V.; Zambad, S.P.; Gupta, R.C.; Deshpande, S.; Chauthaiwale, V.; Dutt, C. Therapeutic treatment with a novel hypoxia-inducible factor hydroxylase inhibitor (TRC160334) ameliorates murine colitis. *Clin. Exp. Gastroenterol.* **2014**, *7*, 13–23. [CrossRef]
20. Kim, Y.I.; Yi, E.J.; Kim, Y.D.; Lee, A.R.; Chung, J.; Ha, H.C.; Cho, J.M.; Kim, S.R.; Ko, H.J.; Cheon, J.H.; et al. Local Stabilization of Hypoxia-Inducible Factor-1alpha Controls Intestinal Inflammation via Enhanced Gut Barrier Function and Immune Regulation. *Front. Immunol.* **2020**, *11*, 609689. [CrossRef]

21. Strowitzki, M.J.; Kimmer, G.; Wehrmann, J.; Ritter, A.S.; Radhakrishnan, P.; Opitz, V.M.; Tuffs, C.; Biller, M.; Kugler, J.; Keppler, U.; et al. Inhibition of HIF-prolyl hydroxylases improves healing of intestinal anastomoses. *JCI Insight* **2021**, *6*, e139191. [CrossRef] [PubMed]
22. De Plaen, I.G.; Tan, X.D.; Chang, H.; Wang, L.; Remick, D.G.; Hsueh, W. Lipopolysaccharide activates nuclear factor kappaB in rat intestine: Role of endogenous platelet-activating factor and tumour necrosis factor. *Br. J. Pharmacol.* **2000**, *129*, 307–314. [CrossRef] [PubMed]
23. Candelli, M.; Franza, L.; Pignataro, G.; Ojetti, V.; Covino, M.; Piccioni, A.; Gasbarrini, A.; Franceschi, F. Interaction between Lipopolysaccharide and Gut Microbiota in Inflammatory Bowel Diseases. *Int. J. Mol. Sci.* **2021**, *22*, 6242. [CrossRef] [PubMed]
24. Kaminsky, L.W.; Al-Sadi, R.; Ma, T.Y. IL-1beta and the Intestinal Epithelial Tight Junction Barrier. *Front. Immunol.* **2021**, *12*, 767456. [CrossRef] [PubMed]
25. Bandarra, D.; Biddlestone, J.; Mudie, S.; Muller, H.A.; Rocha, S. HIF-1alpha restricts NF-kappaB-dependent gene expression to control innate immunity signals. *Dis. Model Mech.* **2015**, *8*, 169–181. [CrossRef]
26. Biddlestone, J.; Bandarra, D.; Rocha, S. The role of hypoxia in inflammatory disease (review). *Int. J. Mol. Med.* **2015**, *35*, 859–869. [CrossRef]
27. Pautz, A.; Art, J.; Hahn, S.; Nowag, S.; Voss, C.; Kleinert, H. Regulation of the expression of inducible nitric oxide synthase. *Nitric Oxide* **2010**, *23*, 75–93. [CrossRef]
28. Kolios, G.; Valatas, V.; Ward, S.G. Nitric oxide in inflammatory bowel disease: A universal messenger in an unsolved puzzle. *Immunology* **2004**, *113*, 427–437. [CrossRef]
29. Soufli, I.; Toumi, R.; Rafa, H.; Touil-Boukoffa, C. Overview of cytokines and nitric oxide involvement in immuno-pathogenesis of inflammatory bowel diseases. *World J. Gastrointest. Pharmacol. Ther.* **2016**, *7*, 353–360. [CrossRef]
30. Berchner-Pfannschmidt, U.; Tug, S.; Kirsch, M.; Fandrey, J. Oxygen-sensing under the influence of nitric oxide. *Cell. Signal.* **2010**, *22*, 349–356. [CrossRef]
31. Bonfili, L.; Gong, C.; Lombardi, F.; Cifone, M.G.; Eleuteri, A.M. Strategic Modification of Gut Microbiota through Oral Bacteriotherapy Influences Hypoxia Inducible Factor-1alpha: Therapeutic Implication in Alzheimer's Disease. *Int. J. Mol. Sci.* **2021**, *23*, 357. [CrossRef]
32. Ceccarelli, G.; Borrazzo, C.; Pinacchio, C.; Santinelli, L.; Innocenti, G.P.; Cavallari, E.N.; Celani, L.; Marazzato, M.; Alessandri, F.; Ruberto, F.; et al. Oral Bacteriotherapy in Patients With COVID-19: A Retrospective Cohort Study. *Front. Nutr.* **2020**, *7*, 613928. [CrossRef] [PubMed]
33. Ceccarelli, G.; Marazzato, M.; Celani, L.; Lombardi, F.; Piccirilli, A.; Mancone, M.; Trinchieri, V.; Pugliese, F.; Mastroianni, C.M.; d'Ettorre, G. Oxygen Sparing Effect of Bacteriotherapy in COVID-19. *Nutrients* **2021**, *13*, 2898. [CrossRef] [PubMed]
34. d'Ettorre, G.; Ceccarelli, G.; Marazzato, M.; Campagna, G.; Pinacchio, C.; Alessandri, F.; Ruberto, F.; Rossi, G.; Celani, L.; Scagnolari, C.; et al. Challenges in the Management of SARS-CoV2 Infection: The Role of Oral Bacteriotherapy as Complementary Therapeutic Strategy to Avoid the Progression of COVID-19. *Front. Med.* **2020**, *7*, 389. [CrossRef] [PubMed]
35. Trinchieri, V.; Marazzato, M.; Ceccarelli, G.; Lombardi, F.; Piccirilli, A.; Santinelli, L.; Maddaloni, L.; Vassalini, P.; Mastroianni, C.M.; d'Ettorre, G. Exploiting Bacteria for Improving Hypoxemia of COVID-19 Patients. *Biomedicines* **2022**, *10*, 1851. [CrossRef]
36. de Rijke, T.J.; Doting, M.H.E.; van Hemert, S.; De Deyn, P.P.; van Munster, B.C.; Harmsen, H.J.M.; Sommer, I.E.C. A Systematic Review on the Effects of Different Types of Probiotics in Animal Alzheimer's Disease Studies. *Front. Psychiatry* **2022**, *13*, 879491. [CrossRef]
37. Derrien, M.; Turroni, F.; Ventura, M.; van Sinderen, D. Insights into endogenous Bifidobacterium species in the human gut microbiota during adulthood. *Trends Microbiol.* **2022**, *30*, 940–947. [CrossRef]
38. Pasolli, E.; De Filippis, F.; Mauriello, I.E.; Cumbo, F.; Walsh, A.M.; Leech, J.; Cotter, P.D.; Segata, N.; Ercolini, D. Large-scale genome-wide analysis links lactic acid bacteria from food with the gut microbiome. *Nat. Commun.* **2020**, *11*, 2610. [CrossRef]
39. Kamada, N.; Chen, G.Y.; Inohara, N.; Nunez, G. Control of pathogens and pathobionts by the gut microbiota. *Nat. Immunol.* **2013**, *14*, 685–690. [CrossRef]
40. Sekirov, I.; Russell, S.L.; Antunes, L.C.; Finlay, B.B. Gut microbiota in health and disease. *Physiol. Rev.* **2010**, *90*, 859–904. [CrossRef]
41. Bonfili, L.; Cecarini, V.; Berardi, S.; Scarpona, S.; Suchodolski, J.S.; Nasuti, C.; Fiorini, D.; Boarelli, M.C.; Rossi, G.; Eleuteri, A.M. Microbiota modulation counteracts Alzheimer's disease progression influencing neuronal proteolysis and gut hormones plasma levels. *Sci. Rep.* **2017**, *7*, 2426. [CrossRef] [PubMed]
42. Bonfili, L.; Cecarini, V.; Cuccioloni, M.; Angeletti, M.; Berardi, S.; Scarpona, S.; Rossi, G.; Eleuteri, A.M. SLAB51 Probiotic Formulation Activates SIRT1 Pathway Promoting Antioxidant and Neuroprotective Effects in an AD Mouse Model. *Mol. Neurobiol.* **2018**, *55*, 7987–8000. [CrossRef] [PubMed]
43. Castelli, V.; d'Angelo, M.; Lombardi, F.; Alfonsetti, M.; Antonosante, A.; Catanesi, M.; Benedetti, E.; Palumbo, P.; Cifone, M.G.; Giordano, A.; et al. Effects of the probiotic formulation SLAB51 in vitro and in vivo Parkinson's disease models. *Aging* **2020**, *12*, 4641–4659. [CrossRef] [PubMed]
44. Cuozzo, M.; Castelli, V.; Avagliano, C.; Cimini, A.; d'Angelo, M.; Cristiano, C.; Russo, R. Effects of Chronic Oral Probiotic Treatment in Paclitaxel-Induced Neuropathic Pain. *Biomedicines* **2021**, *9*, 346. [CrossRef] [PubMed]

45. Nagao, A.; Kobayashi, M.; Koyasu, S.; Chow, C.C.T.; Harada, H. HIF-1-Dependent Reprogramming of Glucose Metabolic Pathway of Cancer Cells and Its Therapeutic Significance. *Int. J. Mol. Sci.* **2019**, *20*, 238. [CrossRef] [PubMed]
46. TeSlaa, T.; Teitell, M.A. Techniques to monitor glycolysis. *Methods Enzymol.* **2014**, *542*, 91–114. [CrossRef]
47. Liu, T.; Zhang, L.; Joo, D.; Sun, S.C. NF-kappaB signaling in inflammation. *Signal Transduct. Target. Ther.* **2017**, *2*, 17023. [CrossRef]
48. Brown, E.; Taylor, C.T. Hypoxia-sensitive pathways in intestinal inflammation. *J. Physiol.* **2018**, *596*, 2985–2989. [CrossRef]
49. Semenza, G.L. Hypoxia-inducible factor 1 (HIF-1) pathway. *Sci. STKE* **2007**, *2007*, cm8. [CrossRef]
50. Wang, R.X.; Henen, M.A.; Lee, J.S.; Vogeli, B.; Colgan, S.P. Microbiota-derived butyrate is an endogenous HIF prolyl hydroxylase inhibitor. *Gut Microbes* **2021**, *13*, 1938380. [CrossRef]
51. Han, S.; Lu, Y.; Xie, J.; Fei, Y.; Zheng, G.; Wang, Z.; Liu, J.; Lv, L.; Ling, Z.; Berglund, B.; et al. Probiotic Gastrointestinal Transit and Colonization After Oral Administration: A Long Journey. *Front. Cell. Infect. Microbiol.* **2021**, *11*, 609722. [CrossRef] [PubMed]
52. Kastl, A.J., Jr.; Terry, N.A.; Wu, G.D.; Albenberg, L.G. The Structure and Function of the Human Small Intestinal Microbiota: Current Understanding and Future Directions. *Cell. Mol. Gastroenterol. Hepatol.* **2020**, *9*, 33–45. [CrossRef]
53. Shao, Y.; Evers, S.S.; Shin, J.H.; Ramakrishnan, S.K.; Bozadjieva-Kramer, N.; Yao, Q.; Shah, Y.M.; Sandoval, D.A.; Seeley, R.J. Vertical sleeve gastrectomy increases duodenal *Lactobacillus* spp. richness associated with the activation of intestinal HIF2alpha signaling and metabolic benefits. *Mol. Metab.* **2022**, *57*, 101432. [CrossRef]
54. Guo, J.; Chakraborty, A.A.; Liu, P.; Gan, W.; Zheng, X.; Inuzuka, H.; Wang, B.; Zhang, J.; Zhang, L.; Yuan, M.; et al. pVHL suppresses kinase activity of Akt in a proline-hydroxylation-dependent manner. *Science* **2016**, *353*, 929–932. [CrossRef]
55. Liu, S.; Zhang, G.; Guo, J.; Chen, X.; Lei, J.; Ze, K.; Dong, L.; Dai, X.; Gao, Y.; Song, D.; et al. Loss of Phd2 cooperates with BRAF(V600E) to drive melanomagenesis. *Nat. Commun.* **2018**, *9*, 5426. [CrossRef]
56. Spinella, F.; Rosano, L.; Del Duca, M.; Di Castro, V.; Nicotra, M.R.; Natali, P.G.; Bagnato, A. Endothelin-1 inhibits prolyl hydroxylase domain 2 to activate hypoxia-inducible factor-1alpha in melanoma cells. *PLoS ONE* **2010**, *5*, e11241. [CrossRef] [PubMed]
57. Cristofori, F.; Dargenio, V.N.; Dargenio, C.; Miniello, V.L.; Barone, M.; Francavilla, R. Anti-Inflammatory and Immunomodulatory Effects of Probiotics in Gut Inflammation: A Door to the Body. *Front. Immunol.* **2021**, *12*, 578386. [CrossRef] [PubMed]
58. Scholz, C.C.; Cavadas, M.A.; Tambuwala, M.M.; Hams, E.; Rodriguez, J.; von Kriegsheim, A.; Cotter, P.; Bruning, U.; Fallon, P.G.; Cheong, A.; et al. Regulation of IL-1beta-induced NF-kappaB by hydroxylases links key hypoxic and inflammatory signaling pathways. *Proc. Natl. Acad. Sci. USA* **2013**, *110*, 18490–18495. [CrossRef] [PubMed]
59. Aki, T.; Funakoshi, T.; Noritake, K.; Unuma, K.; Uemura, K. Extracellular glucose is crucially involved in the fate decision of LPS-stimulated RAW264.7 murine macrophage cells. *Sci. Rep.* **2020**, *10*, 10581. [CrossRef]
60. Riccia, D.N.; Bizzini, F.; Perilli, M.G.; Polimeni, A.; Trinchieri, V.; Amicosante, G.; Cifone, M.G. Anti-inflammatory effects of *Lactobacillus brevis* (CD2) on periodontal disease. *Oral Dis.* **2007**, *13*, 376–385. [CrossRef]
61. Finamore, A.; Roselli, M.; Imbinto, A.; Seeboth, J.; Oswald, I.P.; Mengheri, E. Lactobacillus amylovorus inhibits the TLR4 inflammatory signaling triggered by enterotoxigenic Escherichia coli via modulation of the negative regulators and involvement of TLR2 in intestinal Caco-2 cells and pig explants. *PLoS ONE* **2014**, *9*, e94891. [CrossRef] [PubMed]
62. Mohseni, A.H.; Casolaro, V.; Bermudez-Humaran, L.G.; Keyvani, H.; Taghinezhad, S.S. Modulation of the PI3K/Akt/mTOR signaling pathway by probiotics as a fruitful target for orchestrating the immune response. *Gut Microbes* **2021**, *13*, 1–17. [CrossRef] [PubMed]
63. Sun, L.; Tian, W.; Guo, X.; Zhang, Y.; Liu, X.; Li, X.; Tian, Y.; Man, C.; Jiang, Y. Lactobacillus gasseri JM1 with potential probiotic characteristics alleviates inflammatory response by activating the PI3K/Akt signaling pathway in vitro. *J. Dairy Sci.* **2020**, *103*, 7851–7864. [CrossRef] [PubMed]
64. Ramakrishnan, S.K.; Shah, Y.M. Role of Intestinal HIF-2α in Health and Disease. *Annu. Rev. Physiol.* **2016**, *78*, 301–325. [CrossRef] [PubMed]
65. Shah, Y.M.; Ito, S.; Morimura, K.; Chen, C.; Yim, S.H.; Haase, V.H.; Gonzalez, F.J. Hypoxia-inducible factor augments experimental colitis through an MIF-dependent inflammatory signaling cascade. *Gastroenterology* **2008**, *134*, 2036–2048. [CrossRef] [PubMed]
66. Fernandez-Tome, S.; Marin, A.C.; Ortega Moreno, L.; Baldan-Martin, M.; Mora-Gutierrez, I.; Lanas-Gimeno, A.; Moreno-Monteagudo, J.A.; Santander, C.; Sanchez, B.; Chaparro, M.; et al. Immunomodulatory Effect of Gut Microbiota-Derived Bioactive Peptides on Human Immune System from Healthy Controls and Patients with Inflammatory Bowel Disease. *Nutrients* **2019**, *11*, 2605. [CrossRef]
67. Sadeghi, A.; Ebrahimi, M.; Kharazmi, M.S.; Jafari, S.M. Effects of microbial-derived biotics (meta/pharma/post-biotics) on the modulation of gut microbiome and metabolome; general aspects and emerging trends. *Food Chem.* **2023**, *411*, 135478. [CrossRef]
68. Corrado, C.; Fontana, S. Hypoxia and HIF Signaling: One Axis with Divergent Effects. *Int. J. Mol. Sci.* **2020**, *21*, 5611. [CrossRef]
69. Semenza, G.L. Defining the role of hypoxia-inducible factor 1 in cancer biology and therapeutics. *Oncogene* **2010**, *29*, 625–634. [CrossRef]
70. Semenza, G.L. HIF-1 and tumor progression: Pathophysiology and therapeutics. *Trends Mol. Med.* **2002**, *8*, S62–S67. [CrossRef]
71. Zhong, H.; De Marzo, A.M.; Laughner, E.; Lim, M.; Hilton, D.A.; Zagzag, D.; Buechler, P.; Isaacs, W.B.; Semenza, G.L.; Simons, J.W. Overexpression of hypoxia-inducible factor 1alpha in common human cancers and their metastases. *Cancer Res.* **1999**, *59*, 5830–5835. [PubMed]

72. Rohwer, N.; Cramer, T. Hypoxia-mediated drug resistance: Novel insights on the functional interaction of HIFs and cell death pathways. *Drug Resist. Updates* **2011**, *14*, 191–201. [CrossRef] [PubMed]
73. Lombardi, F.; Augello, F.R.; Palumbo, P.; Mollsi, E.; Giuliani, M.; Cimini, A.M.; Cifone, M.G.; Cinque, B. Soluble Fraction from Lysate of a High Concentration Multi-Strain Probiotic Formulation Inhibits TGF-beta1-Induced Intestinal Fibrosis on CCD-18Co Cells. *Nutrients* **2021**, *13*, 882. [CrossRef] [PubMed]

Disclaimer/Publisher's Note: The statements, opinions and data contained in all publications are solely those of the individual author(s) and contributor(s) and not of MDPI and/or the editor(s). MDPI and/or the editor(s) disclaim responsibility for any injury to people or property resulting from any ideas, methods, instructions or products referred to in the content.

Communication

Analysis of Circulating Food Antigen-Specific T-Cells in Celiac Disease and Inflammatory Bowel Disease

Yasmina Rodríguez-Sillke [1,2], Michael Schumann [1], Donata Lissner [1], Federica Branchi [1], Fabian Proft [1], Ulrich Steinhoff [3], Britta Siegmund [1] and Rainer Glauben [1,*]

[1] Department of Gastroenterology, Infectious Diseases, and Rheumatology, Campus Benjamin Franklin, Charité-University Medicine Berlin, 13125 Berlin, Germany
[2] Institute of Nutrition, University of Potsdam, 14558 Nuthetal, Germany
[3] Institute for Medical Microbiology and Hospital Hygiene, Philipps University of Marburg, 35043 Marburg, Germany
* Correspondence: rainer.glauben@charite.de

Abstract: To demonstrate and analyze the specific T-cell response following barrier disruption and antigen translocation, circulating food antigen-specific effector T-cells isolated from peripheral blood were analyzed in patients suffering from celiac disease (CeD) as well as inflammatory bowel disease (IBD). We applied the antigen-reactive T-cell enrichment (ARTE) technique allowing for phenotypical and functional flow cytometric analyses of rare nutritional antigen-specific T-cells, including the celiac disease-causing gliadin (gluten). For CeD, patient groups, including treatment-refractory cases, differ significantly from healthy controls. Even symptom-free patients on a gluten-free diet were distinguishable from healthy controls, without being previously challenged with gluten. Moreover, frequency and phenotype of nutritional antigen-specific T-cells of IBD patients directly correlated to the presence of small intestinal inflammation. Specifically, the frequency of antigen specific T-cells as well as pro-inflammatory cytokines was increased in patients with active CeD or Crohn's disease, respectively. These results suggest active small intestinal inflammation as key for the development of a peripheral food antigen-specific T-cell response in Crohn's disease and celiac disease.

Keywords: antigen-specific T-cells; celiac disease; gliadin; IBD; food antigens

1. Introduction

Antigen-specific T-cells play a central role in the adaptive immune system, promoting specific acute immune responses and the formation of immunological memory. Analyzing not only frequency, but also phenotype and function of these rare cells, represents not only a critical step towards understanding the mechanisms of adaptive immunity in general, but also in determining the specific immune status of the individual patient or diagnosing infectious or auto-immune diseases. The high diversity of the T-cell receptor, which allows for recognition of billions of different antigens, leads to an extremely low frequency of T-cells, specific for a single peptide-MHC ligand. This holds true even for pathogen-specific memory compartments in the absence of acute infections, for which specific T-cell frequencies in peripheral blood are typically far below 1%, but all the more for the naive repertoire (<0.0005%) [1,2].

Among autoimmune diseases, celiac disease (CeD) represents a model disease, as it turns active once the celiac individual is exposed to dietary gluten. Central to the celiac immune response are gliadin-specific T-cells that convey the small intestinal mucosal remodeling typical for CeD. As gluten has been identified as the disease-causing antigen, elimination of gluten results in regeneration of the duodenal mucosa and consecutive wellbeing of the patient [3,4]. However, diagnosis in CeD patients who are already on a gluten-free diet (GFD) remains challenging. Under a gluten-free diet (GFD), tissue-transglutaminase (tTG) antibodies normalize and the small intestinal villus atrophy regenerates [5]. To date, a burdening re-challenge of patients to gluten is mandatory for a valid diagnosis. However, translocation of nutritional (and pathogenic) antigens due to intestinal barrier breaches is described not exclusively for CeD, but also for inflammatory bowel diseases (IBD) [6,7]. IBD, more specifically Crohn's disease (CD) and ulcerative colitis (UC), are also characterized by a T-cell mediated, chronic inflammation of the intestine [8]. However, when compared with CeD, the specific origin of IBD is yet unknown. CD and UC differ in their inflammation pattern as well as their distribution. While in CD the configuration of inflammation is segmental and affects all layers of the intestinal wall (i.e., transmural inflammation), inflammation in UC is limited to the mucosal and submucosal gut layers and only affects the colon [9]. Although there are first studies connecting GFD to improvement of patient wellbeing [10] and even microbiota composition [11] in IBD, to date, circulating food antigen-specific T-cells have not been analyzed in these patients. Since the small intestine is the primary contact surface for food antigens and hence for the immunological response, we analyzed the specific nutritional T-cell response in the peripheral blood of patients with small intestinal Crohn's disease (CD), celiac disease as well as ulcerative colitis (UC), respectively. To exclude the influence of a non-intestinal inflammation, rheumatoid arthritis patients (RA) were included as control.

We applied antigen-reactive T-cell enrichment (ARTE) [12] technology to determine the specific nutritional effector T-cell response in the peripheral blood. The ARTE technique is based on the stimulation of peripheral blood mononuclear cells (PBMC) with a defined antigen and the subsequent up-regulation of the activation marker $CD154^+$, which is exclusively expressed on antigen-specific $CD4^+$ T-cells [13]. This method permits the detection of the entire antigen-specific $CD4^+$ T-cell response just by adding the antigen of choice directly to PBMC without the need of in-vitro expanding the reacting cells. The subsequent enrichment of $CD154^+$ cells enables further in-depth phenotyping of this rare cell population [14]. Thus, the ARTE technique allows direct ex vivo cytometric—and hence functional—analyses of gluten-specific, but also even rarer food antigen-specific T-cells.

2. Results

2.1. Circulating Gliadin-Specific T-Cells Are Increased in Active Disease with Ileal Inflammation

ARTE technology was applied to all blood samples (Figure 1A) for various food antigens, including controls for antigen-specific T-cell enrichment and T-cell activation. Moreover, we clearly demonstrated the necessity for T-cell enrichment to allow for deeper cell analysis and therefore the advantage of this method over direct staining protocols for rare antigen-specific cell populations (Figure 1B). With the overall frequency of $CD4^+$ T-cells remaining stable in the various disease conditions (Figure 1C), the frequency of gliadin-specific $CD154^+$ T-cells among $CD4^+$ T-cells in PBMC was expectedly highest in active CeD (aCeD), i.e., without GFD, as well as in refractory CeD patients (RCD). aCeD were rare patients as we did not actively initiate a gluten-re-challenge. Moreover, the frequencies were also significantly increased in CeD patients on a GFD without clinical symptoms when compared with healthy controls. Remarkably, a similar frequency to active CeD patients was observed in active CD patients with ileal inflammation (Figure 2A).

The frequency was significantly lower in CD patients in remission, in UC patients, independent of their inflammatory state and in healthy controls. Interestingly, first-degree relatives (FDR) of CeD patients, considered healthy by standard diagnostics, revealed a significant increase in the frequency of gliadin-specific T-cells compared with controls without familiar predisposition of CeD. Of notice, RA as auto-inflammatory control without intestinal inflammation, did not differ from healthy controls (Figure 2A).

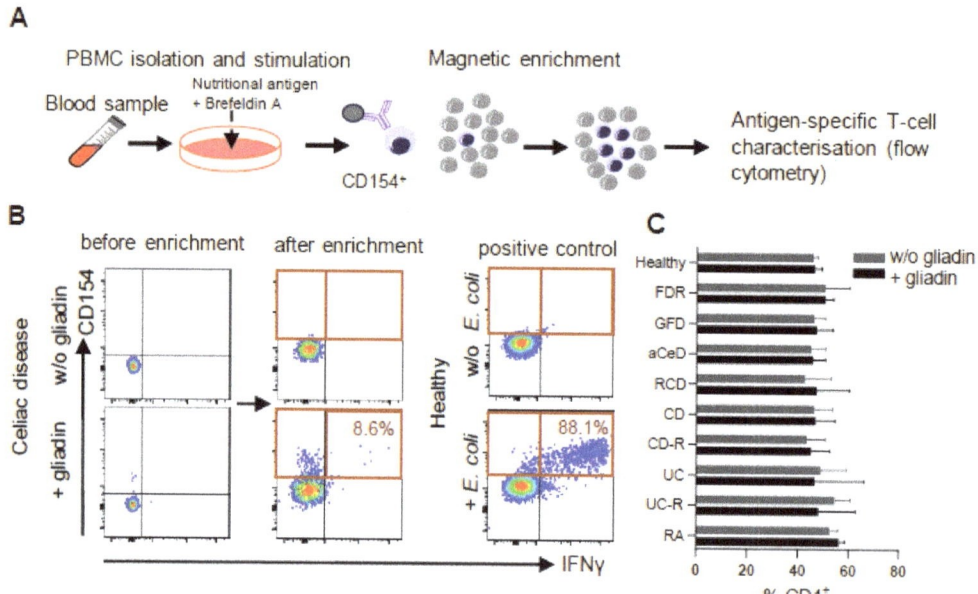

Figure 1. Enrichment of food antigen-specific T-cells. (**A–C**) Peripheral blood mononuclear cells (PBMC) were stimulated with various food antigens, magnetically enriched for CD154 and analyzed by flow cytometry. (**A**) Methodology and (**B**) exemplary density plots of CD154$^+$ T-cell enrichment after stimulation with gliadin or control antigen are shown. (**C**) Frequencies of CD4$^+$ T-cells in PBMC were determined from healthy controls (non-relatives, NR), patients with active Crohn's disease (CD) or ulcerative colitis (UC), or each of these entities in remission (-R), celiac disease patients (CeD) ± gluten-free diet (GFD, aCeD) or refractory (RCD) patients, first degree relatives of CeD patients (FDR) and rheumatoid arthritis patients (RA). Data are shown as median with 95% CI.

Moreover, gliadin-specific CD4$^+$CD154$^+$ T-cells, positive for the small intestinal homing marker α4β1, but not for α4β7, a general gut homing marker, were increased in aCeD patients (Figure 2B), further strengthening the connection of peripheral nutritional antigen-specific T-cells to small intestinal inflammation.

2.2. Pro-Inflammatory Cytokines of Circulating Gliadin-Specific T-Cells

The subsequent functional analysis of the antigen-specific T-cells after gliadin stimulation (Figure 2C,D; Supplementary Figure S2) revealed highest production of the pro-inflammatory cytokines IFNγ, IL-17A and TNFα in cells from aCeD, Refr, and from CD patients with small intestinal involvement. Remarkably, antigen-specific T-cells of first-degree relatives of CeD patients (FDR) presented with higher frequencies of gliadin-specific T-cells and an increased TNFα expression, and were thus comparable to aCeD patients. TNFα-positive CD154$^+$ cells were most discriminative when comparing active and inactive CeD to healthy controls.

2.3. Antigen-Specific Cells for Other Food Antigens Are Also Present in Increased Numbers in Active Disease with Ileal Inflammation

To dissect a sole barrier defect, as it is present in small intestinal CD, from the disease-driving gliadin-reactivity in CeD, we included soybean protein, peanut protein and OVA-peptide in our analysis. In fact, an increased frequency of antigen-specific CD4$^+$ T-cells was exclusively observed in the presence of small intestinal inflammation, namely CD and aCeD. CD patients in remission as well as UC patients independent of their inflammatory state did not differ from healthy controls. Furthermore, CeD patients on GFD, although being highly reactive to gliadin, showed no reaction to other nutritional antigens (Figure 3A,B).

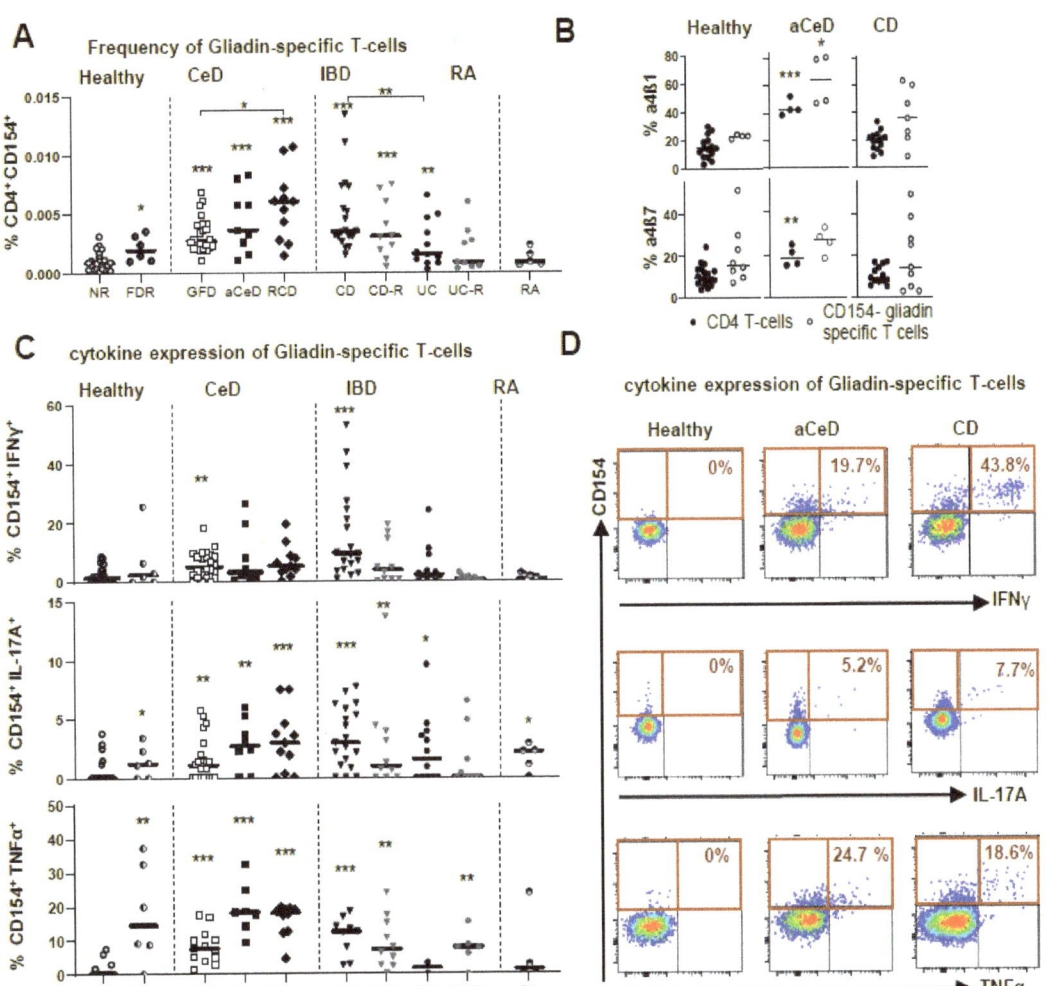

Figure 2. Phenotyping gliadin-specific T-cells. (**A–D**) Peripheral blood mononuclear cells (PBMC) were stimulated with various food antigens, magnetically enriched for CD154 and analyzed by flow cytometry. (**A**) Frequencies of CD154$^+$ cells among CD4$^+$ T-cells in PBMC from healthy controls (non-relatives, NR), patients with active Crohn's disease (CD) or ulcerative colitis (UC), or each of these entities in remission (-R), celiac disease patients (CeD) ± gluten-free diet (GFD, aCeD) or refractory (RCD) patients, first degree relatives of CeD patients (FDR) and rheumatoid arthritis patients (RA) are shown. (**B**) Frequencies of CD4$^+$ T cells and CD4$^+$ CD154$^+$ T cells, positive for integrins α4β1 and α4β7 are shown. (**C**) Frequencies of gliadin-specific IFNγ+, IL-17A+ and TNFα+ cells within CD154$^+$ T-cells in between the patient groups are shown. (**D**) Exemplary dot plots of IFNγ+, IL-17A+ and TNFα+ CD4$^+$CD154$^+$ gliadin-specific T-cells are shown. Data are shown as median. Significance was determined using Mann–Whitney-U-Test. * $p > 0.05$, ** $p > 0.01$, *** $p > 0.001$. Statistically significant differences were calculated in comparison with healthy non-relatives, if not indicated otherwise.

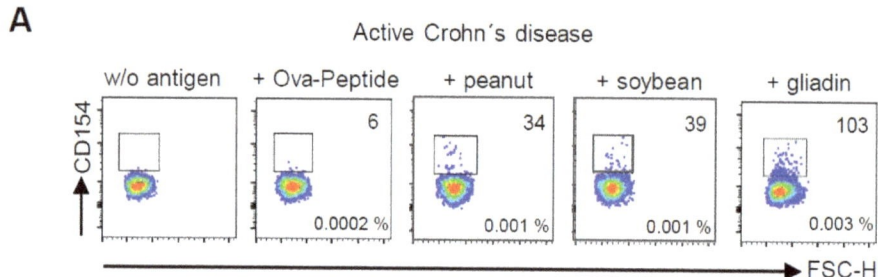

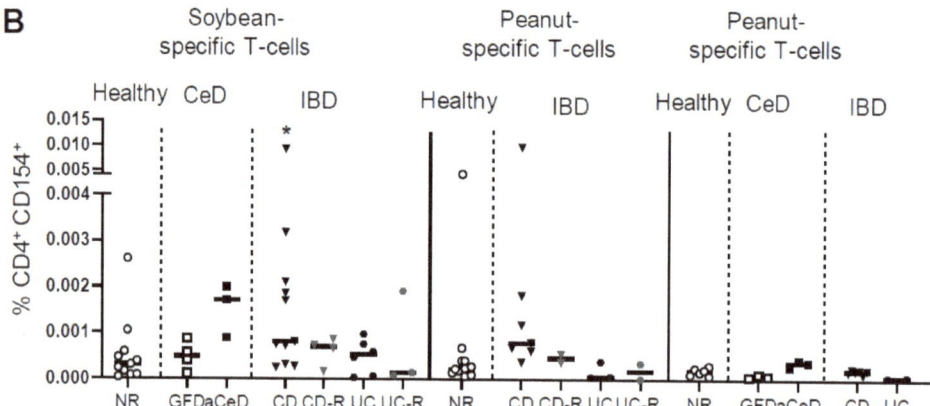

Figure 3. Frequencies of food antigen-specific T-cells. (**A,B**) Peripheral blood mononuclear cells (PBMC) were stimulated with various food antigens, magnetically enriched for CD154 and analyzed by flow cytometry. (**A**) Exemplary dot plots of CD154⁺ T-cell enrichment of indicated nutritional antigens with absolute numbers and frequencies are shown. (**B**) Frequencies of CD154⁺ cells among CD4⁺ T-cells after stimulation with soybean, peanut and OVA-peptide from healthy controls (non-relatives, NR), patients with active Crohn's disease (CD) or ulcerative colitis (UC), or each of these entities in remission (-R), celiac disease patients (CeD) ± gluten-free diet (GFD, aCeD) or refractory (RCD) patients are shown. Data are shown as median. Significance was determined using Mann–Whitney-U-Test. * $p > 0.05$,. Statistically significant differences were calculated in comparison with healthy non-relatives, if not indicated otherwise.

3. Discussion

So far, the published data for ARTE have focused on bacteria- or fungi-specific antigens as well as house dust mites [15–20]. However, this method also allows the study of even rarer food antigen-specific T-cells without in-vitro expansion of the reacting cells and without re-challenging the patients. Therefore, we applied this method to detect rare food antigen-specific T-cells in peripheral blood, in order to analyze antigen reactivity for different clinical subgroups of CeD and IBD patients.

Recently, peripheral gluten-specific CD4⁺ T-cells were analyzed applying HLA-DQ2: gluten tetramers, thus identifying an increase in gluten-specific CD4⁺ T-cells in aCeD [21–25]. However, ARTE, as it was applied in this study, allows for a deeper analysis of the respective specific CD4⁺ T-cells to distinguish different disease states of CeD. To establish diagnosis of CeD in patients who already follow a GFD is challenging, since tTG antibodies under GFD normalize and small intestinal villous atrophy regenerates. This clinical need is growing, given the increasingly popular gluten-free lifestyle in the western world [26,27], or for first degree relatives, who frequently initiate a GFD when a household member is diagnosed with

CeD. For the latter, the high risk of developing CeD has been proven in many studies [28,29] and surveillance for CeD is even recommended for first-degree relatives of a diagnosed patient where carriage of a risk gene has not been excluded [30,31]. Work herein might be the first step towards identifying such cases, without a conventional burdening gluten re-challenge, since characteristic changes in cytokine expression in gliadin-specific CD4$^+$ T-cells in the peripheral blood are present. For the rare subgroup of RCD patients, especially for type I, the specific immunological nature remains unclear. Diagnosis is still based on histopathology alone, while recent studies suggest a heterogeneous composition of different pathologies to be merged under this term. In this respect, the ARTE technique for gliadin-specific T-cells represents a unique research tool for future studies that has the potential to contribute to a subclassification of this disease group. Furthermore, our data reveal a specific immunological phenotype of gliadin-specific CD4$^+$ T-cells in FDR to CeD regarding a hypersensitivity towards gluten, even if diagnosed as healthy, based on their tTG status. It is well-known that FDR harbor a higher genetic risk for developing CeD. As such, it has been shown that FDR reveal an increased intestinal permeability compared with healthy controls CeD [29,32,33]. Composing our data and previously published data on permeability and disease risk to a single picture, one has to emphasize further the necessity to screen FDRs for CeD development, as is already pointed out in various clinical guidelines. By demonstrating an active immune response against the pathogenic antigen, identification and even phenotyping of gluten-reactive T-cells from peripheral blood might represent an interesting alternative diagnostic modality, all the more in pediatric cases, where prevalence is higher, invasive endoscopy is meant to be avoided. Overdiagnosis should not occur to a relevant extent, if diagnostic methodology for CeD is applied and interpreted adequately. Thus, this novel approach could fulfill the clinical need for a noninvasive marker of CeD activity as a clinical and research tool [34].

With regard to IBD, which shares the characteristics of barrier disruption [7] and subsequent intestinal inflammation in the lamina propria, we detected increased levels of gliadin-specific T-cells in the peripheral blood of active CD patients with concurrent small intestinal inflammation, paralleled by the highest frequency of antigen-specific T-cells expressing pro-inflammatory cytokines. This distinct occurrence suggests small intestinal barrier disruption as a major cause for the observed T-cell activation, since these cells express small intestinal homing markers. The homing to the ileum ($\alpha 4 \beta 1$) is described as an essential pathway in CD [35]. Therefore, only in these three patient groups of active small intestinal inflammation, did effector-memory T-cells outnumber the naïve phenotype among gliadin-specific T-cells in the peripheral blood. Furthermore, peripheral T-cells from CD patients with small intestinal inflammation proved to be responsive to other major food antigens [36], while neither active UC, nor CD or UC in remission, showed any reaction. Again, only antigen-specific T-cells from active CeD, but not GFD patients demonstrated similar properties, corroborating on the one hand the leaky barrier of the affected small intestine as the site of food antigen translocation and subsequent T-cell activation. On the other hand, the significant effect of gliadin, but no other food antigen, in the GFD group further confirmed the singular antigen-driven nature of CeD. Nevertheless, based on surveys, it has been suggested that long-term GFD improves gastrointestinal symptoms in active IBD patients [10]. With the present study, we are able to convey cellular and functional data by demonstrating an enhanced gliadin-specific response of pro-inflammatory cytokines towards gliadin for CD patients, which is not found in UC patients. This occurs somewhat in parallel with the detection of anti-*Saccharomyces cerevisiae* antibodies (ASCAs) in CD, but not in UC [37,38], which might reflect the increased small intestinal permeability for peptide antigens found in CD but not in UC. Interestingly and in line with our study, ASCAs were also found in patients suffering from CeD, again suggesting that small intestinal antigen processing might be pivotal [39,40].

This study has a number of limitations that include the small sample size, the monocentric design, the lack of a group of very young patients/children and maybe also the lack of a group of patients suffering from colonic Crohn's disease. Nevertheless, recent genomic data indicate that Crohn's disease of the small intestine is distinct from Crohn's colitis and that small intestinal CD is specifically different from UC [41,42]. Since we aimed to emphasize these very different pathologies, we decided to focus on small intestinal Crohn's and UC. However, a more complete view on this immune pathology including Crohn's colitis might have added the option to recognize, if the differential extent of gliadin-specific T-cells reflects mostly the distribution type of the IBD, or if it is distribution-independent and disease-specific, maybe secondary to the transmural nature of CD.

In summary, our data suggest that small intestinal inflammation is key for the development of a nutritional antigen-specific T-cell response. Therefore, ARTE allows the distinction of CD with small intestinal inflammation from UC and CD in remission by a unique profile of circulating antigen-specific T-cells, and raises the question of whether a well-defined nutritional regimen (e.g., GFD) might have therapeutic potential in the setting of IBD. Hence, based on the analysis of the systemic immune response, an "anti-inflammatory" diet could be developed and monitored. In addition, this technique allows detailed analyses of gliadin-specific T-cells at such a high resolution that even healthy first-degree relatives can be discriminated and might thus provide a novel non-invasive diagnostic tool to identify symptom-free CeD patients on a gluten-free diet.

4. Methods

PBMC from CeD, CD, UC and rheumatoid arthritis patients as well as healthy controls (Tables 1 and 2) were cultured for 6 h in the presence of defined antigens followed by magnetic enrichment of activated $CD154^+$ T-cells (as marker for antigen-specific T-cells) [12] (Figure 1A,B).

Table 1. Patient characteristics: Celiac disease and controls.

		Non-Relative Controls ($n = 24$)	First-Degree Relatives ($n = 6$)	Celiac Disease on GFD ($n = 24$)	Active Celiac Disease ($n = 9$)	Refractory Celiac Disease ($n = 11$)
Age (mean ± SD)		33.3 ± 9.4	34.5 ± 9.5	43.9 ± 16.8	47.3 ± 12.4	61.1 ± 11.6
Female [%]		55	83	80	66	82
tTG (mean ± SD) [U/mL] # [CE]		1.6 ± 0.7 -	1.4 ± 0.4 -	6.3 ± 4.8 -	114.2 ± 70.9 3428.1 ± 1313.7	21.0 ± 27.2 -
Marsh grade at first diagnosis	IIIa IIIc IIIb	-	-	10 9 4	3 3 2	6 2 2
RCD type I /II [%]		-	-	-	-	63.6/36.4

GFD, gluten-free diet; tTG, tissue-transglutaminase. # standard range tTG-IgA [U/mL] < 10 U/mL; [CE] < 20 CE.

Table 2. Patient characteristics: Inflammatory bowel disease and controls.

	Non-Relative Controls ($n = 24$)	Rheumatoid Arthritis ($n = 5$)	Crohn's Disease ($n = 19 + 13$)	Crohn's Disease (Remission) ($n = 10 + 4$)	Ulcerative Colitis ($n = 12 + 7$)	Ulcerative Colitis (Remission) ($n = 9 + 2$)
Age (mean ± SD)	33.3 ± 9.4	49.4 ± 10.8	36.2 ± 9.3	41.4 ± 13.9	41.0 ± 14.9	42.0 ± 15.1
Female [%]	55	67	50	57	37	64
Clinical score:						
HBI	-	-	5.1 ± 2.7	0.5 ± 1.2	-	-
partial Mayo	-	-	-	-	3.9 ± 1.9	1.0 ± 1.0
Montreal classification:						
- A1 < 17 years			0	0	0	0
- A2 17–40 years			23	7	7	6
- A3 > 40 years			9	7	12	5
Crohn's disease						
- L1 ileal			11	4		
- L3 ileocolonic			12	8		
- L4 upper GI			6	2		
Ulcerative colitis						
- E1 proctitis					0	0
- E2 distal UC					8	8
- E3 extensiveUC					10	3

HBI, Harvey–Bradshaw index. n = patients with gliadin stimulation + patients with other food antigen stimulation.

4.1. Patients

PBMC of CD patients with small intestinal manifestation and UC patients with either active disease or remission were analyzed. Activity of disease was analyzed clinically as defined by well-established activity scores including Harvey–Bradshaw Index (HBI) and partial Mayo score (pMayo) [43,44]. Additionally, CeD patients on a GFD for at least one year, newly diagnosed active CeD patients still exposed to gluten (aCeD), or GFD-refractory CeD patients (RCD) were included. Moreover, healthy first-degree relatives to CeD patients (FDR) on a regular diet without symptoms were included. The diagnosis of CeD was based on the presence of tTG antibodies in the serum and characteristic histopathological features in duodenal biopsies (Marsh score > 1). RCD diagnosis was based on the presence of a Marsh III enteropathy and clinical malabsorption in spite of consumption of a gluten-free diet for at least one year. Clonality analysis was performed by PCR of the CDR3 region of the TCR. Detection of a clonal T-cell population and aberrant lymphocytes by immune phenotyping of duodenal tissue allowed for diagnosis of RCD type II. All other refractory cases were diagnosed as RCD type I [45]. HLA-DQ status could not be determined for IBD patients and controls. Additionally, non-intestinal inflammatory control group PBMC from rheumatoid arthritis (RA) patients were analyzed.

4.2. Blood Donors and PBMC Isolation

Peripheral blood samples were obtained from healthy donors and patients of the Charité-Universitätsmedizin Berlin, Medical Department, Division of Gastroenterology, Infectious Diseases and Rheumatology. All blood donors gave informed consent and the study was approved by the ethical committee of the Charité-Universitätsmedizin Berlin. PBMC were freshly isolated from 20 mL blood by density gradient centrifugation (Biocoll; Biochrom, Berlin, Germany). Heparinized whole blood was layered on the Biocoll Separation Solution and centrifuged at $1200 \times g$ for 25 min at 21 °C. PBMC were collected from the interphase, washed and resuspended in RPMI1640 (Gibco, Life Technologies, Darmstadt, Germany) supplemented with 5% human AB-serum (Sigma-Aldrich, St. Louis, MO, USA).

4.3. Antigen-Reactive T-Cell Enrichment

Identification and enrichment of antigen-reactive T-cells was performed by applying the recently described ARTE technique [12]. Briefly, 0.5–1×10^7 PBMC were cultured in RPMI1640 supplemented with 5% human AB-serum and stimulated for 6 h with 1 µg/mL CD40 (Miltenyi Biotec, Bergisch Gladbach, Germany) in the presence or absence of the pepsin-trypsin digested 33-mer gliadin peptide (200 µg/mL) (Sigma-Aldrich), OVA-peptide (Invitrogen), or soybean or peanut extract (200 µg/mL) (Greer Laboratories, Lenoir, North Carolina, United States). For the last 2 h, 1 µg/mL brefeldin A (Sigma-Aldrich) was added. Cells were indirectly labeled with anti-CD154-biotin antibody, followed by anti-biotin MicroBeads (CD154 MicroBead-Kit, Miltenyi Biotec), and magnetically enriched using MS columns (Miltenyi Biotec).

4.4. Flow Cytometric Cell Analysis

Surface staining was performed on the MS column (first panel: Brilliant violet 510™ anti-human CD4; RPA-T4, Brilliant Violet 421™ anti-human CD197 (CCR7); G043H7, PE/Cy7 anti-human CD45RA; HI100; second panel: Brilliant violet 510™ anti-human CD4; PE/Cy7 anti-human CD29/ß1; TS2/16, PE anti-human ß7; FIB504, all from BioLegend (Koblenz, Germany); VioBlue anti-human CD49d/α4, MZ18-24A9, from Miltenyi Biotec (Bergisch Gladbach, Germany); and human FC block, from CSL Behring (Marburg, Germany)). The enriched cell fraction was fixed using eBioscience™, FoxP3 staining buffer (Thermo Fisher Scientific, Waltham, MA, U.S.A.). Intracellular staining was performed: APC anti-human IFNγ; 4S.B3, APC/Cy7 anti-human IL-17A; BL168, PerCP/Cy5.5 anti-human TNFα; MAb11, all from BioLegend; and FITC anti-human CD154 (5C8) from Miltenyi Biotec. Flow cytometry analysis was performed on an FACS Canto II device (BD Bioscience, Heidelberg, Germany). Data were analyzed with FlowJo analysis software (Ashland, OR, U.S.A.) (Supplementary Figure S1).

4.5. Statistics

Statistical analysis was performed using Prism software (GraphPad Software). Significance was determined using Mann–Whitney U-Test as indicated. * $p > 0.05$, ** $p > 0.01$, *** $p > 0.001$.

Supplementary Materials: The following supporting information can be downloaded at: https://www.mdpi.com/article/10.3390/ijms24098153/s1.

Author Contributions: Conceptualization, Y.R.-S., M.S., U.S., B.S. and R.G.; methodology, Y.R.-S., M.S., B.S. and R.G.; formal analysis, Y.R.-S.; investigation, Y.R.-S.; resources, D.L., F.B. and F.P.; writing—original draft preparation, Y.R.-S. and R.G.; writing—review and editing, Y.R.-S., M.S., U.S., B.S. and R.G.; visualization, Y.R.-S. and R.G.; supervision, B.S. and R.G.; All authors have read and agreed to the published version of the manuscript.

Funding: This work was funded by the Deutsche Forschungsgemeinschaft SPP1656 (BS and US), GL 899/1-1 (RG) and TRR241 (BS and MS) as well as the Deutsche Zöliakie-Gesellschaft e.V. (BS, RG and YRS). The APC was funded by the Charité Medizinische Bibliothek.

Institutional Review Board Statement: The study was conducted in accordance with the Declaration of Helsinki and approved by the Ethics Committee of the Charité-Universitätsmedizin Berlin (EA4/014/18, 12 February 2018).

Informed Consent Statement: Informed consent was obtained from all subjects involved in the study.

Data Availability Statement: Primary data will be made available upon request.

Acknowledgments: We thank Inka Freise for her technical assistance and Lea-Maxie Haag for critical reading the manuscript. We thank all of our colleagues from the Gastroenterology and Rheumatology department for providing patient samples.

Conflicts of Interest: The authors declare that the research was conducted in the absence of any commercial or financial relationships that could be construed as a potential conflict of interest.

References

1. Kwok, W.W.; Tan, V.; Gillette, L.; Littell, C.T.; Soltis, M.A.; LaFond, R.B.; Yang, J.; James, E.A.; DeLong, J.H. Frequency of epitope-specific naive CD4(+) T cells correlates with immunodominance in the human memory repertoire. *J. Immunol.* **2012**, *188*, 2537–2544. [CrossRef] [PubMed]
2. Chu, H.H.; Moon, J.J.; Takada, K.; Pepper, M.; Molitor, J.A.; Schacker, T.W.; Hogquist, K.A.; Jameson, S.C.; Jenkins, M.K. Positive selection optimizes the number and function of MHCII-restricted CD4+ T cell clones in the naive polyclonal repertoire. *Proc. Natl. Acad. Sci. USA* **2009**, *106*, 11241–11245. [CrossRef] [PubMed]
3. Schuppan, D.; Junker, Y.; Barisani, D. Celiac disease: From pathogenesis to novel therapies. *Gastroenterology* **2009**, *137*, 1912–1933. [CrossRef] [PubMed]
4. Schuppan, D.; Zimmer, K.P. The diagnosis and treatment of celiac disease. *Dtsch. Arztebl. Int.* **2013**, *110*, 835–846. [CrossRef] [PubMed]
5. Schuppan, D. Current concepts of celiac disease pathogenesis. *Gastroenterology* **2000**, *119*, 234–242. [CrossRef]
6. Odenwald, M.A.; Turner, J.R. Intestinal permeability defects: Is it time to treat? *Clin. Gastroenterol. Hepatol.* **2013**, *11*, 1075–1083. [CrossRef] [PubMed]
7. Martini, E.; Krug, S.M.; Siegmund, B.; Neurath, M.F.; Becker, C. Mend Your Fences: The Epithelial Barrier and its Relationship With Mucosal Immunity in Inflammatory Bowel Disease. *Cell. Mol. Gastroenterol. Hepatol.* **2017**, *4*, 33–46. [CrossRef]
8. Strober, W.; Fuss, I.; Mannon, P. The fundamental basis of inflammatory bowel disease. *J. Clin. Investig.* **2007**, *117*, 514–521. [CrossRef]
9. Neurath, M.F. Targeting immune cell circuits and trafficking in inflammatory bowel disease. *Nat. Immunol.* **2019**, *20*, 970–979. [CrossRef]
10. Herfarth, H.H.; Martin, C.F.; Sandler, R.S.; Kappelman, M.D.; Long, M.D. Prevalence of a gluten-free diet and improvement of clinical symptoms in patients with inflammatory bowel diseases. *Inflamm. Bowel Dis.* **2014**, *20*, 1194–1197. [CrossRef]
11. Bonder, M.J.; Tigchelaar, E.F.; Cai, X.; Trynka, G.; Cenit, M.C.; Hrdlickova, B.; Zhong, H.; Vatanen, T.; Gevers, D.; Wijmenga, C.; et al. The influence of a short-term gluten-free diet on the human gut microbiome. *Genome Med.* **2016**, *8*, 45. [CrossRef] [PubMed]
12. Bacher, P.; Scheffold, A. Flow-cytometric analysis of rare antigen-specific T cells. *Cytometry A* **2013**, *83*, 692–701. [CrossRef] [PubMed]

13. Frentsch, M.; Arbach, O.; Kirchhoff, D.; Moewes, B.; Worm, M.; Rothe, M.; Scheffold, A.; Thiel, A. Direct access to CD4+ T cells specific for defined antigens according to CD154 expression. *Nat. Med.* **2005**, *11*, 1118–1124. [CrossRef] [PubMed]
14. Bacher, P.; Schink, C.; Teutschbein, J.; Kniemeyer, O.; Assenmacher, M.; Brakhage, A.A.; Scheffold, A. Antigen-reactive T cell enrichment for direct, high-resolution analysis of the human naive and memory Th cell repertoire. *J. Immunol.* **2013**, *190*, 3967–3976. [CrossRef]
15. Bacher, P.; Kniemeyer, O.; Schonbrunn, A.; Sawitzki, B.; Assenmacher, M.; Rietschel, E.; Steinbach, A.; Cornely, O.A.; Brakhage, A.A.; Thiel, A.; et al. Antigen-specific expansion of human regulatory T cells as a major tolerance mechanism against mucosal fungi. *Mucosal Immunol.* **2014**, *7*, 916–928. [CrossRef]
16. Bacher, P.; Hohnstein, T.; Beerbaum, E.; Rocker, M.; Blango, M.G.; Kaufmann, S.; Rohmel, J.; Eschenhagen, P.; Grehn, C.; Seidel, K.; et al. Human Anti-fungal Th17 Immunity and Pathology Rely on Cross-Reactivity against Candida albicans. *Cell* **2019**, *176*, 1340–1355.e15. [CrossRef]
17. Bacher, P.; Scheffold, A. Antigen-specific regulatory T-cell responses against aeroantigens and their role in allergy. *Mucosal Immunol.* **2018**, *11*, 1537–1550. [CrossRef]
18. Scheffold, A.; Schwarz, C.; Bacher, P. Fungus-Specific CD4 T Cells as Specific Sensors for Identification of Pulmonary Fungal Infections. *Mycopathologia* **2018**, *183*, 213–226. [CrossRef]
19. Bacher, P.; Steinbach, A.; Kniemeyer, O.; Hamprecht, A.; Assenmacher, M.; Vehreschild, M.J.; Vehreschild, J.J.; Brakhage, A.A.; Cornely, O.A.; Scheffold, A. Fungus-specific CD4(+) T cells for rapid identification of invasive pulmonary mold infection. *Am. J. Respir. Crit. Care Med.* **2015**, *191*, 348–352. [CrossRef]
20. Bacher, P.; Heinrich, F.; Stervbo, U.; Nienen, M.; Vahldieck, M.; Iwert, C.; Vogt, K.; Kollet, J.; Babel, N.; Sawitzki, B.; et al. Regulatory T Cell Specificity Directs Tolerance versus Allergy against Aeroantigens in Humans. *Cell* **2016**, *167*, 1067–1078.e16. [CrossRef]
21. Sarna, V.K.; Lundin, K.E.A.; Morkrid, L.; Qiao, S.W.; Sollid, L.M.; Christophersen, A. HLA-DQ-Gluten Tetramer Blood Test Accurately Identifies Patients With and Without Celiac Disease in Absence of Gluten Consumption. *Gastroenterology* **2018**, *154*, 886–896.e6. [CrossRef] [PubMed]
22. Ben-Horin, S.; Green, P.H.; Bank, I.; Chess, L.; Goldstein, I. Characterizing the circulating, gliadin-specific CD4+ memory T cells in patients with celiac disease: Linkage between memory function, gut homing and Th1 polarization. *J. Leukoc. Biol.* **2006**, *79*, 676–685. [CrossRef] [PubMed]
23. Christophersen, A.; Dahal-Koirala, S.; Chlubnova, M.; Jahnsen, J.; Lundin, K.E.A.; Sollid, L.M. Phenotype-Based Isolation of Antigen-Specific CD4(+) T Cells in Autoimmunity: A Study of Celiac Disease. *Adv. Sci. Weinh* **2022**, *9*, e2104766. [CrossRef] [PubMed]
24. Christophersen, A.; Zuhlke, S.; Lund, E.G.; Snir, O.; Dahal-Koirala, S.; Risnes, L.F.; Jahnsen, J.; Lundin, K.E.A.; Sollid, L.M. Pathogenic T Cells in Celiac Disease Change Phenotype on Gluten Challenge: Implications for T-Cell-Directed Therapies. *Adv. Sci. Weinh* **2021**, *8*, e2102778. [CrossRef] [PubMed]
25. Anderson, R.P.; Goel, G.; Hardy, M.Y.; Russell, A.K.; Wang, S.; Szymczak, E.; Zhang, R.; Goldstein, K.E.; Neff, K.; Truitt, K.E.; et al. Whole blood interleukin-2 release test to detect and characterize rare circulating gluten-specific T cell responses in coeliac disease. *Clin. Exp. Immunol.* **2021**, *204*, 321–334. [CrossRef]
26. Kim, H.S.; Patel, K.G.; Orosz, E.; Kothari, N.; Demyen, M.F.; Pyrsopoulos, N.; Ahlawat, S.K. Time Trends in the Prevalence of Celiac Disease and Gluten-Free Diet in the US Population: Results From the National Health and Nutrition Examination Surveys 2009–2014. *JAMA Intern. Med.* **2016**, *176*, 1716–1717. [CrossRef]
27. Hager, A.S.; Taylor, J.P.; Waters, D.M.; Arendt, E.K. Gluten free beer—A review. *Trends Food Sci. Technol.* **2014**, *36*, 44–54. [CrossRef]
28. Acharya, P.; Kutum, R.; Pandey, R.; Mishra, A.; Saha, R.; Munjal, A.; Ahuja, V.; Mukerji, M.; Makharia, G.K. First Degree Relatives of Patients with Celiac Disease Harbour an Intestinal Transcriptomic Signature that Might Protect them from Enterocyte Damage. *Clin. Transl. Gastroenterol.* **2018**, *9*, 195. [CrossRef]
29. Singh, P.; Arora, S.; Lal, S.; Strand, T.A.; Makharia, G.K. Risk of Celiac Disease in the First- and Second-Degree Relatives of Patients With Celiac Disease: A Systematic Review and Meta-Analysis. *Am. J. Gastroenterol.* **2015**, *110*, 1539–1548. [CrossRef]
30. Hill, I.D.; Dirks, M.H.; Liptak, G.S.; Colletti, R.B.; Fasano, A.; Guandalini, S.; Hoffenberg, E.J.; Horvath, K.; Murray, J.A.; Pivor, M.; et al. Guideline for the diagnosis and treatment of celiac disease in children: Recommendations of the North American Society for Pediatric Gastroenterology, Hepatology and Nutrition. *J. Pediatr. Gastroenterol. Nutr.* **2005**, *40*, 1–19. [CrossRef]
31. Husby, S.; Koletzko, S.; Korponay-Szabo, I.R.; Mearin, M.L.; Phillips, A.; Shamir, R.; Troncone, R.; Giersiepen, K.; Branski, D.; Catassi, C.; et al. European Society for Pediatric Gastroenterology, Hepatology, and Nutrition guidelines for the diagnosis of coeliac disease. *J. Pediatr. Gastroenterol. Nutr.* **2012**, *54*, 136–160. [CrossRef]
32. Vogelsang, H.; Wyatt, J.; Penner, E.; Lochs, H. Screening for celiac disease in first-degree relatives of patients with celiac disease by lactulose/mannitol test. *Am. J. Gastroenterol.* **1995**, *90*, 1838–1842. [PubMed]
33. van Elburg, R.M.; Uil, J.J.; Mulder, C.J.; Heymans, H.S. Intestinal permeability in patients with coeliac disease and relatives of patients with coeliac disease. *Gut* **1993**, *34*, 354–357. [CrossRef] [PubMed]
34. Leffler, D.A.; Schuppan, D. Update on serologic testing in celiac disease. *Am. J. Gastroenterol.* **2010**, *105*, 2520–2524. [CrossRef] [PubMed]

35. Zundler, S.; Fischer, A.; Schillinger, D.; Binder, M.T.; Atreya, R.; Rath, T.; Lopez-Posadas, R.; Voskens, C.J.; Watson, A.; Atreya, I.; et al. The alpha4beta1 Homing Pathway Is Essential for Ileal Homing of Crohn's Disease Effector T Cells In Vivo. *Inflamm. Bowel Dis.* **2017**, *23*, 379–391. [CrossRef]
36. Tordesillas, L.; Berin, M.C.; Sampson, H.A. Immunology of Food Allergy. *Immunity* **2017**, *47*, 32–50. [CrossRef]
37. Main, J.; McKenzie, H.; Yeaman, G.R.; Kerr, M.A.; Robson, D.; Pennington, C.R.; Parratt, D. Antibody to Saccharomyces cerevisiae (bakers' yeast) in Crohn's disease. *BMJ* **1988**, *297*, 1105–1106. [CrossRef]
38. Giaffer, M.H.; Clark, A.; Holdsworth, C.D. Antibodies to Saccharomyces cerevisiae in patients with Crohn's disease and their possible pathogenic importance. *Gut* **1992**, *33*, 1071–1075. [CrossRef]
39. Granito, A.; Zauli, D.; Muratori, P.; Muratori, L.; Grassi, A.; Bortolotti, R.; Petrolini, N.; Veronesi, L.; Gionchetti, P.; Bianchi, F.B.; et al. Anti-Saccharomyces cerevisiae and perinuclear anti-neutrophil cytoplasmic antibodies in coeliac disease before and after gluten-free diet. *Aliment. Pharmacol. Ther.* **2005**, *21*, 881–887. [CrossRef]
40. Granito, A.; Muratori, L.; Muratori, P.; Guidi, M.; Lenzi, M.; Bianchi, F.B.; Volta, U. Anti-saccharomyces cerevisiae antibodies (ASCA) in coeliac disease. *Gut* **2006**, *55*, 296.
41. Kredel, L.I.; Jodicke, L.J.; Scheffold, A.; Grone, J.; Glauben, R.; Erben, U.; Kuhl, A.A.; Siegmund, B. T-cell Composition in Ileal and Colonic Creeping Fat-Separating Ileal from Colonic Crohn's Disease. *J. Crohns Colitis* **2019**, *13*, 79–91. [CrossRef] [PubMed]
42. Cleynen, I.; Boucher, G.; Jostins, L.; Schumm, L.P.; Zeissig, S.; Ahmad, T.; Andersen, V.; Andrews, J.M.; Annese, V.; Brand, S.; et al. Inherited determinants of Crohn's disease and ulcerative colitis phenotypes: A genetic association study. *Lancet* **2016**, *387*, 156–167. [CrossRef] [PubMed]
43. Lewis, J.D.; Chuai, S.; Nessel, L.; Lichtenstein, G.R.; Aberra, F.N.; Ellenberg, J.H. Use of the noninvasive components of the Mayo score to assess clinical response in ulcerative colitis. *Inflamm. Bowel Dis.* **2008**, *14*, 1660–1666. [CrossRef]
44. Harvey, R.F.; Bradshaw, J.M. A simple index of Crohn's-disease activity. *Lancet* **1980**, *1*, 514. [CrossRef]
45. Felber, J.; Aust, D.; Baas, S.; Bischoff, S.; Blaker, H.; Daum, S.; Keller, R.; Koletzko, S.; Laass, M.; Nothacker, M.; et al. Results of a S2k-Consensus Conference of the German Society of Gastroenterolgy, Digestive- and Metabolic Diseases (DGVS) in conjunction with the German Coeliac Society (DZG) regarding coeliac disease, wheat allergy and wheat sensitivity. *Z. Gastroenterol.* **2014**, *52*, 711–743. [CrossRef] [PubMed]

Disclaimer/Publisher's Note: The statements, opinions and data contained in all publications are solely those of the individual author(s) and contributor(s) and not of MDPI and/or the editor(s). MDPI and/or the editor(s) disclaim responsibility for any injury to people or property resulting from any ideas, methods, instructions or products referred to in the content.

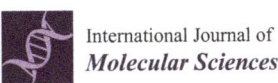

Article

Development of an Inflammation-Triggered In Vitro "Leaky Gut" Model Using Caco-2/HT29-MTX-E12 Combined with Macrophage-like THP-1 Cells or Primary Human-Derived Macrophages

Nguyen Phan Khoi Le [1], Markus Jörg Altenburger [2] and Evelyn Lamy [1,*]

1. Molecular Preventive Medicine, University Medical Center and Faculty of Medicine, University of Freiburg, 79108 Freiburg, Germany; phan.khoi.nguyen.le@uniklinik-freiburg.de
2. Department of Operative Dentistry and Periodontology, University Medical Center and Faculty of Medicine, University of Freiburg, 79108 Freiburg, Germany; markus.altenburger@uniklinik-freiburg.de
* Correspondence: evelyn.lamy@uniklinik-freiburg.de; Tel.: +49-761-270-82150

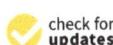

Abstract: The "leaky gut" syndrome describes a damaged (leaky) intestinal mucosa and is considered a serious contributor to numerous chronic diseases. Chronic inflammatory bowel diseases (IBD) are particularly associated with the "leaky gut" syndrome, but also allergies, autoimmune diseases or neurological disorders. We developed a complex in vitro inflammation-triggered triple-culture model using 21-day-differentiated human intestinal Caco-2 epithelial cells and HT29-MTX-E12 mucus-producing goblet cells (90:10 ratio) in close contact with differentiated human macrophage-like THP-1 cells or primary monocyte-derived macrophages from human peripheral blood. Upon an inflammatory stimulus, the characteristics of a "leaky gut" became evident: a significant loss of intestinal cell integrity in terms of decreased transepithelial/transendothelial electrical resistance (TEER), as well as a loss of tight junction proteins. The cell permeability for FITC-dextran 4 kDa was then increased, and key pro-inflammatory cytokines, including TNF-alpha and IL-6, were substantially released. Whereas in the M1 macrophage-like THP-1 co-culture model, we could not detect the release of IL-23, which plays a crucial regulatory role in IBD, this cytokine was clearly detected when using primary human M1 macrophages instead. In conclusion, we provide an advanced human in vitro model that could be useful for screening and evaluating therapeutic drugs for IBD treatment, including potential IL-23 inhibitors.

Keywords: leaky gut; inflammatory bowel disease (IBD); triple-culture; Caco-2; HT29-MTX-E12; THP-1; monocyte-derived macrophage; inflammation; TEER; FITC-dextran 4 kDa (FD4); pro-inflammatory cytokines

Citation: Le, N.P.K.; Altenburger, M.J.; Lamy, E. Development of an Inflammation-Triggered In Vitro "Leaky Gut" Model Using Caco-2/HT29-MTX-E12 Combined with Macrophage-like THP-1 Cells or Primary Human-Derived Macrophages. *Int. J. Mol. Sci.* **2023**, *24*, 7427. https://doi.org/10.3390/ijms24087427

Academic Editor: Susanne M. Krug

Received: 24 March 2023
Revised: 12 April 2023
Accepted: 15 April 2023
Published: 18 April 2023

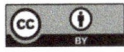

Copyright: © 2023 by the authors. Licensee MDPI, Basel, Switzerland. This article is an open access article distributed under the terms and conditions of the Creative Commons Attribution (CC BY) license (https://creativecommons.org/licenses/by/4.0/).

1. Introduction

The "leaky gut", also known as increased intestinal permeability, describes a damaged (leaky) intestinal barrier caused by the loose tight junctions of intestinal epithelial cell walls. This phenomenon results in the passage of harmful substances such as pathogens and toxic digestive metabolites from the gut into the bloodstream, and then consequently causes systemic inflammation and immune system activation. An increased intestinal permeability has been considered to play an important role in the development and progression of numerous chronic diseases [1–3]. Autoimmune diseases [4,5], food sensitivities and allergies [6,7], asthma [8], neurological conditions [9–11], autism spectrum disorder [12,13], and gut-related disorders like chronic inflammatory bowel disease (IBD) [14–16] have been reported in association with a "leaky gut". IBD is an umbrella term that is used mainly to describe two chronic inflammatory conditions of the gastrointestinal (GI) tract: ulcerative colitis (UC) and Crohn's disease (CD). In 2017, about seven million people were suffering from IBD worldwide [17], with the prevalence surpassing 0.3% of the general population in North America, Oceania, and many European countries. Moreover, IBD has become a global disease in the twenty-first century with rising incidence and prevalence in many regions, particularly in the emerging economies of South America, Eastern Europe, Asia, and Africa [18]. As there is currently no specific cause and cure for IBD, it presents a tremendous financial burden globally due to the substantial direct costs of medical care and the indirect costs related to disability and missed work [19].

To better understand underlying mechanisms and ultimately identify effective treatment options, many researchers have established various cell-based in vitro models of IBD. For decades, the Caco-2 cell line, a heterogeneous human epithelial colorectal adenocarcinoma cell line, has undoubtedly become the most widely accepted in vitro cell model to study the intestinal absorption of drugs, cell membrane permeability, and inflammatory response [20–26]. When growing as a confluent monolayer on inserts, Caco-2 cells differentiate and demonstrate morphological and functional characteristics of small intestinal absorptive cells such as tight junctions, and a brush border with well-developed microvilli on the apical surface [27]. Furthermore, Caco-2 cells also express typical enzymes of normal small-intestinal villus cells, such as disaccharidases and peptidases [28].

On the other hand, this single-cell Caco-2 model has been criticized by many authors, because it lacks mucus production. Based on the Caco-2 cell model, many modifications and improvements have followed [29]. One of the most important enhancements was combining it with the mucin-secreting HT29-MTX-E12 goblet cell line [30]. The proportion of goblet cells among epithelial cell types ranges from 10% in the small intestine to 24% in the distal colon [31]. Therefore, the Caco-2/HT29-MTX-E12 co-culture model then better resembled the human small intestine. In the in vitro system, the presence of mucus can act as an interactive barrier, limiting the free diffusion of small compounds to the cells, and thus helping to avoid overestimation of the permeability of such compounds [32]. Moreover, an increasing number of studies reported that the disruption of bidirectional communication between the intestinal mucus barrier and gut microbiota plays a critical role in the development and progression of several inflammatory conditions such as IBD [33,34].

In IBD, intestinal macrophages become activated, and contribute to chronic intestinal inflammation [35–37]. Intestinal macrophages in the subepithelial lamina propria (LP) are the most abundant mononuclear phagocytes in the body and play a critical role in maintaining intestinal homeostasis. Thus, some researchers have started to combine intestinal cell lines with human macrophage-like cells (e.g., differentiated monocytic THP-1 cells), or monocyte-derived macrophages from peripheral blood mononuclear cells (PBMCs) [38–40]. However, each of these IBD models has its disadvantages, because of either (1) the lack of mucus-producing cells [41–44], (2) a spatial distance between the intestinal cells and macrophages [45–47], or (3) being specifically adapted for buoyant particles [48].

In this study, we developed a complex in vitro triple-culture model of the human intestine, consisting of differentiated human intestinal Caco-2 cells, HT29-MTX-E12 mucus-producing goblet cells (90:10 ratio), cultured on inserts in close contact with either differentiated human macrophage-like THP-1 cells, or primary human monocyte-derived macrophages obtained from PBMCs of healthy donors. The combination of human cell line-derived intestinal cells and macrophages provides a more biological and physiological representation of the complex interactions between the intestinal epithelium and the immune system in health and IBD.

2. Results

2.1. Establishment of an Inflammation-Triggered, Triple-Culture In Vitro "Leaky Gut" Model Using Caco-2/HT29-MTX-E12 Co-Culture and Macrophage-like THP-1 Cells

A graphic description of the cell culture and the setup of the inflammation-triggered, triple-culture in vitro "leaky gut" model is demonstrated in Figure 1.

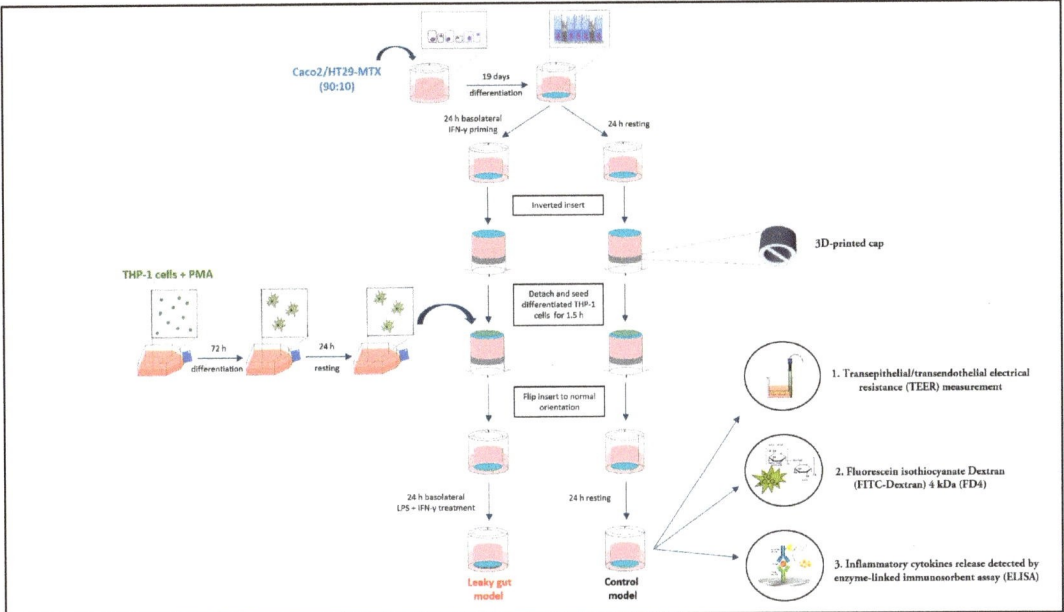

Figure 1. Schematic diagram of the inflammation-triggered, triple-culture in vitro "leaky gut" model. 19-day-differentiated Caco-2/HT29-MTX-E12 co-cultures were either rested in fresh medium (control), or primed for 24 h with IFN-γ. On the following day, a custom-designed three dimension (3D)-printed cap was carefully placed into the insert of the cultures to confine the medium, before placing the insert upside down in a Petri dish. After that, phorbol 12-myristate 13-acetate (PMA)-differentiated macrophage-like THP-1 cells, or primary monocyte-derived macrophages were transferred on the bottom side of the inverted inserts for 1.5 h, before flipping it back to the regular orientation. Then, for generating the inflammation-mediated "leaky gut" condition, macrophages were activated for 24 h by adding a combination of LPS and IFN-γ. At the same time, for the control model, macrophages were rested in medium for this time.

2.2. Custom-Designed Three Dimension (3D)-Printed Cap for Medium Confinement in the Insert

A cap was 3D designed (Figure 2A–C) to fit into the insert and sealed the setup by friction. The base of the cap was shaped conically to eliminate possible air pockets when the cap was inserted into the insert (Figure 2D,E).

2.3. Characterization of 21-Day-Differentiated Caco-2/HT29-MTX-E12 (90:10 Ratio) Co-Culture

The development of cell monolayer integrity of the Caco-2/HT29-MTX-E12 co-culture during the 21-day incubation was determined by transepithelial/transendothelial electrical resistance (TEER) measurement, which is a widely accepted quantitative technique to assess the integrity of cellular barriers in cell culture models [49]. As presented in Figure 3A, the TEER value of HT29-MTX-E12 cells increased from $18 \pm 9\ \Omega \cdot cm^2$ to $128 \pm 18\ \Omega \cdot cm^2$ between day 3 to 21 of cultivation. In contrast, the TEER values of the Caco-2 monoculture, and the Caco-2/HT29-MTX-E12 co-culture reached $660 \pm 31\ \Omega \cdot cm^2$ and $605 \pm 29\ \Omega \cdot cm^2$ on day 21, respectively. Therefore, in this study, only co-cultures of Caco-2/HT29-MTX-E12 with TEER values above $300\ \Omega \cdot cm^2$ were used in further experiments.

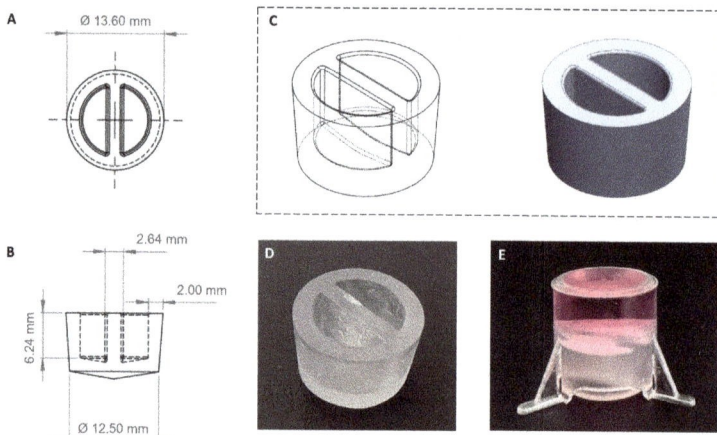

Figure 2. Custom-designed 3D-printed cap. The design sketches of the cap are: top view (**A**), front view (**B**), and 3D view (**C**). The dimensions of this cap (**D**) were determined to fit into the insert perfectly to safely confine the medium within the insert during the macrophage adherence procedure (**E**).

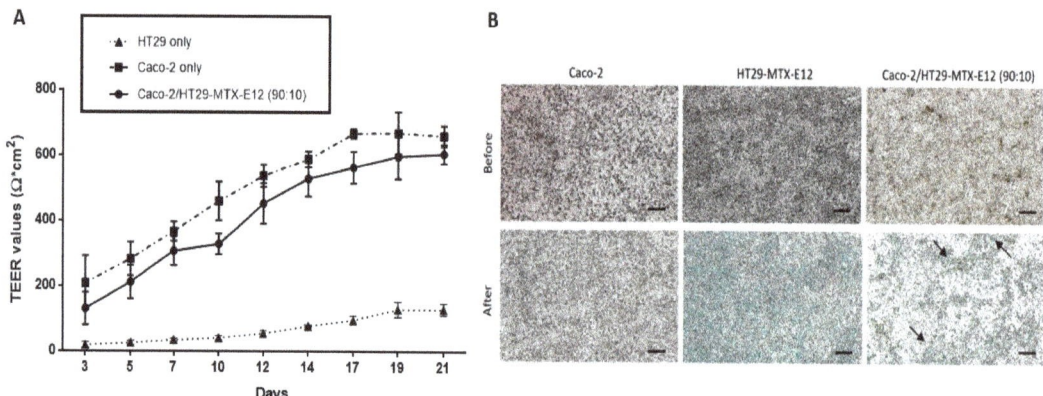

Figure 3. Characterization of the Caco-2/HT29-MTX-E12 (90:10 ratio) co-culture during 21 days of cultivation. (**A**) Transepithelial-transendothelial electrical resistance (TEER) values of Caco-2, HT29-MTX-E12, and Caco-2/HT29-MTX-E12 (90:10) cell cultures. Values are shown as mean ± standard deviation (SD) ($n \geq 3$). (**B**) Representative microscopy images of cell layers were obtained before and after staining with Alcian blue for mucus production (evident by blue color and black arrows). Scale bar = 100 μm.

To determine the presence of mucus on the cell surface, the cell layers of 21-day cultured Caco-2, HT29-MTX-E12, and Caco-2/HT29-MTX-E12 (90:10 ratio) were stained with Alcian blue. Figure 3B shows that the Caco-2 monoculture did not exhibit Alcian blue staining. In contrast, as expected, the surface of HT29-MTX-E12 cells was covered by mucus production, while it was randomly dispersed throughout the cell layer of the Caco-2/HT29-MTX-E12 co-culture.

2.4. Increased Intestinal Permeability in Caco-2/HT29-MTX-E12 Co-Culture Induced by IFN-γ Priming

A previous study has reported that IFN-γ priming resulted in the expression of TNF receptor 2, which was crucial for the subsequent induction of TNF-α-induced intestinal epithelial barrier dysfunction, caused by LPS [50]. Therefore, the Caco-2/HT29-MTX-E12 co-culture was primed here with IFN-γ for 24 h, before the addition of the LPS-stimulated macrophage-like THP-1 cells, or primary monocyte-derived macrophages. As shown in Figure 4, IFN-γ priming resulted in a significant drop in the TEER value (Figure 4A) and an increase in permeability (Figure 4B) as signs of barrier integrity loss. Compared to the untreated co-culture (SC), there was a TEER reduction of 25% and a permeability increase of around 18%.

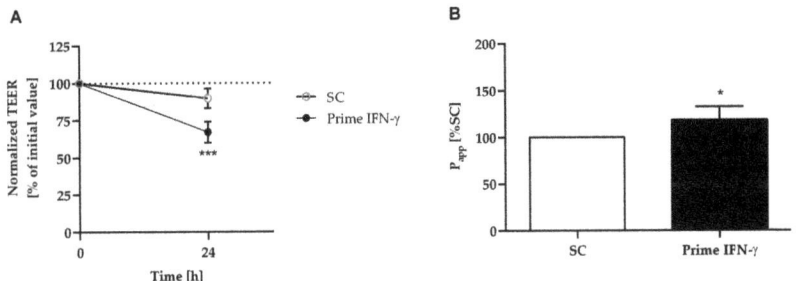

Figure 4. IFN-γ priming on the Caco-2/HT29-MTX-E12 co-culture. After 24 h incubation with 50 ng/mL IFN-γ, TEER (**A**) and permeability value (P_{app}) (**B**) of Caco-2/HT29-MTX-E12 co-cultures were measured. TEER values were expressed as a percentage of the initial TEER value (100%). Permeability was expressed as fold change of the untreated control (SC) used as a reference. Bars are the means ± SD ($n \geq 3$). * $p < 0.05$, or *** $p < 0.001$ were considered significantly different versus SC.

2.5. Characterization of the Inflammation-Triggered, Triple-Culture "Leaky Gut" Model

After 6 h and 24 h co-incubation with stimulated macrophage-like THP-1 cells, the intestinal barrier function of the Caco-2/HT29-MTX-E12 epithelial cell layer was assessed by measuring TEER (Figure 5A) and FITC-Dextran 4 kDa (FD4) paracellular transmission (Figure 5B). As seen in Figure 5A, within 6 h, the TEER of the "leaky gut" model decreased to 85% from the initial value, and further to 77% after 24 h. The paracellular flux of FD4 across the cellular layer showed a significantly increased permeability under "leaky gut" conditions, which was up to 41% and further to 71% higher than the control model after 6 h and 24 h, respectively (Figure 5B).

In comparison to the control model, significant release of the cytokines IL-6 and TNF-α, (insignificant for IL-1β), was observed in the "leaky gut" model after 6 h (Figure 5C), and 24 h (Figure 5D). As seen in Figure 5C, after 6 h, the mean concentration of IL-6 and TNF-α in the "leaky gut" model were 66 ± 8 pg/mL and 163 ± 72 pg/mL, respectively. Those were significantly higher than levels of IL-6 and TNF-α in the control model (6 ± 8 pg/mL and 41 ± 22 pg/mL, respectively). However, there was no significant difference in IL-1β production between the "leaky gut" and control models (16 ± 8 pg/mL and 57 ± 50 pg/mL, respectively). Figure 5D also shows the significantly higher levels of IL-6 and TNF-α in the "leaky gut" model (77 ± 26 pg/mL and 91 ± 41 pg/mL, respectively), as compared to the control model (11 ± 4 pg/mL and 30 ± 17 pg/mL, respectively) after 24 h cultivation. Again, there was no significant difference in IL-1β production between the "leaky gut" and control models after 24 h (7 ± 5 pg/mL and 20 ± 13 pg/mL, respectively).

The significant increased permeability highly corresponded to a significant production of zonulin, a proposed regulator of the permeability of the intestinal barrier [51], in the "leaky gut" model after 6 h (Figure 5E) and 24 h (Figure 5F). As seen in Figure 5E, within 6 h, the mean concentration of zonulin in both compartments of the "leaky gut" model (2043 ± 464 pg/mL) was nearly 25-fold higher than in the control model (83 ± 143 pg/mL). After 24 h, the mean concentration of zonulin in both compartments of the "leaky gut" model (1982 ± 260 pg/mL) was around 1.3-fold higher than the control model (1664 ± 29 pg/mL) (Figure 5F).

As shown in Figure 5E,F, while there was no change in Tight Junction Protein-1 (TJP1) between the "leaky gut" and control models after 6 h (24 ± 7 pg/mL and 22 ± 8 pg/mL, respectively) and 24 h (141 ± 12 pg/mL and 147 ± 6 pg/mL, respectively), the amount of released occludin in the "leaky gut" model increased from 66 ± 13 pg/mL at 6 h to 104 ± 49 pg/mL at 24 h. On the other hand, the amount of occludin in the control model decreased from 54 ± 15 pg/mL (6 h) to 51 ± 60 pg/mL (24 h).

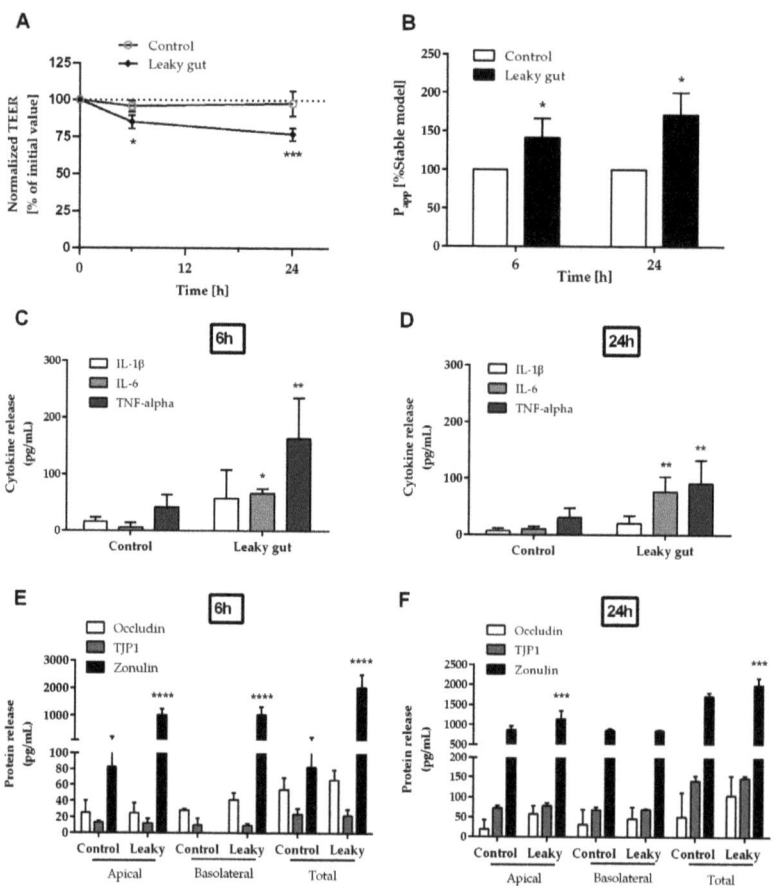

Figure 5. Characterization of the in vitro "leaky gut" model. Intestinal barrier function of the triple cell culture was assessed by (**A**) TEER and (**B**) permeability value (P_{app}) after 6 h and 24 h incubation. The secretion of the key pro-inflammatory cytokines IL-1β, IL-6, and TNF-α in the basolateral compartment were quantified after (**C**) 6 h and (**D**) 24 h. The release of Occludin, Tight Junction Protein-1 (TJP1), and Zonulin in the apical, and basolateral compartment were measured after (**E**) 6 h and (**F**) 24 h. Data are given as mean ± SD ($n \geq 3$). * $p < 0.05$, ** $p < 0.01$, *** $p < 0.001$, **** $p < 0.0001$ as compared to the control model.

2.6. Comparison of Different Modifications on the "Leaky Gut" Model Using Macrophage-like THP-1 Cells

A previous study has described that increased intestinal permeability is correlated with increased levels of LPS in intestinal tissue and plasma [52]. Therefore, the "leaky gut" model was additionally treated with 100 ng/mL LPS in the apical compartment for 24 h. As shown in Figure 6, this modification resulted in a significant TEER drop of 30% (Figure 6A) and a permeability increase of 28% (Figure 6B) compared to the control model.

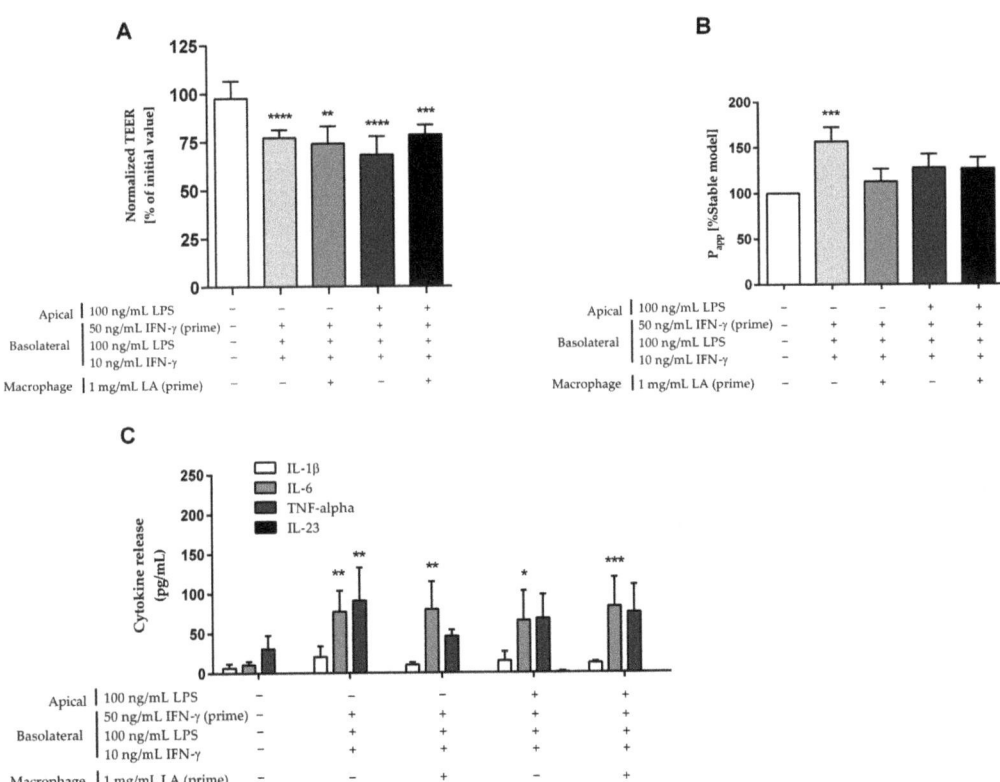

Figure 6. Comparison of different modifications on the "leaky gut" model using macrophage-like THP-1 cells ("−": non-treatment, "+": treatment). Intestinal barrier function was assessed by (**A**) TEER and (**B**) permeability value (P_{app}) as compared to the control model. (**C**) The secretion of key pro-inflammatory cytokines IL-1β, IL-6, IL-23, and TNF-α was quantified in the basolateral compartment of the models after 24 h cultivation. Bars are mean ± SD ($n \geq 3$). * $p < 0.05$, ** $p < 0.01$, *** $p < 0.001$, **** $p < 0.0001$ as compared to the control model.

The cytokine interleukin-23 (IL-23), which is primarily produced by macrophages and dendritic cells in response to microbial stimulation, has been considered a key promoter of chronic intestinal inflammation, especially in IBD [53]. However, we could not detect IL-23 secretion in our model (Figure 6C). Lactic acid (LA) was reported as a stimulator of IL-23 production in PBMCs exposed to bacterial LPS [54]. Therefore, we pre-treated macrophage-like THP-1 cells with 1 mg/mL LA for 24 h before setting up the triple-culture. This modification showed a significant TEER reduction of approximately 24% (Figure 6A) and a permeability rise of 13% (Figure 6B) compared to the control model. The combination of the two modifications (apical treatment with LPS and LA priming) also resulted in a significant TEER decrease of 20%, and a permeability increase of 27% as compared to the control model.

As described in Figure 6C, similar to the inflamed model, a significant secretion of IL-6 was found after additional modifications by using apical treatment of 100 ng/mL LPS (66 ± 37 pg/mL), or 24 h-priming of macrophage-like THP-1 cells with 1 mg/mL LA (79 ± 35 pg/mL), or the combination of these (83 ± 37 pg/mL) as compared to the control model (11 ± 4 pg/mL). There were similar levels in the production of IL-1β, TNF-α, and especially IL-23 between the modified "leaky gut" and control models.

2.7. Comparison of Different Modifications on the "Leaky Gut" Model Using Primary Human-Derived Macrophages

To better reflect the properties of primary macrophages in vivo, we replaced the THP-1 cell line in our model with primary monocyte-derived macrophages from human PBMCs. The experiments were then carried out as with the macrophage-like THP-1 cells.

The additional treatment with 100 ng/mL LPS in the apical compartment of the "leaky gut" model resulted in a significant TEER drop of 24% (Figure 7A) and a permeability increase of approximately 30% (Figure 7B) as compared to the control model.

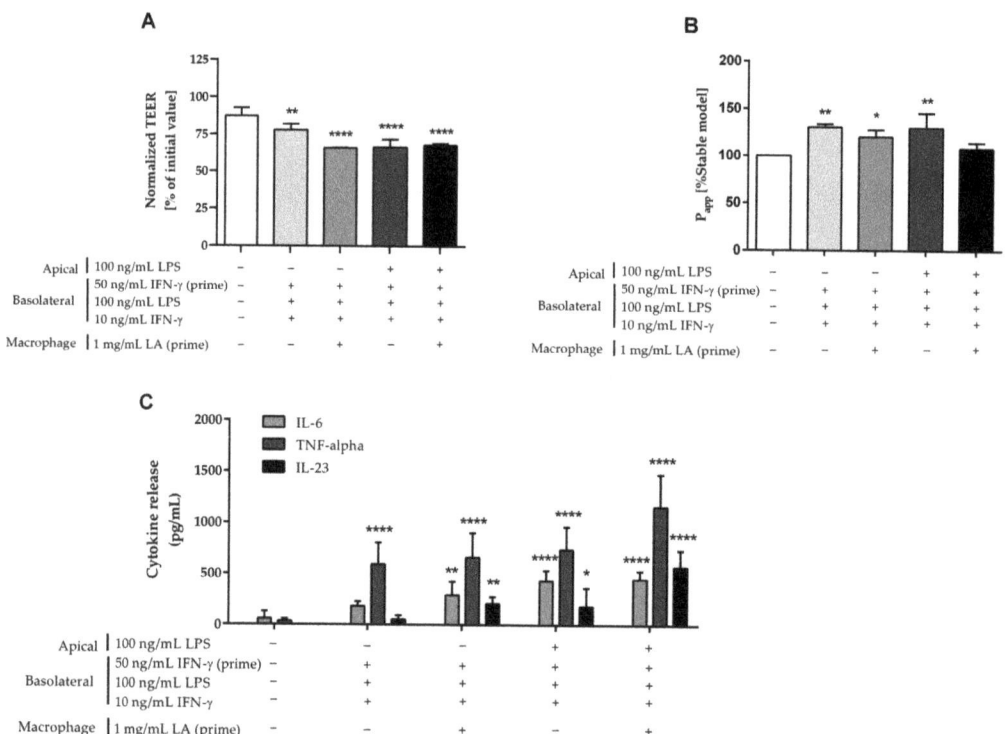

Figure 7. Comparison of the modifications on the "leaky gut" model using primary human-derived macrophages ("−": non-treatment, "+": treatment). Intestinal barrier function in comparison to the control model was assessed after 24 h by (**A**) TEER and (**B**) permeability values. (**C**) The secretion of key pro-inflammatory cytokines IL-6, IL-23, and TNF-α in the basolateral compartment of control and "leaky gut" models were quantified after 24 h. Bars are mean ± SD ($n \geq 3$). * $p < 0.05$, ** $p < 0.01$, **** $p < 0.0001$ as compared to the control model.

Similarly, 1 mg/mL LA pre-treatment of primary monocyte-derived macrophages for 24 h also caused a significant TEER reduction of 25% (Figure 7A), and a permeability rise of

20% (Figure 7B) in comparison with the control model. The combination of the two above modifications (apical treatment with LPS and LA priming) also resulted in a significant TEER decrease of 22%, but the permeability only slightly increased by 8% as compared to the control model.

As shown in Figure 7C, additional modifications with the apical treatment of 100 ng/mL LPS (433 ± 102 pg/mL), or 24 h-priming of macrophages with 1 mg/mL LA (290 ± 130 pg/mL), or the combination of these two modifications (451 ± 80 pg/mL) all produced a significant secretion of IL-6 in comparison with the control model (58 ± 70 pg/mL). Similarly, the substantial secretion in TNF-α was also seen by the apical treatment of 100 ng/mL LPS (741 ± 223 pg/mL), 24 h-priming macrophage with 1 mg/mL LA (662 ± 240 pg/mL), and the combination of these two modifications (1163 ± 314 pg/mL) as compared to the control model (34 ± 21 pg/mL). In contrast to macrophage-like THP-1 cells, the apical treatment with 100 ng/mL LPS (184 ± 180 pg/mL), or 24 h-priming of macrophages with 1 mg/mL LA (209 ± 65 pg/mL), or the combination of these two modifications (577 ± 161 pg/mL) resulted in a strong, significant secretion of IL-23 when compared to the control model (0 pg/mL).

3. Discussion

IBD is a chronic gastrointestinal inflammatory disease with unclear causes and pathogenesis. However, it is thought that a complex sequence of interactions among genetic, microbial, immunological, and environmental factors results in an abnormal and exaggerated immune response of the commensal microbiota, finally resulting in the induction of intestinal inflammation [55–58].

Various in vitro models have been developed to understand IBD's etiology, pathology, and potential treatment options. Most of them used the Caco-2 cell line, because differentiated Caco-2 cells can reflect many features of mature enterocytes in the intestinal epithelium, such as a brush border with microvilli, tight junction formation, production of characteristic digestive enzymes, and transporters [27]. Importantly, Caco-2 cells showed the ability to produce a range of inflammatory cytokines such as IL-6, IL-8, IL-1β, and TNF-α, that may contribute to inflammatory conditions in IBD [59]. Different studies have also utilized this cell line to evaluate novel molecules for potential therapeutic treatment/management of UC. For example, it was demonstrated, that rhamnogalacturonan accelerated wound healing, decreased epithelial barrier dysfunction, and suppressed IL-1 induced IL-8 production in Caco-2 cells [60]. Another study by Liang et al. reported that the corn protein hydrolysate down-regulated the secretion of IL-8 production in TNF-α induced inflammation in Caco-2 cells [61].

Nevertheless, the most significant limitation of the monolayer Caco-2 cell culture system was the lack of a mucus layer, which serves as a physical and chemical barrier in the intestinal epithelium against luminal contents involving digestive enzymes, food particles, microbiota and microbial compounds, as well as host-secreted products such as bile acids [62]. Hence, previous studies co-cultured Caco-2 cells with the mucus-secreting goblet HT29-MTX-E12 cell line to provide a closer physiological model of the human intestinal epithelium [63–65]. Many recent studies have widely used the optimal 90:10 ratio of Caco-2/HT29-MTX cells, because it better represented the in vivo situation of the human small intestine regarding the proportion of absorptive enterocytes and mucin-producing goblet cells [66–69]. Therefore, we applied this combination of Caco-2/HT29-MTX-E12 co-culture conditions for our "leaky gut" model system to closely mimic the cell composition and functionality of the intestinal epithelium. In our model, the mucin secreted by the HT29-MTX cells does not appear to completely cover the whole surface of the intestinal cells after 21 days of co-culture. A healthy mucosal barrier contributes to the prevention of pathogens invasion and defects therein have been implicated in several intestinal pathologies. Thus, depending on the application of our in vitro model, this might be considered as a limitation or advantage.

Macrophages in the lamina propria of the small intestine are one of the most prevalent populations of leukocytes in the body. They play a crucial role in maintaining intestinal homeostasis and intestinal inflammation emergence [70]. Several investigations have demonstrated that intestinal macrophages become activated and promote the occurrence and development of IBD [35,37,71]. Over the last decade, to better replicate the in vivo physiology of IBD, in vitro IBD models have been established using a combination of Caco-2 cells and macrophage-like differentiated THP-1 cells, for example, Kämpfer et al. (2017) [46]. IFN-γ priming of Caco-2 cells together with the stimulation of differentiated THP-1 cells by LPS and IFN-γ, induced an inflammation-like response in their diseased intestine model, evident by intestinal barrier disruption and pro-inflammatory cytokine release. Based on this model of Kämpfer, co-culture models with differentiated Caco-2 cells and PMA-differentiated THP-1 cells in the presence of inflammatory stimulators (e.g., LPS with/without IFN-γ) have been used to evaluate the potential immunomodulatory and anti-inflammatory effects of phytochemicals [43,72,73], marine natural products [74–76], bacterial β-glucans [77], siRNA-based nanomedicine [42], bovine milk-derived extracellular vesicles [78], and probiotic bacteria [41].

Some IBD studies used an advanced in vitro triple-culture model composed of Caco-2 cells, HT29-MTX-(E12) cells, and PMA-differentiated macrophage-like THP-1 cells. The combination of two intestine cell lines (Caco-2/HT29-MTX) with differentiated THP-1 cells was first introduced by Kaulmann et al. (2016) to study the anti-inflammatory and antioxidant effects of plums and cabbages [79]. Busch et al. (2021) suggested that this advanced in vitro triple-culture model was a promising approach for studying the toxicological effects of ingested micro- and nano-plastic particles [80]. An adverse and pro-inflammatory role of the NLRP3 inflammasome in IBD has been described by using this triple-culture model [81].

However, this model system cannot reflect the anatomical distribution of lamina propria macrophages in humans, which are close to the epithelial monolayer of intestinal cells [70]. Thus, Calatayud et al. co-cultured Caco-2, HT29-MTX, and differentiated THP-1 cells in close contact [38]. In contrast to our model, they used Type I collagen from a rat tail to support THP-1 adhering to the membrane. Even though the presence of coated collagen could increase cell attachment and viability [82], it may potentially impact TEER measurements indirectly because the phenotyping properties of THP-1 cells were modified by the surrounding extracellular matrix (i.e., collagen Type I). Teplicky et al. have demonstrated that cell doubling times (i.e., cell proliferation) and mean diameters (i.e., cell size) of THP-1 cells in collagen Type I were slightly increased when compared to cells cultured in normal medium [83]. Furthermore, the biological activity of collagen-coated immune cells and the detection of released pro-inflammatory cytokines might also be affected [84]. Another study by Busch et al. (2021) also used a triple-culture model with close contact between intestinal cells (Caco-2/HT29-MTX-E12) and differentiated macrophage-like THP-1 cells [48]. They seeded Caco-2/HT29-MTX-E12 cells on the bottom side of the insert, while differentiated macrophage-like THP-1 cells were cultured on the top side of the insert. Due to the experimental design of their model, it is only suitable for studies with buoyant particles, which float in cell culture media due to their density of less than 1 g/cm^3.

A significant increase in zonulin production could be observed in our "leaky gut" model when compared to the control model. Intestinal epithelial cell tight junctions are a multi-protein complex that support the integrity of the physical intestinal barrier by regulating the paracellular movement between the internal environment and external antigens or bacterial products [85,86]. It has been demonstrated that impaired tight junction proteins present an early event of IBD [87,88]. In fact, elevated levels of zonulin have been detected in both serum [89–91] and fecal [92,93] samples of IBD patients and it is used as biomarker of intestinal permeability of the small intestine [94,95]. Therefore, on this point our approach of a "leaky gut" model provides in vitro to in vivo concordance.

Cytokines play a critical role in the immunopathogenesis of IBD, where they regulate various aspects of the inflammatory response [96–98]. In patients with IBD, pro-

and anti-inflammatory cytokines have been demonstrated to be produced in the inflamed mucosa by various immune cells such as macrophages, dendritic cells (DCs), neutrophils, natural killer (NK) cells, intestinal epithelial cells (IECs), innate lymphoid cells (ILCs), mucosal effector T cells (T helper 1 (T_H1), T_H2 and T_H17), and regulatory T (T_{reg}) cells [99]. In particular, the translocation of commensal bacteria and microbial products from the gut lumen into the bowel wall resulting from an impaired cell barrier function ("leaky gut") leads to inflammatory macrophage (M1 phenotype) stimulation, and consequent production of high levels of pro-inflammatory cytokines such as IL-1, IL-6, IL18, TNF-α, IL-23, and IL-17. These cytokines directly or indirectly result in the injury or necrosis of the intestinal epithelial cells, which then promotes the pathogenesis of IBD [35]. Being critical mediators in the development of IBD, pro-inflammatory cytokines are considered effective therapeutic targets [100,101]. Anti-TNF-α therapy is the first biologic approved, and currently the most effective treatment for IBD, including infliximab, golimumab, adalimumab, and certolizumab pegol, which have been demonstrated good clinical efficacy [102]. However, approximately 20% of IBD patients are primary non-responders [103], and over 30% eventually lose response to anti-TNF drugs [104]. Blocking of lamina propria macrophages-produced IL-6 with monoclonal antibodies (e.g., tocilizumab, PF-0423691) is here considered as alternative treatment for IBD, but serious side effects have been reported for these anti-IL-6 drugs [32].

More recent data have demonstrated, that the pro-inflammatory IL-23 was a critical promoter of the pathogenesis of IBD, because it stimulates and influences the differentiation and proliferation of pathogenic T helper type 17 (T_h17) cells. This in turn further induces inflammatory cytokines [53,105,106]. Therefore, targeting the IL-23 pathway is another important way for drug development of IBD [107]. Currently, only ustekinumab has been approved for the treatment of both CD and UC patients, but several IL-23p19 antagonists (e.g., risankizumab, brazikumab, mirikizumab) are in phase II or III development programs and give promising results. Our "leaky gut" model showed a significant increase in IL-6 and TNF-α upon activation. Interestingly, we could also achieve the substantial secretion of IL-23 by additional modifications using primary human-derived macrophages, but not by using macrophage-like THP-1 cells. Since the exact mechanism by which lactic acid stimulates macrophages to release IL-23 is not fully understood, one possible reason for this difference could be correlated to the genetic and phenotypic differences between macrophage-like THP-1 cells, and primary blood macrophages. Compared to primary blood macrophages belonging to a non-malignant and non-proliferating cell type, THP-1 cells are leukemia monocytic cells with genetic and functional differences. Furthermore, concerning LPS responses, THP-1 cells express much lower levels of monocyte differentiation antigen CD14 in comparison to primary monocytes [108]. The detection of IL-23 has not yet been described in any other intestinal inflamed model before, thus our "leaky gut" model provides a promising new in vitro platform for drug investigation of IBD treatment, especially IL-23 pathway inhibitors.

4. Materials and Methods

4.1. Chemicals

Fetal calf serum (FCS), GlutaMAX™ supplement, Roswell Park Memorial Institute (RPMI)-1640, Dulbecco's Modified Eagle's medium (DMEM) with low glucose, trypsin-EDTA (0.5%), trypsin (2.5%) solution, phosphate-buffered saline (PBS, without Ca^{2+} and Mg^{2+}), Non-Essential Amino Acid (NEAA), penicillin/streptomycin solution (10,000 U/mL and 10,000 µg/mL), StemPro™ Accutase™, and Hank's Balanced Salt Solution (HBSS) were purchased from Gibco™, Life Technologies GmbH (Darmstadt, Germany). Lipopolysaccharide (LPS, from Escherichia coli O111:B4), phorbol 12-myristate 13-acetate (PMA), fluorescein isothiocyanate (FITC)-Dextran, Alcian blue 8GX solution (1% in 3% acetic acid) were from Sigma Aldrich (Taufkirchen, Germany). IFN-γ (human recombinant) was purchased from STEMCELL technologies GmbH (Köln, Germany). Macrophage colony-stimulating factor (M-CSF) was purchased from Peprotech (Hamburg, Germany).

Paraformaldehyde (PFA) solution of 4% in PBS was purchased from Santa Cruz Biotechnology (Heidelberg, Germany).

4.2. Cell Culture

The human colon carcinoma Caco-2 (ACC169) and HT29-MTX-E12-E12 cell lines were obtained from the German Collection of Microorganisms and Cell Cultures (DSMZ, Braunschweig, Germany) and European Collection of Authenticated Cell Cultures (Porton Down, UK), respectively. The cells were cultured separately in flasks in DMEM supplemented with 10% (v/v) FCS, 1% (v/v) NEAA, 100 U/mL penicillin, and 100 µg/mL streptomycin at 37 °C in a humidified incubator with a 5% CO_2/95% air atmosphere. The culture medium was changed every 2–3 days and cells were regularly split at 90% confluence.

The THP-1 cell line was cultured in a flask in RPMI-1640 supplemented with 10% (v/v) FCS, 1% GlutaMAX™, 100 U/mL penicillin, and 100 µg/mL streptomycin at 37 °C in a humidified incubator with a 5% CO_2/95% air atmosphere. THP-1 cells were maintained at a concentration between 0.2 to 1×10^6 cells/mL.

4.3. Isolation and Cultivation of Human PBMCs

Human PBMCs were isolated from buffy coats of healthy volunteers at the University Medical Center in Freiburg, Germany by centrifugation on a LymphoPrep™ gradient (density: 1.077 g/cm^3, 20 min, 500× g). Isolated PBMCs were cultured in complete RPMI 1640 medium supplemented with 10% heat-inactivated FCS, 2 mM L-glutamine, 100 U/mL penicillin, and 100 µg/mL streptomycin at 37 °C in a humidified incubator with a 5% CO_2/95% air atmosphere.

4.4. Co-Culture of Caco-2 and HT29-MTX-E12-E12 on Inserts

Monocultures of Caco-2 and HT29-MTX-E12 cells were harvested with Trypsin-EDTA and seeded on the apical chamber side of 12-well ThinCert® inserts (0.4 µm PET pore membrane, Greiner Bio-One, Frickenhausen, Germany) in an optimal proportion of 90:10, respectively, to reach a final density of 1×10^5 cells/cm^2/insert. Cells were co-cultured for 19–21 days in a humidified incubator with a 5% CO_2/95% air atmosphere with medium (0.5 mL on the apical side and 1.5 mL on the basolateral side) changed every 2–3 days.

4.5. Macrophage Differentiation from THP-1 Cell Line and Peripheral Blood Primary Monocytes

THP-1 monocytes were seeded at 2×10^5 cells/mL in a 75 cm^2 flask and differentiated into macrophages by 72 h treated with 20 ng/mL PMA in a 5% CO_2/95% air atmosphere incubator at 37 °C. After differentiation, the PMA-containing medium was discarded and the macrophage-like differentiated THP-1 were rested in fresh medium for 24 h.

Primary monocytes were purified from isolated PBMCs by using the culture plastic adherence technique: 2×10^6 isolated PBMCs/mL in complete medium were seeded into a 75 cm^2 culture flask and then monocytes were allowed to adhere at 37 °C in a 5% CO_2/95% air atmosphere incubator. After 24 h incubation, non-adherent cells were removed from the flask. For macrophage differentiation, the adherent cells (mainly monocytes) were fed with the complete medium containing 50 ng/mL recombinant human M-CSF for additional 6 days in a 5% CO_2/95% air atmosphere at 37 °C. The medium was then replaced every 3 days with fresh complete medium, supplemented with 50 ng/mL M-CSF. After that, monocyte-derived macrophages were rested in fresh medium for 24 h.

4.6. Fabrication of 3D-Printed Cap for Insert

The caps were fabricated with a FormLabs 3+ 3D printer and BioMed Clear Resin, a USP class VI material used for medical devices that complies with ISO 18562. To avoid possible cross-contamination of the used materials, the caps were fabricated in an ISO 13485-certified laboratory with a printer that was solely used for the respective material. After printing, the caps were washed (Form Wash) and cured (Form Cure) according to the manufacturer's instructions (all devices and materials were purchased from FormLabs

GmbH, Berlin, Germany). The .stl file of the cap can be downloaded as supplemental material from the journal's homepage.

4.7. Experimental Setup of the Inflammation-Triggered "Leaky Gut" Model

The control and inflammation-triggered or "leaky gut" Caco-2/HT29-MTX-E12-E12/THP-1 triple-culture was established as illustrated in Figure 1. Firstly, 19-day-differentiated Caco-2/HT29-MTX-E12-E12 epithelial cells in the apical compartment were either rested in fresh medium (control model) or primed with 50 ng/mL IFN-γ for the inflammation-triggered model in 24 h before the triple-culture. On the next day, the medium from the basolateral side of the insert was completely discarded. The medium from the apical part was replaced with fresh medium, and a specially 3D-printed constructed cap was carefully placed into the insert (see Figure 2) to avoid the leakage of the medium during the following immune cell adherence procedure. The insert was placed upside down in a Petri dish. Then THP-1-differentiated macrophages (2×10^5 cells), or primary monocyte-derived macrophages (4×10^4 cells), which were initially detached from the 75 cm^2 culture flask with 50 ng/mL accutase, were transferred on the bottom side of the inverted inserts, for 1.5 h at 37 °C in a 5% CO$_2$ incubator. After immune cell adherence, the inserts were put back into 12-well plates in regular orientation before the specially 3D-printed constructed caps were carefully removed from the inserts. After medium removal, fresh medium was added to the upper and lower compartments of the insert. Macrophages from the control triple-culture were rested in fresh medium, while macrophages from the inflammation-triggered triple-culture were activated by 100 ng/mL LPS in combination with 10 ng/mL IFN-γ for 24 h at 37 °C in a humidified incubator with a 5% CO$_2$/95% air atmosphere.

To further optimize the "leaky gut" model, the treatment procedures involved some additional modifications. Condition 1: macrophage-like THP-1 cells were primed with 1 mg/mL lactic acid (LA) in 24 h before triple culture. Condition 2: the apical compartment was simultaneously treated with 100 ng/mL LPS during macrophage activation in the basolateral compartment. Condition 3: combination of conditions 1 and 2.

4.8. Transepithelial Electrical Resistance Measurement

The cell monolayer integrity of the Caco-2/HT29-MTX-E12 co-culture on an insert was investigated using transepithelial electrical resistance (TEER) measurement. This measurement was performed by using an EVOM epithelial volt-ohmmeter equipped with a 'chopstick' electrode (STX-2) (Millicell® ERS, Millipore, Bedford, MA, USA). Before measurement, cells were stabilized at room temperature, while the electrode was sterilized with 70% ethanol and preconditioned in growth media. The measurement was performed in triplicates, and immediately after medium replacement. The final TEER value (TEER $_{final}$) was corrected by subtracting the blank resistance (R $_{blank}$) of the semipermeable membrane only (an insert without cells) from the resistance across the sample (R $_{sample}$) before multiplying it by the effective growth area (A) of the insert.

$$\text{TEER}_{final} \, [\Omega \times cm^2] = (R_{sample} - R_{blank}) \, [\Omega] \times A \, [cm^2]$$

Co-culture inserts with TEER values over 300 Ω·cm^2 were used for further experiments. TEER results were expressed as a percentage of the initial TEER value.

4.9. Alcian Blue Staining

Alcian Blue stain was used to visualize acidic epithelial and connective tissue mucins that were produced by HT29-MTX-E12 cells in the co-culture model. Briefly, Caco-2/HT29-MTX-E12 co-culture (90:10 ratio) was cultured at a density of 1×10^5 cells/cm^2/insert on 12-well plates for 21 days. After 21-day incubation, culture media were removed and cells were washed twice with pre-warmed PBS before they were fixed with 4% paraformaldehyde (PFA) for 30 min at room temperature. Next, PFA was aspirated and cells were rinsed with PBS twice before they were stained with 1% alcian blue in 3% acetic acid. After 30 min incubation at room temperature, extra alcian blue was removed by two-time washing with PBS. The stained mucus was visualized by an inverted microscope (Fluorescence microscope Biozero BZ 8100E, Keyence GmbH, Neu-Isenburg, Germany).

4.10. Permeability Studies

Paracellular permeability of the intestinal epithelium layer was determined using FITC-Dextran with a molecular weight of 4 kDa (FD4). Briefly, 250 µL FD4 solution (1 mg/mL in HBSS), and 800 µL HBSS was added to the apical and basolateral compartment, respectively. After 2 h incubation at 37 °C, 150 µL from the basolateral side were transferred to a black 96-well plate (Greiner Bio-One, Frickenhausen, Germany). HBSS and FD4 solution were used as a negative and positive control, respectively. Fluorescence intensity was measured at excitation and emission wavelengths of 490 and 520 nm, respectively, by using a plate reader (TECAN infinite M200, Tecan tranding AG, Männedorf, Switzerland). Permeability coefficient (P_{app}) was calculated by using the following equation:

$$P_{app} = \frac{dQ}{dt} \times \frac{1}{A \times C_0}$$

Defined as:
P_{app} = apparent permeability coefficient [cm/s].
dQ/dt = rate of appearance of FD4 on the basolateral side [µg/s].
A = surface area of the monolayer [cm^2].
C_0 = initial FD4 concentration in the apical side [µg/mL].

4.11. Tight Junction Proteins and Their Regulator Quantification

Cells were stimulated as described above. Secreted tight junction proteins (Occludin, Tight Junction Protein 1) and their regulator (Zonulin) in the supernatant were quantified by using specific ELISA kits (AssayGenie, Dublin, Ireland) according to the manufacturer's instructions. Results were standardized by comparison with a standard curve.

4.12. Cytokine Level Measurement

Cells were stimulated as described above. Secreted proinflammatory cytokines (IL-1β, IL-6, IL-23, and TNF-α) in the supernatant of the lower compartment were evaluated by using specific ELISA kits (Thermo Scientific, Darmstadt, Germany) according to the manufacturer's instructions. Results were standardized by comparison with a standard curve.

4.13. Statistical Analysis

Results are expressed as the means ± standard deviation (SD) of at least three independent experiments. When comparing between two groups, Student's unpaired t test was used. For experiments involving more than three groups, results were analyzed either by two-way ANOVA or two-way ANOVA followed by Tukey's multiple comparison tests. Data were analyzed using the GraphPad Prism version 6.07 software (GraphPad Software Inc., San Diego, CA, USA). Results were considered statistically significant when $p < 0.05$.

5. Conclusions

In conclusion, we described the establishment of a complex "leaky gut" model using epithelial cells (i.e., Caco-2), and mucus-secreting cells (i.e., HT29-MTX-E12) in close contact with activated immune cells (i.e., differentiated macrophage-like THP-1 cells or primary monocyte-derived macrophage) to simulate pathophysiological mechanisms of intestinal inflammation. Modifications on the original "leaky gut" model using primary human-derived macrophages, with either the additionally apical LPS treatment, or the LA pretreatment of macrophages, further increased at least one of the "leaky gut" characteristics in our model. In particular, the expression of IL-23 could present a further advantage of this in vitro model. Even though there is no single model that can mimic all complex aspects of

IBD, we could address some limitations of previously established models. Therefore, our in vitro "leaky gut" model can provide a promising pre-clinical tool for novel IBD-related drug development and serve as an alternative system to in vivo animal testing.

Supplementary Materials: The supporting information can be downloaded at: https://www.mdpi.com/article/10.3390/ijms24087427/s1.

Author Contributions: E.L. and N.P.K.L. conceived and designed the study and experiments. N.P.K.L. and M.J.A. designed and carried out the experiments. N.P.K.L. and E.L. prepared the graphs and analyzed the data. N.P.K.L., E.L. and M.J.A. wrote the paper. All authors have read and agreed to the published version of the manuscript.

Funding: N.P.K.L. was funded by the German Academic Exchange Service (DAAD) through a Research Grant—Doctoral Programmes in Germany. The article processing charge was funded by the Baden-Württemberg Ministry of Science, Research and Art and the University of Freiburg in the funding program Open Access Publishing.

Institutional Review Board Statement: The experiments using human blood samples were conducted in accordance with the Declaration of Helsinki, and approved by the Ethics Committee of the University of Freiburg (protocol code 597/14 and 22-1466-S1, 17 January 2023).

Informed Consent Statement: Written informed consent was obtained from all subjects involved in the study.

Data Availability Statement: Not applicable.

Acknowledgments: The authors are especially thankful to Marie Czogalla for her support in the experiment of Alcian blue staining.

Conflicts of Interest: The authors declare no conflict of interest.

References

1. Fukui, H. Increased Intestinal Permeability and Decreased Barrier Function: Does It Really Influence the Risk of Inflammation? *Inflamm. Intest. Dis.* **2016**, *1*, 135–145. [CrossRef]
2. Leech, B.; McIntyre, E.; Steel, A.; Sibbritt, D. Risk factors associated with intestinal permeability in an adult population: A systematic review. *Int. J. Clin. Pract.* **2019**, *73*, e13385. [CrossRef]
3. Vanuytsel, T.; Tack, J.; Farre, R. The Role of Intestinal Permeability in Gastrointestinal Disorders and Current Methods of Evaluation. *Front. Nutr.* **2021**, *8*, 717925. [CrossRef] [PubMed]
4. Fasano, A. Leaky gut and autoimmune diseases. *Clin. Rev. Allergy Immunol.* **2012**, *42*, 71–78. [CrossRef] [PubMed]
5. Mu, Q.; Kirby, J.; Reilly, C.M.; Luo, X.M. Leaky Gut As a Danger Signal for Autoimmune Diseases. *Front. Immunol.* **2017**, *8*, 598. [CrossRef] [PubMed]
6. Akdis, C.A. Does the epithelial barrier hypothesis explain the increase in allergy, autoimmunity and other chronic conditions? *Nat. Rev. Immunol.* **2021**, *21*, 739–751. [CrossRef] [PubMed]
7. Perrier, C.; Corthesy, B. Gut permeability and food allergies. *Clin. Exp. Allergy* **2011**, *41*, 20–28. [CrossRef]
8. Farshchi, M.K.; Azad, F.J.; Salari, R.; Mirsadraee, M.; Anushiravani, M. A Viewpoint on the Leaky Gut Syndrome to Treat Allergic Asthma: A Novel Opinion. *J. Evid. Based Complement. Altern. Med.* **2017**, *22*, 378–380. [CrossRef]
9. Fiorentino, M.; Sapone, A.; Senger, S.; Camhi, S.S.; Kadzielski, S.M.; Buie, T.M.; Kelly, D.L.; Cascella, N.; Fasano, A. Blood-brain barrier and intestinal epithelial barrier alterations in autism spectrum disorders. *Mol. Autism.* **2016**, *7*, 49. [CrossRef]
10. Kohler, O.; Krogh, J.; Mors, O.; Benros, M.E. Inflammation in Depression and the Potential for Anti-Inflammatory Treatment. *Curr. Neuropharmacol.* **2016**, *14*, 732–742. [CrossRef]
11. Obrenovich, M.E.M. Leaky Gut, Leaky Brain? *Microorganisms* **2018**, *6*, 107. [CrossRef] [PubMed]
12. Kushak, R.I.; Buie, T.M.; Murray, K.F.; Newburg, D.S.; Chen, C.; Nestoridi, E.; Winter, H.S. Evaluation of Intestinal Function in Children With Autism and Gastrointestinal Symptoms. *J. Pediatr. Gastroenterol. Nutr.* **2016**, *62*, 687–691. [CrossRef] [PubMed]
13. Yitik Tonkaz, G.; Esin, I.S.; Turan, B.; Uslu, H.; Dursun, O.B. Determinants of Leaky Gut and Gut Microbiota Differences in Children with Autism Spectrum Disorder and Their Siblings. *J. Autism. Dev. Disord.* **2022**, 1–14. [CrossRef] [PubMed]
14. Jaworska, K.; Konop, M.; Bielinska, K.; Hutsch, T.; Dziekiewicz, M.; Banaszkiewicz, A.; Ufnal, M. Inflammatory bowel disease is associated with increased gut-to-blood penetration of short-chain fatty acids: A new, non-invasive marker of a functional intestinal lesion. *Exp. Physiol.* **2019**, *104*, 1226–1236. [CrossRef] [PubMed]
15. Michielan, A.; D'Inca, R. Intestinal Permeability in Inflammatory Bowel Disease: Pathogenesis, Clinical Evaluation, and Therapy of Leaky Gut. *Mediators. Inflamm.* **2015**, *2015*, 628157. [CrossRef]

16. Vindigni, S.M.; Zisman, T.L.; Suskind, D.L.; Damman, C.J. The intestinal microbiome, barrier function, and immune system in inflammatory bowel disease: A tripartite pathophysiological circuit with implications for new therapeutic directions. *Therap. Adv. Gastroenterol.* **2016**, *9*, 606–625. [CrossRef]
17. Collaborators, G.B.D.I.B.D. The global, regional, and national burden of inflammatory bowel disease in 195 countries and territories, 1990-2017: A systematic analysis for the Global Burden of Disease Study 2017. *Lancet Gastroenterol. Hepatol.* **2020**, *5*, 17–30. [CrossRef]
18. Kaplan, G.G.; Ng, S.C. Understanding and Preventing the Global Increase of Inflammatory Bowel Disease. *Gastroenterology* **2017**, *152*, 313–321. [CrossRef]
19. Kaplan, G.G. The global burden of IBD: From 2015 to 2025. *Nat. Rev. Gastroenterol. Hepatol.* **2015**, *12*, 720–727. [CrossRef]
20. Angelis, I.D.; Turco, L. Caco-2 cells as a model for intestinal absorption. *Curr. Protoc. Toxicol.* **2011**, *47*, 20.6.1–20.6.15. [CrossRef]
21. Cheng, K.C.; Li, C.; Uss, A.S. Prediction of oral drug absorption in humans–from cultured cell lines and experimental animals. *Expert. Opin. Drug Metab. Toxicol.* **2008**, *4*, 581–590. [CrossRef] [PubMed]
22. Liu, X.; Zheng, S.; Qin, Y.; Ding, W.; Tu, Y.; Chen, X.; Wu, Y.; Yanhua, L.; Cai, X. Experimental Evaluation of the Transport Mechanisms of PoIFN-alpha in Caco-2 Cells. *Front. Pharmacol.* **2017**, *8*, 781. [CrossRef] [PubMed]
23. Narayani, S.S.; Saravanan, S.; Ravindran, J.; Ramasamy, M.S.; Chitra, J. In vitro anticancer activity of fucoidan extracted from Sargassum cinereum against Caco-2 cells. *Int. J. Biol. Macromol.* **2019**, *138*, 618–628. [CrossRef] [PubMed]
24. Sevin, E.; Dehouck, L.; Fabulas-da Costa, A.; Cecchelli, R.; Dehouck, M.P.; Lundquist, S.; Culot, M. Accelerated Caco-2 cell permeability model for drug discovery. *J. Pharmacol. Toxicol. Methods* **2013**, *68*, 334–339. [CrossRef]
25. Shah, P.; Jogani, V.; Bagchi, T.; Misra, A. Role of Caco-2 cell monolayers in prediction of intestinal drug absorption. *Biotechnol. Prog.* **2006**, *22*, 186–198. [CrossRef]
26. Wang, Y.; Chen, X. QSPR model for Caco-2 cell permeability prediction using a combination of HQPSO and dual-RBF neural network. *RSC Adv.* **2020**, *10*, 42938–42952. [CrossRef]
27. Smetanova, L.; Stetinova, V.; Svoboda, Z.; Kvetina, J. Caco-2 cells, biopharmaceutics classification system (BCS) and biowaiver. *Acta. Medica.* **2011**, *54*, 3–8.
28. Simon-Assmann, P.; Turck, N.; Sidhoum-Jenny, M.; Gradwohl, G.; Kedinger, M. In vitro models of intestinal epithelial cell differentiation. *Cell Biol. Toxicol.* **2007**, *23*, 241–256. [CrossRef]
29. Panse, N.; Gerk, P.M. The Caco-2 Model: Modifications and enhancements to improve efficiency and predictive performance. *Int. J. Pharm.* **2022**, *624*, 122004. [CrossRef]
30. Martinez-Maqueda, D.; Miralles, B.; Recio, I. HT29 Cell Line. In *The Impact of Food Bioactives on Health: In Vitro and Ex Vivo Models*; Verhoeckx, K., Cotter, P., Kleiveland, C., Mackie, A., Swiatecka, D., Eds.; Springer: Cham, Switzerland, 2015; pp. 113–124. [CrossRef]
31. Corfield, A.P.; Carroll, D.; Myerscough, N.; Probert, C.S. Mucins in the gastrointestinal tract in health and disease. *Front. Biosci.* **2001**, *6*, D1321–D1357. [CrossRef]
32. Boegh, M.; Nielsen, H.M. Mucus as a barrier to drug delivery—Understanding and mimicking the barrier properties. *Basic Clin. Pharmacol. Toxicol.* **2015**, *116*, 179–186. [CrossRef] [PubMed]
33. Fang, J.; Wang, H.; Zhou, Y.; Zhang, H.; Zhou, H.; Zhang, X. Slimy partners: The mucus barrier and gut microbiome in ulcerative colitis. *Exp. Mol. Med.* **2021**, *53*, 772–787. [CrossRef] [PubMed]
34. Fernandez-Tome, S.; Ortega Moreno, L.; Chaparro, M.; Gisbert, J.P. Gut Microbiota and Dietary Factors as Modulators of the Mucus Layer in Inflammatory Bowel Disease. *Int. J. Mol. Sci.* **2021**, *22*, 10224. [CrossRef] [PubMed]
35. Han, X.; Ding, S.; Jiang, H.; Liu, G. Roles of Macrophages in the Development and Treatment of Gut Inflammation. *Front. Cell Dev. Biol.* **2021**, *9*, 625423. [CrossRef]
36. Hine, A.M.; Loke, P. Intestinal Macrophages in Resolving Inflammation. *J. Immunol.* **2019**, *203*, 593–599. [CrossRef]
37. Na, Y.R.; Stakenborg, M.; Seok, S.H.; Matteoli, G. Macrophages in intestinal inflammation and resolution: A potential therapeutic target in IBD. *Nat. Rev. Gastroenterol. Hepatol.* **2019**, *16*, 531–543. [CrossRef] [PubMed]
38. Calatayud, M.; Dezutter, O.; Hernandez-Sanabria, E.; Hidalgo-Martinez, S.; Meysman, F.J.R.; Van de Wiele, T. Development of a host-microbiome model of the small intestine. *FASEB J.* **2019**, *33*, 3985–3996. [CrossRef] [PubMed]
39. Kämpfer, A.A.; Shah, U.K.; Chu, S.L.; Busch, M.; Büttner, V.; He, R.; Rothen-Rutishauser, B.; Schins, R.P.; Jenkins, G.J. Inter-laboratory comparison of an intestinal triple culture to confirm transferability and reproducibility. *In Vitro Model.* **2022**, 1–9. [CrossRef]
40. Ponce de Leon-Rodriguez, M.D.C.; Guyot, J.P.; Laurent-Babot, C. Intestinal in vitro cell culture models and their potential to study the effect of food components on intestinal inflammation. *Crit. Rev. Food Sci. Nutr.* **2019**, *59*, 3648–3666. [CrossRef]
41. Foey, A.; Habil, N.; Strachan, A.; Beal, J. Lacticaseibacillus casei Strain Shirota Modulates Macrophage-Intestinal Epithelial Cell Co-Culture Barrier Integrity, Bacterial Sensing and Inflammatory Cytokines. *Microorganisms* **2022**, *10*, 2087. [CrossRef]
42. Hartwig, O.; Loretz, B.; Nougarede, A.; Jary, D.; Sulpice, E.; Gidrol, X.; Navarro, F.; Lehr, C.M. Leaky gut model of the human intestinal mucosa for testing siRNA-based nanomedicine targeting JAK1. *J. Control Release* **2022**, *345*, 646–660. [CrossRef] [PubMed]
43. Kordulewska, N.K.; Topa, J.; Tanska, M.; Cieslinska, A.; Fiedorowicz, E.; Savelkoul, H.F.J.; Jarmolowska, B. Modulatory Effects of Osthole on Lipopolysaccharides-Induced Inflammation in Caco-2 Cell Monolayer and Co-Cultures with THP-1 and THP-1-Derived Macrophages. *Nutrients* **2020**, *13*, 123. [CrossRef] [PubMed]

44. Schnur, S.; Wahl, V.; Metz, J.K. Inflammatory bowel disease addressed by Caco-2 and monocyte-derived macrophages: An opportunity for an in vitro drug screening assay. *In Vitro Model.* **2022**, *1*, 363–383. [CrossRef]
45. Kampfer, A.A.M.; Busch, M.; Buttner, V.; Bredeck, G.; Stahlmecke, B.; Hellack, B.; Masson, I.; Sofranko, A.; Albrecht, C.; Schins, R.P.F. Model Complexity as Determining Factor for In Vitro Nanosafety Studies: Effects of Silver and Titanium Dioxide Nanomaterials in Intestinal Models. *Small* **2021**, *17*, e2004223. [CrossRef] [PubMed]
46. Kampfer, A.A.M.; Urban, P.; Gioria, S.; Kanase, N.; Stone, V.; Kinsner-Ovaskainen, A. Development of an in vitro co-culture model to mimic the human intestine in healthy and diseased state. *Toxicol. In Vitro* **2017**, *45*, 31–43. [CrossRef]
47. Marescotti, D.; Lo Sasso, G.; Guerrera, D.; Renggli, K.; Ruiz Castro, P.A.; Piault, R.; Jaquet, V.; Moine, F.; Luettich, K.; Frentzel, S.; et al. Development of an Advanced Multicellular Intestinal Model for Assessing Immunomodulatory Properties of Anti-Inflammatory Compounds. *Front. Pharmacol.* **2021**, *12*, 639716. [CrossRef]
48. Busch, M.; Kampfer, A.A.M.; Schins, R.P.F. An inverted in vitro triple culture model of the healthy and inflamed intestine: Adverse effects of polyethylene particles. *Chemosphere* **2021**, *284*, 131345. [CrossRef]
49. Srinivasan, B.; Kolli, A.R.; Esch, M.B.; Abaci, H.E.; Shuler, M.L.; Hickman, J.J. TEER measurement techniques for in vitro barrier model systems. *J. Lab. Autom.* **2015**, *20*, 107–126. [CrossRef]
50. Wang, F.; Graham, W.V.; Wang, Y.; Witkowski, E.D.; Schwarz, B.T.; Turner, J.R. Interferon-gamma and tumor necrosis factor-alpha synergize to induce intestinal epithelial barrier dysfunction by up-regulating myosin light chain kinase expression. *Am. J. Pathol.* **2005**, *166*, 409–419. [CrossRef]
51. Fasano, A. Intestinal permeability and its regulation by zonulin: Diagnostic and therapeutic implications. *Clin. Gastroenterol. Hepatol.* **2012**, *10*, 1096–1100. [CrossRef]
52. Andreasen, A.S.; Krabbe, K.S.; Krogh-Madsen, R.; Taudorf, S.; Pedersen, B.K.; Moller, K. Human endotoxemia as a model of systemic inflammation. *Curr. Med. Chem.* **2008**, *15*, 1697–1705. [CrossRef] [PubMed]
53. Sewell, G.W.; Kaser, A. Interleukin-23 in the Pathogenesis of Inflammatory Bowel Disease and Implications for Therapeutic Intervention. *J. Crohns. Colitis.* **2022**, *16*, ii3–ii19. [CrossRef] [PubMed]
54. Witkin, S.S.; Alvi, S.; Bongiovanni, A.M.; Linhares, I.M.; Ledger, W.J. Lactic acid stimulates interleukin-23 production by peripheral blood mononuclear cells exposed to bacterial lipopolysaccharide. *FEMS Immunol. Med. Microbiol.* **2011**, *61*, 153–158. [CrossRef] [PubMed]
55. Ananthakrishnan, A.N.; Bernstein, C.N.; Iliopoulos, D.; Macpherson, A.; Neurath, M.F.; Ali, R.A.R.; Vavricka, S.R.; Fiocchi, C. Environmental triggers in IBD: A review of progress and evidence. *Nat. Rev. Gastroenterol. Hepatol.* **2018**, *15*, 39–49. [CrossRef]
56. Khor, B.; Gardet, A.; Xavier, R.J. Genetics and pathogenesis of inflammatory bowel disease. *Nature* **2011**, *474*, 307–317. [CrossRef]
57. Liu, T.C.; Stappenbeck, T.S. Genetics and Pathogenesis of Inflammatory Bowel Disease. *Annu. Rev. Pathol.* **2016**, *11*, 127–148. [CrossRef]
58. Wallace, K.L.; Zheng, L.B.; Kanazawa, Y.; Shih, D.Q. Immunopathology of inflammatory bowel disease. *World J. Gastroenterol.* **2014**, *20*, 6–21. [CrossRef]
59. Andrews, C.; McLean, M.H.; Durum, S.K. Cytokine Tuning of Intestinal Epithelial Function. *Front. Immunol.* **2018**, *9*, 1270. [CrossRef]
60. Maria-Ferreira, D.; Nascimento, A.M.; Cipriani, T.R.; Santana-Filho, A.P.; Watanabe, P.D.S.; Sant Ana, D.M.G.; Luciano, F.B.; Bocate, K.C.P.; van den Wijngaard, R.M.; Werner, M.F.P.; et al. Rhamnogalacturonan, a chemically-defined polysaccharide, improves intestinal barrier function in DSS-induced colitis in mice and human Caco-2 cells. *Sci. Rep.* **2018**, *8*, 12261. [CrossRef]
61. Liang, Q.; Ren, X.; Chalamaiah, M.; Ma, H. Simulated gastrointestinal digests of corn protein hydrolysate alleviate inflammation in caco-2 cells and a mouse model of colitis. *J. Food Sci. Technol.* **2020**, *57*, 2079–2088. [CrossRef]
62. Johansson, M.E.; Larsson, J.M.; Hansson, G.C. The two mucus layers of colon are organized by the MUC2 mucin, whereas the outer layer is a legislator of host-microbial interactions. *Proc. Natl. Acad. Sci. USA* **2011**, *108* (Suppl. S1), 4659–4665. [CrossRef] [PubMed]
63. Chen, X.M.; Elisia, I.; Kitts, D.D. Defining conditions for the co-culture of Caco-2 and HT29-MTX cells using Taguchi design. *J. Pharmacol. Toxicol. Methods* **2010**, *61*, 334–342. [CrossRef] [PubMed]
64. Lozoya-Agullo, I.; Araujo, F.; Gonzalez-Alvarez, I.; Merino-Sanjuan, M.; Gonzalez-Alvarez, M.; Bermejo, M.; Sarmento, B. Usefulness of Caco-2/HT29-MTX and Caco-2/HT29-MTX/Raji B Coculture Models To Predict Intestinal and Colonic Permeability Compared to Caco-2 Monoculture. *Mol. Pharm.* **2017**, *14*, 1264–1270. [CrossRef] [PubMed]
65. Pan, F.; Han, L.; Zhang, Y.; Yu, Y.; Liu, J. Optimization of Caco-2 and HT29 co-culture in vitro cell models for permeability studies. *Int. J. Food Sci. Nutr.* **2015**, *66*, 680–685. [CrossRef]
66. Barnett, A.M.; Roy, N.C.; Cookson, A.L.; McNabb, W.C. Metabolism of Caprine Milk Carbohydrates by Probiotic Bacteria and Caco-2:HT29(-)MTX Epithelial Co-Cultures and Their Impact on Intestinal Barrier Integrity. *Nutrients* **2018**, *10*, 949. [CrossRef]
67. Garcia-Rodriguez, A.; Vila, L.; Cortes, C.; Hernandez, A.; Marcos, R. Effects of differently shaped TiO$_2$NPs (nanospheres, nanorods and nanowires) on the in vitro model (Caco-2/HT29) of the intestinal barrier. *Part. Fibre. Toxicol.* **2018**, *15*, 33. [CrossRef]
68. Hu, W.; Feng, P.; Zhang, M.; Tian, T.; Wang, S.; Zhao, B.; Li, Y.; Wang, S.; Wu, C. Endotoxins Induced ECM-Receptor Interaction Pathway Signal Effect on the Function of MUC2 in Caco2/HT29 Co-Culture Cells. *Front. Immunol.* **2022**, *13*, 916933. [CrossRef]
69. Le, N.P.K.; Herz, C.; Gomes, J.V.D.; Forster, N.; Antoniadou, K.; Mittermeier-Klessinger, V.K.; Mewis, I.; Dawid, C.; Ulrichs, C.; Lamy, E. Comparative Anti-Inflammatory Effects of Salix Cortex Extracts and Acetylsalicylic Acid in SARS-CoV-2 Peptide and LPS-Activated Human In Vitro Systems. *Int. J. Mol. Sci.* **2021**, *22*, 6766. [CrossRef]

70. Bain, C.C.; Mowat, A.M. Macrophages in intestinal homeostasis and inflammation. *Immunol. Rev.* **2014**, *260*, 102–117. [CrossRef]
71. Geremia, A.; Arancibia-Carcamo, C.V. Innate Lymphoid Cells in Intestinal Inflammation. *Front. Immunol.* **2017**, *8*, 1296. [CrossRef]
72. Liu, L.; Lu, Y.; Xu, C.; Chen, H.; Wang, X.; Wang, Y.; Cai, B.; Li, B.; Verstrepen, L.; Ghyselinck, J.; et al. The Modulation of Chaihu Shugan Formula on Microbiota Composition in the Simulator of the Human Intestinal Microbial Ecosystem Technology Platform and its Influence on Gut Barrier and Intestinal Immunity in Caco-2/THP1-Blue Cell Co-Culture Model. *Front. Pharmacol.* **2022**, *13*, 820543. [CrossRef] [PubMed]
73. Stevens, Y.; de Bie, T.; Pinheiro, I.; Elizalde, M.; Masclee, A.; Jonkers, D. The effects of citrus flavonoids and their metabolites on immune-mediated intestinal barrier disruption using an in vitro co-culture model. *Br. J. Nutr.* **2022**, *128*, 1917–1926. [CrossRef] [PubMed]
74. Ji, Y.K.; Lee, S.M.; Kim, N.H.; Tu, N.V.; Kim, Y.N.; Heo, J.D.; Jeong, E.J.; Rho, J.R. Stereochemical Determination of Fistularins Isolated from the Marine Sponge Ecionemia acervus and Their Regulatory Effect on Intestinal Inflammation. *Mar. Drugs* **2021**, *19*, 170. [CrossRef] [PubMed]
75. Kim, Y.N.; Ji, Y.K.; Kim, N.H.; Van Tu, N.; Rho, J.R.; Jeong, E.J. Isoquinolinequinone Derivatives from a Marine Sponge (Haliclona sp.) Regulate Inflammation in In Vitro System of Intestine. *Mar. Drugs* **2021**, *19*, 90. [CrossRef] [PubMed]
76. Lee, S.M.; Kim, N.H.; Lee, S.; Kim, Y.N.; Heo, J.D.; Rho, J.R.; Jeong, E.J. (10Z)-Debromohymenialdisine from Marine Sponge Stylissa sp. Regulates Intestinal Inflammatory Responses in Co-Culture Model of Epithelial Caco-2 Cells and THP-1 Macrophage Cells. *Molecules* **2019**, *24*, 3394. [CrossRef]
77. Notararigo, S.; Varela, E.; Otal, A.; Antolin, M.; Guarner, F.; Lopez, P. Anti-Inflammatory Effect of an O-2-Substituted (1-3)-beta-D-Glucan Produced by Pediococcus parvulus 2.6 in a Caco-2 PMA-THP-1 Co-Culture Model. *Int. J. Mol. Sci.* **2022**, *23*, 1527. [CrossRef]
78. Mecocci, S.; Ottaviani, A.; Razzuoli, E.; Fiorani, P.; Pietrucci, D.; De Ciucis, C.G.; Dei Giudici, S.; Franzoni, G.; Chillemi, G.; Cappelli, K. Cow Milk Extracellular Vesicle Effects on an In Vitro Model of Intestinal Inflammation. *Biomedicines* **2022**, *10*, 570. [CrossRef]
79. Kaulmann, A.; Legay, S.; Schneider, Y.J.; Hoffmann, L.; Bohn, T. Inflammation related responses of intestinal cells to plum and cabbage digesta with differential carotenoid and polyphenol profiles following simulated gastrointestinal digestion. *Mol. Nutr. Food Res.* **2016**, *60*, 992–1005. [CrossRef]
80. Busch, M.; Bredeck, G.; Kampfer, A.A.M.; Schins, R.P.F. Investigations of acute effects of polystyrene and polyvinyl chloride micro- and nanoplastics in an advanced in vitro triple culture model of the healthy and inflamed intestine. *Environ. Res.* **2021**, *193*, 110536. [CrossRef]
81. Busch, M.; Ramachandran, H.; Wahle, T.; Rossi, A.; Schins, R.P.F. Investigating the Role of the NLRP3 Inflammasome Pathway in Acute Intestinal Inflammation: Use of THP-1 Knockout Cell Lines in an Advanced Triple Culture Model. *Front. Immunol.* **2022**, *13*, 898039. [CrossRef]
82. Park, B.U.; Park, S.M.; Lee, K.P.; Lee, S.J.; Nam, Y.E.; Park, H.S.; Eom, S.; Lim, J.O.; Kim, D.S.; Kim, H.K. Collagen immobilization on ultra-thin nanofiber membrane to promote in vitro endothelial monolayer formation. *J. Tissue Eng.* **2019**, *10*, 2041731419887833. [CrossRef] [PubMed]
83. Teplicky, T.; Mateasik, A.; Balazsiova, Z.; Kajo, K.; Vallova, M.; Filova, B.; Trnka, M.; Cunderlikova, B. Phenotypical modifications of immune cells are enhanced by extracellular matrix. *Exp. Cell. Res.* **2021**, *405*, 112710. [CrossRef] [PubMed]
84. Vaday, G.G.; Lider, O. Extracellular matrix moieties, cytokines, and enzymes: Dynamic effects on immune cell behavior and inflammation. *J. Leukoc. Biol.* **2000**, *67*, 149–159. [CrossRef]
85. Turner, J.R. Intestinal mucosal barrier function in health and disease. *Nat. Rev. Immunol.* **2009**, *9*, 799–809. [CrossRef] [PubMed]
86. Zihni, C.; Mills, C.; Matter, K.; Balda, M.S. Tight junctions: From simple barriers to multifunctional molecular gates. *Nat. Rev. Mol. Cell Biol.* **2016**, *17*, 564–580. [CrossRef]
87. Lechuga, S.; Ivanov, A.I. Disruption of the epithelial barrier during intestinal inflammation: Quest for new molecules and mechanisms. *Biochim. Biophys. Acta Mol. Cell Res.* **2017**, *1864*, 1183–1194. [CrossRef] [PubMed]
88. Lee, B.; Moon, K.M.; Kim, C.Y. Tight Junction in the Intestinal Epithelium: Its Association with Diseases and Regulation by Phytochemicals. *J. Immunol. Res.* **2018**, *2018*, 2645465. [CrossRef] [PubMed]
89. Caviglia, G.P.; Dughera, F.; Ribaldone, D.G.; Rosso, C.; Abate, M.L.; Pellicano, R.; Bresso, F.; Smedile, A.; Saracco, G.M.; Astegiano, M. Serum zonulin in patients with inflammatory bowel disease: A pilot study. *Minerva. Med.* **2019**, *110*, 95–100. [CrossRef]
90. Wang, X.; Memon, A.A.; Palmer, K.; Hedelius, A.; Sundquist, J.; Sundquist, K. The association of zonulin-related proteins with prevalent and incident inflammatory bowel disease. *BMC Gastroenterol.* **2022**, *22*, 3. [CrossRef]
91. Lacombe, L.A.C.; Matiollo, C.; Rosa, J.S.D.; Felisberto, M.; Dalmarco, E.M.; Schiavon, L.L. Factors Associated with Circulating Zonulin in Inflammatory Bowel Disease. *Arq. Gastroenterol.* **2022**, *59*, 238–243. [CrossRef]
92. Szymanska, E.; Wierzbicka, A.; Dadalski, M.; Kierkus, J. Fecal Zonulin as a Noninvasive Biomarker of Intestinal Permeability in Pediatric Patients with Inflammatory Bowel Diseases-Correlation with Disease Activity and Fecal Calprotectin. *J. Clin. Med.* **2021**, *10*, 3905. [CrossRef] [PubMed]
93. Malickova, K.; Francova, I.; Lukas, M.; Kolar, M.; Kralikova, E.; Bortlik, M.; Duricova, D.; Stepankova, L.; Zvolska, K.; Pankova, A.; et al. Fecal zonulin is elevated in Crohn's disease and in cigarette smokers. *Pract. Lab. Med.* **2017**, *9*, 39–44. [CrossRef] [PubMed]

94. Fasano, A. Zonulin, regulation of tight junctions, and autoimmune diseases. *Ann. N. Y. Acad. Sci.* **2012**, *1258*, 25–33. [CrossRef]
95. Sturgeon, C.; Fasano, A. Zonulin, a regulator of epithelial and endothelial barrier functions, and its involvement in chronic inflammatory diseases. *Tissue Barriers* **2016**, *4*, e1251384. [CrossRef]
96. Bevivino, G.; Monteleone, G. Advances in understanding the role of cytokines in inflammatory bowel disease. *Expert Rev. Gastroenterol. Hepatol.* **2018**, *12*, 907–915. [CrossRef]
97. Guan, Q.; Zhang, J. Recent Advances: The Imbalance of Cytokines in the Pathogenesis of Inflammatory Bowel Disease. *Mediat. Inflamm.* **2017**, *2017*, 4810258. [CrossRef] [PubMed]
98. Nakase, H.; Sato, N.; Mizuno, N.; Ikawa, Y. The influence of cytokines on the complex pathology of ulcerative colitis. *Autoimmun. Rev.* **2022**, *21*, 103017. [CrossRef] [PubMed]
99. Neurath, M.F. Cytokines in inflammatory bowel disease. *Nat. Rev. Immunol.* **2014**, *14*, 329–342. [CrossRef]
100. Caviglia, G.P.; Ribaldone, D.G.; Nicolosi, A.; Pellicano, R. Cytokines and Biologic Therapy in Patients with Inflammatory Bowel Diseases. *Gastroenterol. Insights* **2021**, *12*, 443–445. [CrossRef]
101. Friedrich, M.; Pohin, M.; Powrie, F. Cytokine Networks in the Pathophysiology of Inflammatory Bowel Disease. *Immunity* **2019**, *50*, 992–1006. [CrossRef]
102. Berns, M.; Hommes, D.W. Anti-TNF-alpha therapies for the treatment of Crohn's disease: The past, present and future. *Expert Opin. Investig. Drugs* **2016**, *25*, 129–143. [CrossRef] [PubMed]
103. Ford, A.C.; Sandborn, W.J.; Khan, K.J.; Hanauer, S.B.; Talley, N.J.; Moayyedi, P. Efficacy of biological therapies in inflammatory bowel disease: Systematic review and meta-analysis. *Am. J. Gastroenterol.* **2011**, *106*, 644–659. [CrossRef] [PubMed]
104. Ungar, B.; Kopylov, U. Advances in the development of new biologics in inflammatory bowel disease. *Ann. Gastroenterol.* **2016**, *29*, 243–248. [CrossRef] [PubMed]
105. Bunte, K.; Beikler, T. Th17 Cells and the IL-23/IL-17 Axis in the Pathogenesis of Periodontitis and Immune-Mediated Inflammatory Diseases. *Int. J. Mol. Sci.* **2019**, *20*, 3394. [CrossRef] [PubMed]
106. Schmitt, H.; Neurath, M.F.; Atreya, R. Role of the IL23/IL17 Pathway in Crohn's Disease. *Front. Immunol.* **2021**, *12*, 622934. [CrossRef] [PubMed]
107. Noviello, D.; Mager, R.; Roda, G.; Borroni, R.G.; Fiorino, G.; Vetrano, S. The IL23-IL17 Immune Axis in the Treatment of Ulcerative Colitis: Successes, Defeats, and Ongoing Challenges. *Front. Immunol.* **2021**, *12*, 611256. [CrossRef]
108. Bosshart, H.; Heinzelmann, M. THP-1 cells as a model for human monocytes. *Ann. Transl. Med.* **2016**, *4*, 438. [CrossRef]

Disclaimer/Publisher's Note: The statements, opinions and data contained in all publications are solely those of the individual author(s) and contributor(s) and not of MDPI and/or the editor(s). MDPI and/or the editor(s) disclaim responsibility for any injury to people or property resulting from any ideas, methods, instructions or products referred to in the content.

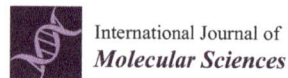

Article

Proteolytic Activity of the Paracaspase MALT1 Is Involved in Epithelial Restitution and Mucosal Healing

Leonie Wittner [1,†], Lukas Wagener [1,†], Jakob J. Wiese [2], Iris Stolzer [1], Susanne M. Krug [3], Elisabeth Naschberger [4], Rene Jackstadt [5], Rudi Beyaert [6], Raja Atreya [1,7,8,9], Anja A. Kühl [8,9,10], Gregor Sturm [11], Miguel Gonzalez-Acera [1], Jay V. Patankar [1,8,9], Christoph Becker [1,7,8,9], Britta Siegmund [2,8,9], Zlatko Trajanoski [8,9,11], Beate Winner [7,12,13], Markus F. Neurath [1,6,8,9], Michael Schumann [2,8,9] and Claudia Günther [1,7,8,9,*]

1. Department of Medicine 1, Friedrich-Alexander University Erlangen-Nürnberg, 91054 Erlangen, Germany; leonie.wittner@mail.de (L.W.); lukas.wagener@fau.de (L.W.); iris.stolzer@uk-erlangen.de (I.S.); raja.atreya@uk-erlangen.de (R.A.); miguel.gonzalezacera@uk-erlangen.de (M.G.-A.); jay.patankar@uk-erlangen.de (J.V.P.); christoph.becker@uk-erlangen.de (C.B.); markus.neurath@uk-erlangen.de (M.F.N.)
2. Department of Gastroenterology, Rheumatology and Infectious Diseases, Charité-Universitätsmedizin Berlin, Campus Benjamin Franklin, 12203 Berlin, Germany; jakob.wiese@charite.de (J.J.W.); britta.siegmund@charite.de (B.S.); michael.schumann@charite.de (M.S.)
3. Clinical Physiology/Nutritional Medicine, Charité-Universitätsmedizin Berlin, Campus Benjamin Franklin, 12203 Berlin, Germany; susanne.m.krug@charite.de
4. Division Molecular and Experimental Surgery, Friedrich-Alexander University Erlangen-Nürnberg, 91054 Erlangen, Germany; elisabeth.naschberger@uk-erlangen.de
5. Cancer Progression and Metastasis Group, German Cancer Research Center (DKFZ), 69120 Heidelberg, Germany; r.jackstadt@hi-stem.de
6. VIB—UGent Center for Inflammation Research, Department of Biomedical Molecular Biology, Ghent University, 9052 Ghent, Belgium; rudi.beyaert@irc.vib-ugent.be
7. Deutsches Zentrum Immuntherapie, Friedrich-Alexander University Erlangen-Nürnberg, 91054 Erlangen, Germany; beate.winner@fau.de
8. IBDome Consortium, 91054 Erlangen, Germany; anja.kuehl@charite.de (A.A.K.); zlatko.trajanoski@i-med.ac.at (Z.T.)
9. IBDome Consortium, 12203 Berlin, Germany
10. iPATH.Berlin-Core Unit, Charité-Universitätsmedizin Berlin, Campus Benjamin Franklin, 12203 Berlin, Germany
11. Biocenter, Institute of Bioinformatics, Medical University of Innsbruck, 6020 Innsbruck, Austria; gregor.sturm@i-med.ac.at
12. Department of Stem Cell Biology, Friedrich-Alexander University Erlangen-Nürnberg, 91054 Erlangen, Germany
13. Center of Rare Diseases (ZSEER), University Hospital Erlangen, Friedrich-Alexander University Erlangen-Nürnberg, 91054 Erlangen, Germany
* Correspondence: c.guenther@uk-erlangen.de
† These authors contributed equally to this work.

Abstract: The paracaspase MALT1 is a crucial regulator of immune responses in various cellular contexts. Recently, there is increasing evidence suggesting that MALT1 might represent a novel key player in mucosal inflammation. However, the molecular mechanisms underlying this process and the targeted cell population remain unclear. In this study, we investigate the role of MALT1 proteolytic activity in the context of mucosal inflammation. We demonstrate a significant enrichment of MALT1 gene and protein expression in colonic epithelial cells of UC patients, as well as in the context of experimental colitis. Mechanistically we demonstrate that MALT1 protease function inhibits ferroptosis, a form of iron-dependent cell death, upstream of NF-κB signaling, which can promote inflammation and tissue damage in IBD. We further show that MALT1 activity contributes to STAT3 signaling, which is essential for the regeneration of the intestinal epithelium after injury. In summary, our data strongly suggests that the protease function of MALT1 plays a critical role in the regulation of immune and inflammatory responses, as well as mucosal healing. Understanding the mechanisms by which MALT1 protease function regulates these processes may offer novel therapeutic targets for the treatment of IBD and other inflammatory diseases.

Keywords: ulcerative colitis; mucosal wound healing; ferroptosis

1. Introduction

Ulcerative colitis (UC) is a chronically relapsing inflammatory disease starting in the rectum and extending throughout the colon. Patients suffer from abdominal pain, rectal bleeding, and diarrhea. The underlying etiology is multifactorial and is associated with genetic predisposition, environmental risk factors, imbalanced microbial composition, dysregulated immune responses, and intestinal epithelial barrier dysfunction [1,2]. In this multifactorial setting, the intestinal epithelium is a single epithelial layer that serves as a selective permeable barrier between the intestinal lumen and the underlying immune cell compartment and thus maintains mucosal homeostasis [3]. Deregulated cell death in the intestinal epithelium is a critical driver of barrier dysfunction and subsequent inflammation [4–8]. Among the different types of inflammatory cell death, ferroptosis has been recently described as an important regulated cell death pathway contributing to the pathogenesis of UC. In the intestinal epithelium, ferroptotic cell death is mediated by ER-stress and can be inhibited by phosphorylation of the NF-κB subunit p65 [6].

NF-κB signaling has been well characterized in the context of intestinal inflammation, infection and cancer, where it can exert both detrimental and protective functions. Especially during mucosal wound healing, it has been reported that NF-κB mediates proliferative and pro-survival gene expression and thereby is considered to play an important protective function. Under steady state conditions, the NF-κB subunit p65 mediates anti-apoptotic signaling and preserves intestinal stem cell homeostasis. In the context of epithelial injury, p65 is highly expressed especially at wound edges to induce cell migration and mucosal healing [9]. Accordingly, loss of p65 in the intestinal epithelium is associated with severe mucosal injury and susceptibility to experimental colitis triggered by deregulated intestinal proliferation [10]. Activity of the NF-κB essential modulator (NEMO) is required for NF-κB activation in response to inflammatory stimuli. Intestinal epithelial cell (IEC) specific deletion of NEMO negatively affects epithelial barrier function through excessive activation of TNF-mediated apoptosis in colonocytes associated with severe chronic inflammation [11].

The paracaspase MALT1 (mucosa-associated lymphoid tissue lymphoma translocation protein 1) is an upstream signaling component of NF-κB with high therapeutic potential. Although these data implicate a potential role of MALT1 in orchestrating mucosal immune response, inflammation and tumorigenesis, the role of MALT1 scaffolding and proteolytic activity in the pathogenesis of mucosal inflammation has not been addressed. So far it is known, that various immunoreceptors of the innate and adaptive immune response activate MALT1, which is best characterized in the context of T cell receptor (TCR) and B cell receptor (BCR) mediated lymphocyte development, activation and proliferation [12–14]. It is further involved in ITAM- (immunoreceptor tyrosine-based activation motif) coupled natural killer (NK) cell receptor signaling [15] and in non-hematopoietic cells in epidermal growth factor receptor (EGFR) signaling [16] and G protein-coupled receptor (GPCR) signaling [17]. For a long time MALT1 was believed to function as a scaffold protein, providing an assembly platform for NF-κB activation. Besides its scaffold function, MALT1 was described as a paracaspase carrying a proteolytic activity. The protease activity of MALT1 facilitates optimal NF-κB and AP-1 activation by proteolytic cleavage of negative regulators, such as A20, CYLD and RELB. Other MALT1 substrates regulate mRNA stability (Regnase-1, Roquin-1) [18–20]. Upon surface receptor activation, CARMA/CARD, BCL10 and MALT1 form the CBM complex serving as a protein assembly platform for NF-κB activation [17,21]. TRAF6 (TNF receptor associated factor 6) and NEMO are further recruited to the CBM complex to induce a NF-κB activation cascade in response to TCR, BCR and GPCR activation [21–23]. Mutations in genes belonging to the CBM complex and consequent loss of MALT1 function are associated with human combined immunodeficiency [14,24].

Symptoms of human MALT1 deficiency include severe inflammation of the esophagus accompanied by absence of naïve and memory B cell populations and functional B and T cell defects [14]. In line with this, mice expressing a genetically inactivated MALT1 protease variant display immune defects including a reduction in the regulatory T cell and CD4$^+$ T cell compartment. They develop a progressive systemic inflammation early, driven by an altered T cell compartment and accompanied by lymphocyte infiltration in various organs also affecting the gastrointestinal tract [12,25]. Protease mutant mice further display an elevated disease burden in experimental DSS colitis compared to wild-type controls [26]. Accordingly, several lines of evidence indicate that MALT1 protease might play an important role in maintaining mucosal homeostasis and that dysfunction or deregulation contributes to the development and maintenance of intestinal inflammation.

While MALT1 protease has been proposed as a therapeutic target in acute colitis [27], its role in mucosal healing remains unclear. Disruption of epithelial barrier function and thus loss of intestinal homeostasis is a key feature of inflammatory bowel disease (IBD). Therefore, the recovery process requires thorough wound healing, which is also mediated by proliferative and pro-survival NF-κB signaling. The objective of this study was to identify if and how the MALT1 protease is involved in NF-κB mediated wound healing in response to intestinal epithelial injury.

2. Results

2.1. Epithelial MALT1 Is Upregulated in Ulcerative Colitis Patients

In order to investigate the role of MALT1 in the context of chronic intestinal inflammation, we initially analyzed *MALT1* expression patterns in IBD patients. An RNA-seq dataset from colonic tissue of non-IBD, Crohn's disease (CD) and ulcerative colitis (UC) patients revealed significantly increased *MALT1* gene expression in the colon of UC patients (Figure 1A), which was confirmed by quantification of whole colon RNA lysates derived from a cohort of UC patients and healthy controls (Figure 1B). Similarly, analysis of the PROTECT cohort (GSE109142), an RNA-seq dataset of rectal biopsies derived from newly-diagnosed pediatric UC patients prior to therapeutic intervention [28], revealed a 1.5 fold upregulation of *MALT1* and even stronger upregulation of *CARD9* (2.9 fold change), *CARD11* (2.5 fold change), *CARD14* (3.4 fold change), and *p100/p52* (2.9 fold change) (Figure 1C), additional members of the CBM signalosome. Within the CARD family, *CARD14* was particularly upregulated in UC patients and correlated positively with disease severity. Accordingly, moderate-to-severe inflammation was associated with higher *CARD14* expression than mild inflammation. (Figure 1D) We further confirmed an increase in MALT1 on a protein level, which was most prominent in intestinal epithelial cells, as demonstrated by immunofluorescence co-staining with the epithelial cell marker E-cadherin in colonic UC sections (Figure 1E). This increase was also confirmed by quantification of the immunofluorescence signal (Figure 1F). Together, this suggests a potential contribution of epithelial MALT1 to the pathogenesis of UC.

2.2. Malt1 Expression Is Upregulated in Response to Mucosal Injury

To study the expression of *Malt1* during the onset, progression and resolution of mucosal inflammation, we investigated *Malt1* expression in an RNA-seq dataset from a murine experimental dextran sodium sulfate (DSS) colitis time course. We detected significantly elevated expression levels in fully inflamed colonic tissue, which subsided during the resolution of the inflammation (Figure 2A). In line with this, *Card9* expression, an essential regulator of intestinal epithelial wound healing in the context of colitis [29] and member of the CBM signalosome, was significantly upregulated during intestinal inflammation. We further observed significantly elevated expression levels of the MALT1 effector proteins *pP100/p52* and *Relb* during high inflammation and resolution, respectively (Figure 2A). We additionally compared *Malt1* expression levels in an RNA-seq dataset from a murine wound healing time course. Under these experimental conditions, *Malt1* and *Card11* were significantly upregulated at 48 h after wounding, indicating a potential contribution to epithelial proliferation and mucosal healing. Early upregulation of *Bcl10* and *Card9* further suggests a role for the CBM complex in mucosal wound healing, that potentially induces classical as well as alternative NF-κB signaling as shown by consistent upregulation of *p65* and *p100/p52* (Figure 2B).

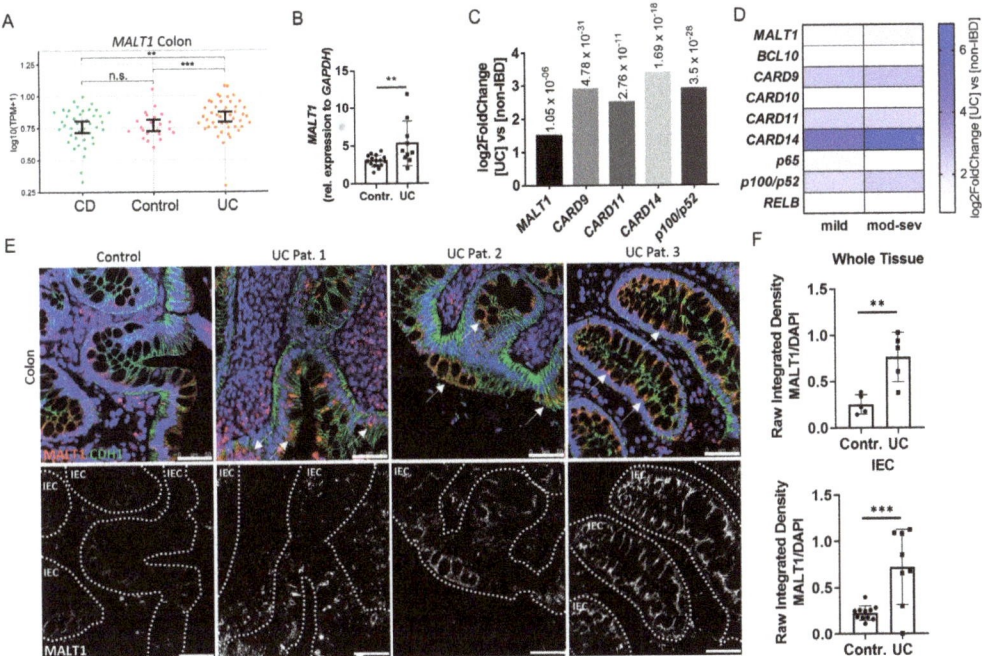

Figure 1. Increased intestinal epithelial *MALT1* expression in UC patients. (**A**) RNA-seq expression levels of *MALT1* in colon tissue samples derived from Crohn's disease (CD) (n = 41) and ulcerative colitis (UC) (n = 46) patients and controls (n = 22). *p* values are derived from a two-tailed Wilcoxon test. Error bars represent 95% confidence intervals of the mean. (**B**) Quantitative real-time PCR of *MALT1* mRNA expression levels in whole colon biopsies derived from control individuals (n = 16) and UC patients (n = 10). ** $p < 0.01$ in unpaired two-tailed *t*-test, error bars represent mean ± SD, 95% CI. (**C**) RNA-seq expression analysis of significantly altered CBM complex (*MALT1, CARD9, -11, -14*) and NF-κB genes (*p100/p52*) in colon biopsies derived from treatment-naïve UC patients (n = 206) and non-IBD controls (n = 20). *p* values are indicated with the fold change. ANOVA for multiple comparisons, error bars represent mean ± SD, 95% CI. (**D**) RNA-seq expression analysis of CBM complex (*MALT1, BCL10, CARD9–11, -14*) and NF-κB (*p65, p100/p52, RELB*) genes in mild (n = 53) and moderate–severe (mod–sev, n = 152) inflamed treatment-naïve UC patients and non-IBD controls (n = 20). (**E**) Representative images of colon cross sections from control individuals and UC patients immunohistochemically stained with antibodies against E-Cadherin (CDH1, green) and MALT1 (red), nuclei were counterstained with Hoechst 33342 (blue) (upper panel). High MALT1 expressing intestinal epithelial areas are indicated with arrows. Representation of MALT1 single channel (white), intestinal epithelial cells (IEC) are indicated with dashed lines (lower panel) (scale bar: 50 µm). (**F**) Quantification of MALT1 expression normalized to Hoechst intensity in whole colon tissue and IECs. n.s. (not significant), ** $p < 0.01$, *** $p < 0.001$ in unpaired two-tailed *t*-test, error bars represent mean ± SD, 95% CI.

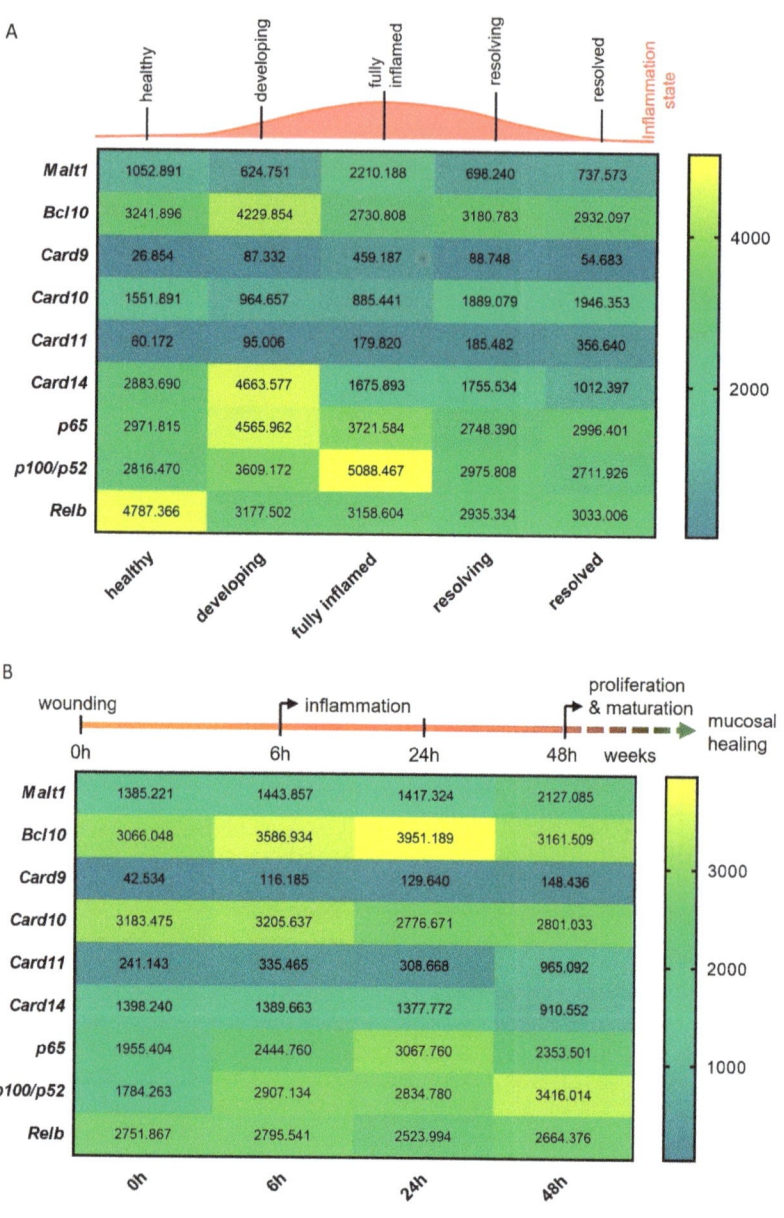

Figure 2. MALT1-mediated signaling is activated during experimental colitis and epithelial damage. (**A**,**B**) RNA-seq expression analyses of CBM complex genes (*Malt1*, *Bcl10*, *Card9–11*, *-14*) and NF-κB subunit genes (*p65*, *p100/p52*, *Relb*) during (**A**) a murine DSS colitis time course (n = 3) and (**B**) a murine colon wound healing time course (n = 3).

In summary these data point to a central role of MALT1 in orchestrating inflammatory signaling in response to mucosal injury, potentially promoting NF-κB signaling activation in response to inflammation to foster mucosal healing.

2.3. MALT1 Protease Is Necessary for Cell Proliferation and Viability

The scaffold function of MALT1 has been proposed as a therapeutic target in experimental colitis [27]. To study a specific contribution of the MALT1 protease to mucosal healing, we used the small molecule inhibitor MI-2, targeting specifically the paracaspase domain of MALT1 [30]. The effect of MALT1 protease inhibition on colorectal cancer (CRC) cell proliferation and survival was analyzed in vitro using the cell lines Caco2, HT-29, and HCT116 (Figure 3A). Impaired proliferation was observed in MI-2 dose escalation studies as the inhibitor concentrations increased, and this was accompanied by an increase in the mean Sytox Orange intensities, indicating an increase in cell death (Figure 3B). Thus, high MI-2 concentrations were sufficient to induce cell death in each cell line. As Caco2, HT-29, and HCT116 cells express different MALT1 protein levels (Figure 3A), each cell line displayed cell line-specific dose responses to MALT1 protease inhibition, correlating with the protein level. Accordingly, low MALT1 protein expressing Caco2 cells displayed low sensitivity towards MI-2 treatment. In contrast, HT-29 and HCT116 cells expressing higher MALT1 protein levels likewise showed higher sensitivity towards MI-2 (Figure 3A,B). The necessity of MALT1 proteolytic activity for cell proliferation was further confirmed in a Caco2 wound healing assay, where MI-2 treatment significantly delayed the gap closure at 48 h compared to mock treated cells (Figure 3C). Moreover, we demonstrated that MALT1 protease inhibition affects murine VAKPT (VillinCre, Apc, Kras, P53, Alk5 (TGF-b-signaling)) and human patient-derived tumor (CRC-tumoroids) organoid spheroid-formation. In response to MI-2, fewer organoids arose from single cells, which were also smaller in size than control organoids (Figure 3D,E). Inhibitor specificity was confirmed using murine small intestinal organoids carrying a specific deletion of *Malt1* in intestinal epithelial cells (*Malt1*$^{\Delta IEC}$). *Malt1*$^{\Delta IEC}$ organoids were protected from MI-2 induced impairment of cell viability (Figure S1A). In line with its important function as NF-κB regulator, we observed a significant decrease in gene expression of the NF-κB target gene *Nos2* (nitric oxide synthase 2) in intestinal organoids in response to MI-2 stimulation (Figure S1B). These data indicate a pivotal role of the MALT1 protease in promoting cell proliferation and viability which may have a beneficial effect on epithelial restitution and mucosal healing in response to intestinal inflammation.

2.4. MALT1 Protease Inhibition Causes Ferroptosis In Vitro

Having shown that MALT1 proteolytic activity promotes epithelial cell proliferation and is necessary for cell viability, we next performed a cell death screen to evaluate the effects of MALT1 inhibition on cell viability and to elucidate which cell death pathway is regulated by MALT1 protease. We found that treatment with MI-2 caused a significant decrease in cell viability and that the addition of the ferroptosis inhibitor liproxstatin-1 [31] was sufficient to rescue Caco2 cells from MI-2 induced cell death (Figure 4A). In contrast none of the other cell death inhibitors targeting apoptosis or regulated necrosis was able to block MI-2 induced toxicity, suggesting that the MALT1 protease is an inhibitor of ferroptosis. As expected, MI-2 failed to induce cell death in Caco2 *MALT1* knockout (KO) cells and HCT116 *MALT1* KO cells, which likewise exposed low Sytox green levels (Figure 4B). In contrast, MI-2 treated wild-type (WT) Caco2 and HCT116 cells exhibited the highest Sytox green intensity and cell death starting around 18 h post stimulation, which was completely rescued by additional liproxstatin-1 treatment (Figure 4B). These data suggest that MALT protease functions upstream of NF-κB to inhibit ferroptosis.

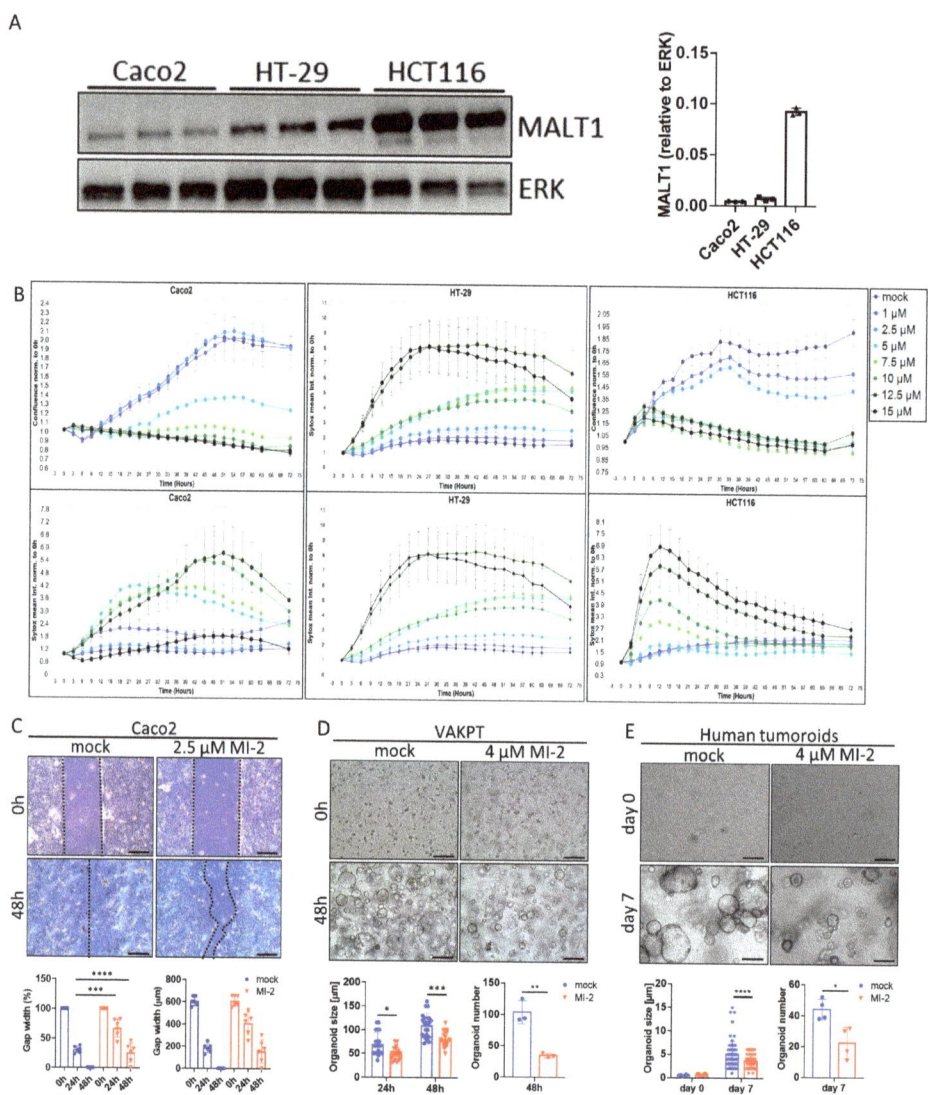

Figure 3. MALT1 proteolytic activity controls cell proliferation and viability. (**A**) Western blot analysis and protein volume quantification of MALT1 protein levels in Caco2, HT-29 and HCT116 cells. ERK was used as a loading control. (**B**) Live cell analysis of Caco2, HT-29 and HCT116 cells stimulated with indicated MI-2 concentrations. Cell confluence (upper panel) and Sytox orange intensity (lower panel) indicate cell growth and cell death over time (hours). (**C**) Scratch assay of Caco2 cells stimulated with 2.5 µM MI-2. Cell growth was monitored for 48 h, gap width was measured every 24 h for quantification (scale bar: 200 µm). *** $p < 0.001$, **** $p < 0.0001$ in ANOVA for multiple comparisons, error bars represent mean ± SD, 95% CI. (**D,E**) Tumor organoid formation assays using (**D**) murine tumor organoids (VAKPT) and (**E**) human tumor organoids (CRC patients). Single tumor cells were stimulated with 4 µM MI-2 and monitored over time (scale bar: 200 µm). * $p < 0.05$, ** $p < 0.01$, *** $p < 0.001$, **** $p < 0.0001$ in ANOVA for multiple comparisons and in unpaired two-tailed t-test; error bars represent mean ± SD, 95% CI.

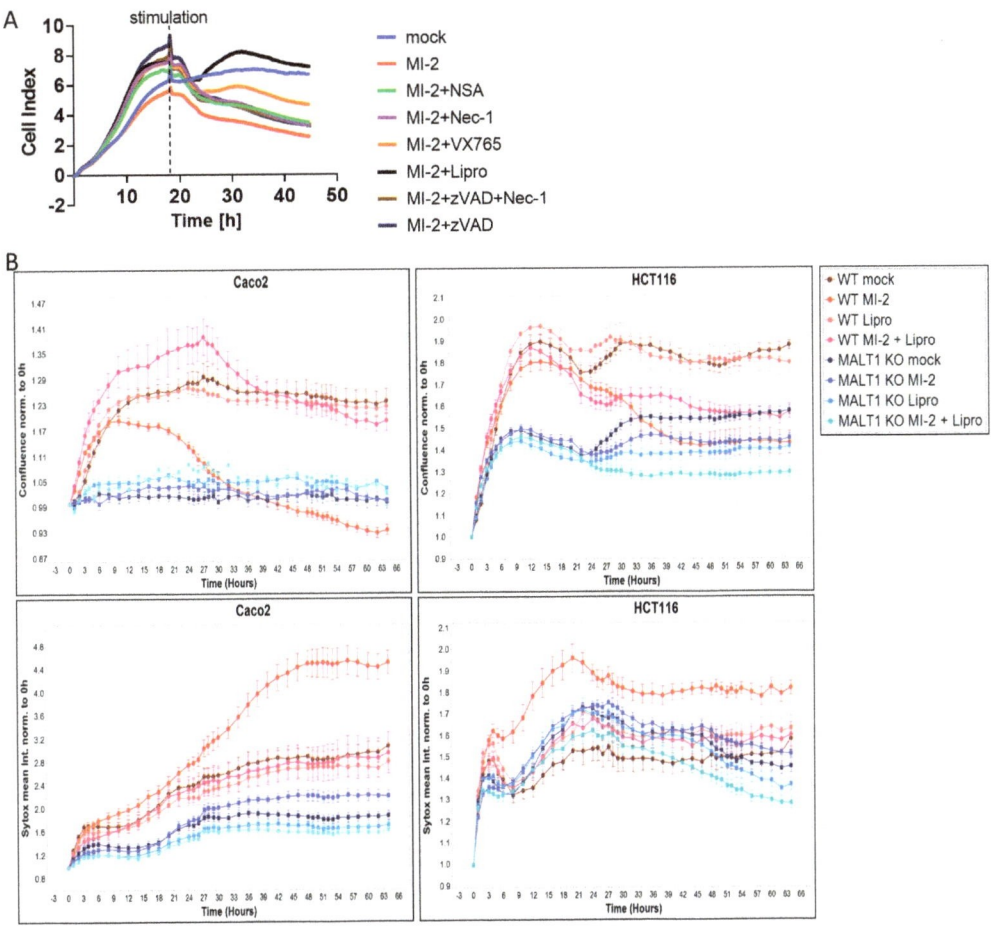

Figure 4. MALT1 protease negatively regulates ferroptosis in vitro. (**A**) Cell death screen of Caco2 cells stimulated with 13.5 µM MI-2, 0.5 µM necrosulfonamide (NSA), 10 µM necrostatin-1 (Nec-1), 20 µM VX-765, 20 µM z-VAD-FMK (zVAD) and 0.2 µM liproxstatin-1 (Lipro). (**B**) Live cell analysis of Caco2 and HCT116 cells stimulated with 13.5 µM MI-2 and 0.2 µM liproxstatin-1 (Lipro). Cell confluence (upper panel) and Sytox green intensity (lower panel) indicate cell growth and cell death over time (hours).

2.5. MALT1 Protease Inhibition Impairs Intestinal Barrier Function In Vitro

The intestinal epithelial barrier is a crucial defense mechanism of the gut, which separates the luminal contents from the mucosal immune system. Tight junctions are specialized structures between adjacent epithelial cells that seal the epithelial monolayer and regulate paracellular transport as well as the exchange between environmental factors within the gut lumen and the mucosal immune system located within the lamina propria. Pathophysiological alterations within this structural part of the epithelium can severely compromise mucosal barrier function which may trigger an inflammatory reaction [32]. To investigate the impact of MALT1 proteolytic activity on tight junction biology, we used the Caco2-brush border epithelial (bbe) cell line to establish a single-cell monolayer on a permeable support membrane. The cells were treated with MI-2 at various concentrations. The effect of pharmacological MALT1 protease inhibition on cell–cell contacts was visualized by immunofluorescence staining for the tight junction-associated protein Zonula occludens-1 (ZO-1) using live cell imaging with confocal microscopy (Figure 5A). Already at the lowest inhibitor concentration (0.5 µM), ZO-1 was relocated from the cell–cell border and accumulated within the cytoplasm of the cell. This effect was even more prominent with increasing concentrations of MI-2. Consequently, cells started to die, and the cell layer was disintegrated. Similar, tight junction proteins of the Claudin family were rearranged in Caco2-bbe cells upon MALT1 protease inhibition, leading to cell layer disintegration and cell death (Figure 5B). Rapid and dose-dependent decrease in the trans-epithelial electrical resistance (TEER) in response to MI-2 treatment confirmed the pathophysiological effect of MI-2 on tight junction biology and barrier function (Figure 5C). These data strongly suggest that MALT1 protease activity is important for maintaining the integrity of the intestinal epithelial barrier function, an essential step during mucosal healing. MALT1 inhibition disrupts the localization of the tight junction protein ZO-1 and leads to a loss of tight junction density, resulting in impaired barrier function. In contrast to the suggested therapeutic effect of MI-2 on acute colitis [27], these findings suggest that MALT1 inhibitors may have unintended effects on the intestinal epithelial barrier function.

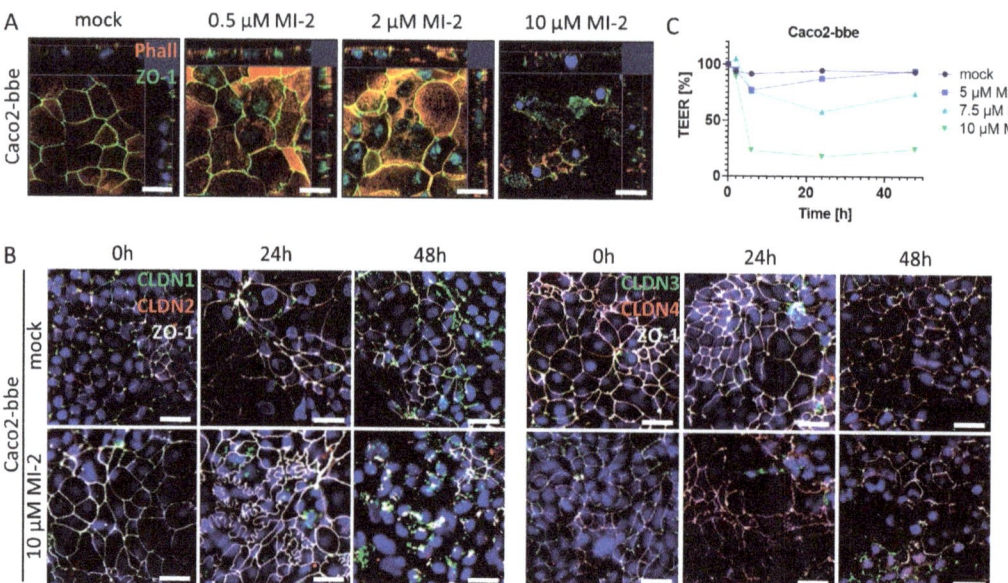

Figure 5. MALT1 proteolytic activity supports epithelial tight junctions. (**A**) Representative images of Caco2-bbe cell monolayers stimulated with indicated MI-2 concentrations 48 h after stimulation immunocytochemically stained with antibody against ZO-1 (green) and phalloidin-594 dye (Phall, red), nuclei were counterstained with Hoechst 33342 (blue) (scale bar: 50 µm). (**B**) Representative images of 10 µM MI-2 stimulated Caco2-bbe cell monolayers over time. Monolayers were immunocytochemically stained with antibodies against ZO-1 (white) and in the left panel claudin-1 (green), claudin-2 (red) and in the right panel claudin-3 (green), claudin-4 (red), nuclei were counterstained with Hoechst 33342 (blue) (scale bar: 50 µm). (**C**) TEER measurement of MI-2 stimulated Caco2-bbe cells.

2.6. MALT1 Protease Promotes pSTAT3 Mediated Mucosal Wound Healing in Experimental Colitis

To further study the role of the MALT1 protease in barrier function and mucosal wound healing in vivo, acute colitis was induced in C57BL/6J mice using 2% DSS. During mucosal recovery, mice were treated daily with 25 mg/kg MI-2 (Figure 6A). In line with previous results from Bornancin et al. [33] and Monajemi et al. [34], MI-2 treated mice displayed signs of persisting intestinal inflammation, which included shortened colon length and a delay in mucosal healing (Figure 6B). Further, these mice showed a higher and persistent disease activity during endoscopic analysis on day 13 (Figure 6C). This was accompanied by severe epithelial tissue destruction as shown in histological colon cross sections, confirmed by an elevated histological pathology score which includes evaluation of the integrity of the intestinal epithelium, mucosal inflammation, and changes of the submucosa (immune cell infiltration, edema formation) (Figure 6C). Wound-associated intestinal epithelial cells are characterized by expression of the tight junction protein claudin-4 (CLDN4) [35]. While *Cldn4* gene expression did not change due to MALT1 protease inhibition, we observed less CLDN4 protein localized at epithelial lesions as shown by immunofluorescence staining and a decreased CLDN4 protein level in whole colon tissue protein lysates in response to MI-2 treatment (Figure 6D,E). Consistent with our in vitro studies, this implies a potential role for MALT1 protease function in regulating epithelial tight junction biology to enhance the maintenance of the mucosal barrier and to provide intestinal homeostasis. Significantly increased colonic *Ifit1* mRNA expression as well as decreased expression levels of the proliferation marker *Mki67* and the essential mucosal wound healing factor *Tjp1* [36] supported the finding that inhibition of MALT1 protease during mucosal recovery affected cell proliferation in the intestinal epithelium, which finally delayed the wound healing process. Further, *Nos2* gene expression was significantly downregulated in response to MI-2 treatment indicating impaired NF-κB signaling in the absence of MALT1 proteolytic activity (Figure 6F). In line with our observation that MALT1 protease function can inhibit ferroptosis, MI-2 treatment in vivo was accompanied by strongly increased expression levels of pro-ferroptotic acyl-CoA synthetase long-chain family member 4 (*Acsl4*) (Figure 6F) promoting enrichment of polyunsaturated fatty acids in cellular membranes, which in turn enhances lipid peroxidation and ferroptosis [37]. This identifies the MALT1 protease as a potential negative regulator of ferroptosis in the intestinal epithelium in the context of mucosal healing. Further, interleukin (IL) 22 dependent epithelial signal transducer and activator of transduction 3 (STAT3) activation has been reported to promote mucosal wound healing [38]. *Stat3* gene expression levels were significantly downregulated in MI-2 treated mice. In line with this, the gene expression of *Birc5* (baculoviral IAP repeat-containing 5), a STAT3 target gene whose activity benefits wound healing by inducing angiogenesis [39] and has been reported to promote proliferation of LGR5[+] stem cells and transit amplifying cells in adult intestinal tissue [40], was significantly reduced (Figure 6G). Immunofluorescence staining further revealed that epithelial STAT3 Tyr705 phosphorylation, which is associated with cell proliferation, survival and self-renewal [41], was almost absent in these mice, while in control animals about 70% of epithelial cells expressed pSTAT3 (Figure 6H).

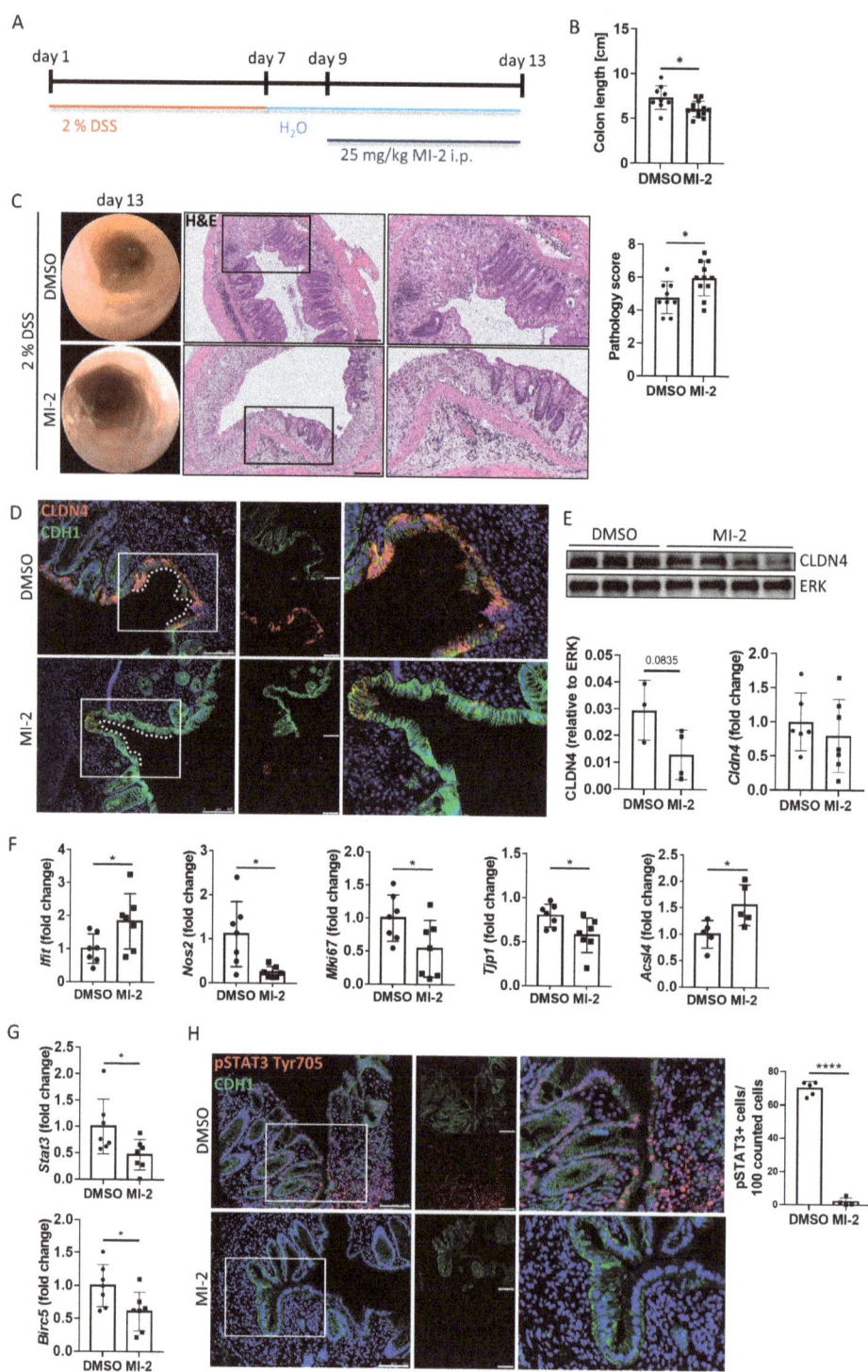

Figure 6. MALT1 protease mediated pSTAT3 signaling promotes mucosal wound healing in vivo. (**A**) C57BL/6J mice received 2% DSS in the drinking water for 7 days to induce acute colitis. A daily dose of 25 mg/kg MI-2 inhibited MALT1 proteolytic activity during mucosal recovery (day 9–13) (n = 13). Control mice (n = 9) were injected with DMSO. Mice were analyzed on day 13. Experiments were repeated three times with similar results. * $p < 0.05$ in unpaired two-tailed t-test; error bars represent mean ± SD, 95% CI. (**B**) Colon length measurement in cm. (**C**) Representative images of endoscopic analysis and H&E staining of colonic cross sections on day 13 (scale bar: 200 μm). Pathology score of endoscopic analysis. * $p < 0.05$ in unpaired two-tailed t-test; error bars represent mean ± SD, 95% CI. (**D**) Representative images of colonic cross sections stained immunohistochemically with antibodies against claudin-4 (red) and E-cadherin (CDH1, green), nuclei were counterstained with Hoechst 33342 (blue) (scale bar: 100 μm). (**E**) Western blot analysis and protein volume quantification of claudin-4 protein levels in whole colon tissue. ERK was used as a loading control. Quantitative real-time PCR of *Cldn4* gene expression levels. (**F,G**) Quantitative real-time analysis of (**F**) intestinal inflammation (DMSO n = 7, MI-2 n = 7) and ferroptosis associated genes (DMSO n = 5, MI-2 n = 5) and (**G**) wound healing associated genes (DMSO n = 7, MI-2 n = 7). * $p < 0.05$ in unpaired two-tailed t-test; error bars represent mean ± SD, 95% CI. (**H**) Representative colonic cross sections stained immunohistochemically with antibodies against pSTAT3 Tyr705 (red) and E-cadherin (CDH1, green), nuclei were counterstained with Hoechst 33342 (blue) (scale bar: 100 μm). Quantification of pSTAT3 positive cells in the intestinal epithelium. **** $p < 0.0001$ in unpaired two-tailed t-test; error bars represent mean ± SD, 95% CI.

These data indicate a comprehensive role for the MALT1 protease in regulating mucosal wound healing during experimental colitis. As a potential negative regulator of ferroptosis in colonic tissue and regulator of wound-associated epithelial CLDN4, it supports the maintenance of the epithelial barrier and mucosal homeostasis. In addition, it mediates STAT3 activation in epithelial cells, which in turn induces mucosal healing.

2.7. MALT1 Regulates STAT3-Mediated Wound Healing and Ferroptosis during Active UC

Genome-wide expression analysis of DSS treated mice carrying a specific deletion of *Stat3* in the intestinal epithelium (*Stat3*$^{\Delta IEC}$) revealed a gene set that under inflammatory conditions is regulated by this transcription factor (GSE15955). Within this gene set, a wound healing and cellular stress response associated cluster was identified [38]. RNA-seq analysis of human UC colon tissue demonstrated a positive correlation of these wound healing associated and STAT3-regulated genes with *MALT1* gene expression levels during active colitis (Figure 7A). This further strengthens the hypothesis that in the context of colitis, MALT1 might promote the activation of STAT3.

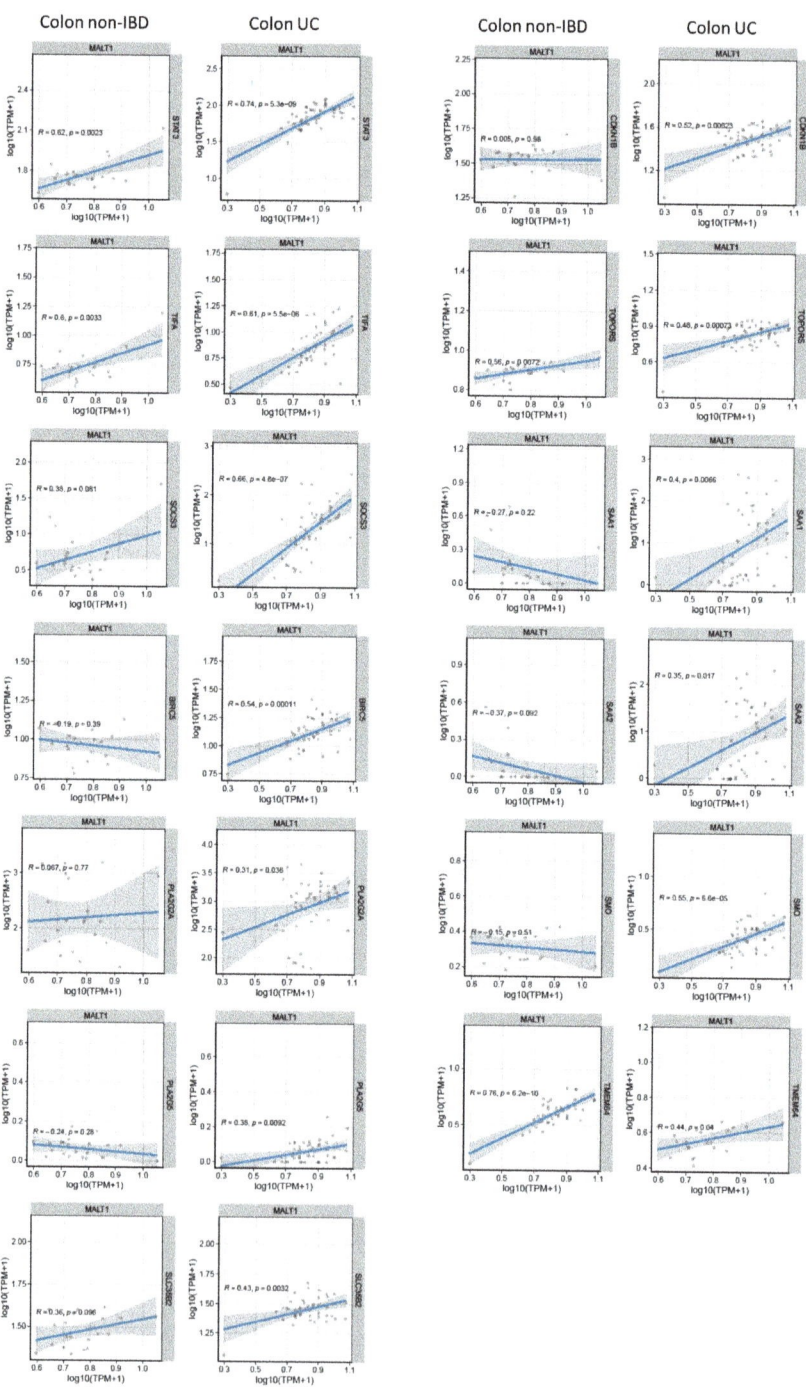

Figure 7. MALT1 gene expression levels correlate with wound healing associated gene expression in UC. RNA-seq correlation analysis of *MALT1* and STAT3-regulated wound healing associated genes.

3. Discussion

Ulcerative colitis (UC) is a chronic inflammatory bowel disease characterized by inflammation of the colon and rectum. Mucosal healing, or the restoration of the intestinal barrier function, is an important therapeutic goal in UC, as it can improve symptoms and prevent disease progression. Disruption of the intestinal barrier can lead to the translocation of bacteria and other microorganisms across the intestinal mucosa, which can exacerbate inflammation and contribute to disease severity. Resolving inflammation and promoting mucosal healing can help to prevent this translocation and to improve outcomes in UC [42,43].

We detected a significant enrichment of MALT1 gene and protein expression in the colon of UC patients, particularly in intestinal epithelial cells. Analysis of a DSS time course RNA-seq dataset further revealed increased expression of *Malt1* and the CBM complex protein *Card9* during active colitis. Together this indicates a specific contribution of MALT1 to the disease, which has also been proposed before and has identified MALT1 as a potential therapeutic target in IBD [27]. However, whether MALT1 is also involved in recovery from intestinal inflammation remains unclear. In this study we identified the MALT1 protease as a central regulator of colitis associated mucosal healing (Figure 8).

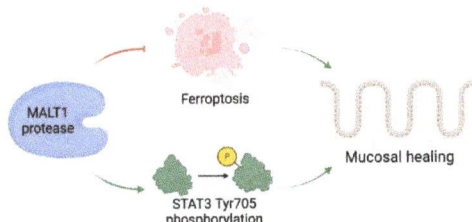

Figure 8. The role of MALT1 protease during mucosal wound healing. The proteolytic activity of MALT1 contributes to mucosal healing by blocking ferroptosis and promoting STAT3 activation in the intestinal epithelium. Created in Biorender.com.

Our data show that MALT1 proteolytic activity is necessary for the maintenance of intestinal homeostasis. It supports the intestinal barrier by regulating tight junctions and promotes epithelial cell proliferation. These properties facilitate a rapid repair of epithelial injuries which in turn has anti-inflammatory effects. The assignment of proliferative and pro-repair capacities to the MALT1 protease strongly advise against MALT1 as a therapeutic target in the context of mucosal inflammation.

MALT1 plays a key role in the activation of NF-κB signaling, a critical pathway in immune and inflammatory responses. In 2020 Wu et al. demonstrated that NF-κB regulates ferroptosis in intestinal epithelial cells. They further demonstrated that ferroptosis is involved in IEC death in the context of UC, and that ferroptosis is a potential therapeutic target for UC. Mechanistically they proved that phosphorylated p65 in the intestinal epithelium significantly inhibited ferroptosis and thus contributed to the resolution of the inflammation [6]. Here, we could further expand these analyses by demonstrating that MALT1, as an upstream regulator of NF-κB signaling, and might also control ferroptosis during intestinal inflammation. The pro-ferroptotic gene *ACSL4* has been shown to be three-fold upregulated in intestinal mucosal biopsies derived from IBD patients and was identified as a ferroptosis-related hub gene in UC, making it a key protein in disease development [44,45]. Here we show that the MALT1 protease inhibits *Acsl4* expression during recovery from experimental colitis in mice. ACSL4 promotes biosynthesis and enrichment of long chain polyunsaturated fatty acids (PUFA) in cellular membranes. As lipid peroxidation occurs more frequently at PUFAs, this facilitates ferroptosis and induces lesions in the intestinal epithelium [37]. Accordingly, MALT1 proteolytic activity negatively regulates ferroptosis by limiting *Acsl4* expression during mucosal wound healing.

STAT3 expression has been reported to be upregulated during active inflammation and clinical remission in mucosal biopsies from UC patients, indicating a potential contribution of STAT3 to mucosal wound healing [46]. Moreover, mice lacking STAT3 in intestinal epithelial cells display a severe defect of epithelial restitution further demonstrating that intestinal epithelial STAT3 activation regulates immune homeostasis in the gut by promoting IL-22-dependent mucosal wound healing [38]. Here we demonstrate that in mice, expression and STAT3 Tyr705 phosphorylation might be regulated by MALT1 proteolytic activity during mucosal healing. Pharmacological inhibition of the MALT1 protease during recovery from experimental colitis significantly reduced *Stat3* expression levels as well as STAT3 activation in the intestinal epithelium, which in turn might have promoted the delay in mucosal healing. In addition, expression of previously identified STAT3-regulated wound healing-associated genes [38] correlated positively with *MALT1* expression in colonic tissue derived from UC patients. These data suggest that the MALT1 protease promotes STAT3-mediated wound healing during colitis.

We conclude that MALT1 protease function plays a critical role in the regulation of immune and inflammatory responses, as well as mucosal healing by inhibition of inflammation-associated ferroptosis and positive regulation of the STAT3 axis. Understanding the mechanisms by which MALT1 protease function regulates these processes may offer novel therapeutic targets for the treatment of IBD and other inflammatory diseases. Further studies are needed to determine whether it may be a therapeutic target in IBD.

4. Material and Methods

4.1. Human Samples

All studies with human material were approved by the ethics committee of the University Hospital of Erlangen (# 49_20B, 159_15 B), or the ethics committee of Charité—Universitätsmedizin Berlin (no. EA4/015/13). The diagnosis of inflammatory bowel disease was based on clinical, endoscopical and histological findings. Disease activity was evaluated based on the Harvey Bradshaw Index.

4.2. Animals and Housing

Malt1^{fl} mice were kindly provided by R. Beyaert and were described earlier [47]. *Malt1*$^{\Delta IEC}$ mice were generated by crossing *Malt1*^{fl} mice to *Villin-Cre* mice which were described earlier [48,49]. Mice were screened regularly according to FELASA guidelines. Experimental protocols were approved by the Institutional Animal Care and Use Committee of the Regierung von Unterfranken.

4.3. DSS Colitis

Mice received 2% dextran sodium sulfate (DSS) (MP Biomedicals, Santa Ana, CA, USA, Cat. No. 160110) in sterilized tap water for six days to induce acute colitis followed by drinking water for nine days. From recovery day three to nine mice were daily injected intraperitoneally with 25 mg/kg MI-2 (Selleckchem, Houston, TX, USA, Cat. No. S7429) in 5% DMSO + 30% PEG-300 + 5% Tween-20 + aqua injectable.

Colitis development was monitored using a high-resolution video mini-endoscopic system. Colitis pathology was graded according to the murine endoscopic index of colitis severity (MEICS) involving evaluation of colon wall thickening, changes of the vascular pattern, fibrin visibility, granularity of the mucosal surface, and stool consistency [50].

4.4. Histology and Immunohistochemistry

Formalin-fixed and paraffin-embedded tissue cross sections were stained with Mayer's haematoxylin and eosin (H&E). Immunofluorescence staining of tissue sections was performed using the TSA cyanine 3 system (Akoya Biosciences, Marlborough, MA, USA, Cat. No. SKU NEL704A001KT) according to the manufacturer's instructions. Primary antibodies were incubated overnight at 4 °C: MALT1 (Abcam, Boston, MA, USA, Cat. No. 33921), claudin-4 (Invitrogen, Waltham, MA, USA, Cat. No. 36-4800), p65 (Cell Signaling, Danvers,

MA, USA, Cat. No. 8242), pSTAT3 Tyr705 (Cell Signaling, Cat. No. 9145), E-Cadherin (BD, Franklin Lakes, NJ, USA, Cat. No. 612130). Secondary anti-rabbit (Dianova, Hamburg, Germany, Cat. No. 111-065-144) was incubated for 1 h at room temperature. Hoechst (Invitrogen, Cat. No. 33342) was used for staining nuclei. Images were taken using the confocal fluorescence LEICA TCS SP5 II microscope, or a LEICA DMI 4000B microscope together with the LEICA DFC360 FX or LEICA DFC420 C camera and the corresponding imaging software.

4.5. Organoid Culture

Intestinal crypts were isolated from the mouse small intestine and cultured in organoid medium supplemented with murine recombinant EGF, noggin and R-spondin for at least seven days to enable organoid formation according to Sato et al. [51]. Human tumor organoids were cultured in Advanced DMEM/F-12 (Gibco, Waltham, MA, USA, Cat. No. 12634028) supplemented with R-spondin, noggin, 1X B27, 1.25 mM N-acetylcystein, 50 µg/mL Primocin, 500 nM A83-01, 10 µM SB202190, 50 ng/mL human recombinant EGF. Murine tumor organoids (VAKPT) were cultured in Advanced DMEM/F-12 supplemented with 1X B27, 1 mM N-acetylcysteine, 50 ng/mL murine recombinant EGF and 0.5 nM dexamethasone. Organoid growth was monitored by light microscopy. Organoids were stimulated with 4 µM or 30 µM MI-2 (Selleckchem, Cat. No. S7429) and stained with propidium iodide staining solution (BD Pharmingen, San Diego, CA, USA, Cat. No. 556463). Time-lapse microscopy was performed using the EVOS M7000 Imaging System.

4.6. Organoid Formation Assay

Human and murine tumor organoids were dissociated into single cells in 1X TrypLE Select (Gibco, Cat. No. A12177-01) + PBS, filtered using a 40 µM cell strainer and plated in Matrigel (Corning, Corning, NY, USA, Cat. No. 356231). Single cells were treated with 4 µM MI-2 (Selleckchem, Cat. No. S7429) in organoid medium. Time-lapse microscopy was performed using the EVOS M7000 Imaging System. VAKPT organoids were kindly provided by Rene Jackstadt.

4.7. Cell Culture

Caco2 and HT-29 cells were cultured in DMEM (1X) + GlutaMAX (Gibco, Cat. No. 31966-021) supplemented with 1% penicillin/streptomycin (Sigma-Aldrich, St. Louis, MO, USA, Cat. No. P4333) and 10% FCS (Sigma-Aldrich, Cat. No. F7524). For Caco2-bbe cells the medium was additionally supplemented with non-essential amino acids (- L-glutamine) (Sigma-Aldrich, Cat. No. M7145) and 100 mM HEPES (Sigma-Aldrich H0887). HCT116 cells were cultured in McCoy's 5A medium (Sigma-Aldrich, Cat. No. M4892) supplemented with 1% penicillin/streptomycin and 10% FCS. All cell lines used in this study were obtained from the American Type Culture Collection (ATCC).

Cells were stimulated with 13.5 µM MI-2 (Selleckchem, Cat. No. S7429), 0.5 µM NSA (Merck, Darmstadt, Germany, Cat. No. 432531-71-0), 10 µM necrostatin-1 (Enzo, Farmingdale, NY, USA, Cat. No. BML-AP309), 20 µM VX-765 (Selleckchem, Cat. No. S2228), 20 µM z-VAD-FMK (MedChemExpress, Monmouth Junction, NJ, USA, Cat. No. HY-16658B), 0.2 µM liproxstatin-1 (Biomol, Hamburg, Germany, Cat. No. Cay17730) and 30 µM mepazine (MedChemExpress, Cat. No. HY-121282A). Proliferation assays were performed using the Agilent xCELLigence System or Sartorius Incucyte SX5. For Incucyte analysis cells were stained with SYTOX green nucleic acid stain (Thermo Fisher, Waltham, MA, USA, Cat. No. S7020).

4.8. Immunocytochemistry

Confluent Caco2-bbe cells on transwell inserts (Millicell®, Cell culture inserts, 0.4 µm PCF, Merck Millipore Ltd., Carrigtwohill, Ireland; Cat. No. PIHP01250) were fixed with 1% PFA (Roth, Karlsruhe, Germany, Cat. No. 0964.2) in PBS$^{+Mg/Ca}$, permeabilized using 0.5% Triton X 100 (Roth, Cat. No. 3051.3) in PBS$^{+Mg/Ca}$, blocked with 6% goat serum

(Sigma-Aldrich, Cat. No. G9023) + 1% BSA (Sigma-Aldrich, Cat. No. F7524) in PBS$^{+Mg/Ca}$ and incubated with the following primary antibodies: claudin-1 (Invitrogen, Cat. No. 51-9000), claudin-2 (Invitrogen, Cat. No. 51-6100), claudin-3 (Invitrogen, Cat. No. 34-1700), claudin-4 (Invitrogen, Cat. No. 32-9400), ZO-1 (Invitrogen Cat. No. 339194), phalloidin-594 (Dyomics, Jena, Germany, Cat. No. 594-33). Goat anti-mouse (Invitrogen, Cat. No. A32728), Goat anti-mouse (Invitrogen, Cat. No. A32723) and Goat anti-rabbit (Invitrogen, Cat. No. A32731) were used as secondary antibodies. Hoechst (Invitrogen, Cat. No. 33342) was used for staining of nuclei.

4.9. Transepithelial Electrical Resistance (TEER) Assay

Caco2-bbe cells were seeded on transwell inserts (Millicell®, cell culture inserts, 0.4 μm PCF, Merck Millipore Ltd., Cat. No. PIHP01250) in cell culture medium. Confluent cells were exposed to MI-2 (Selleckchem, Cat. No. S7429) from basolateral and apical sides. To determine epithelial barrier function, TEER was measured at 37 °C using chopstick electrodes and an Ohmmeter (EVOM, WPI, Sarasota, FL, USA). The electrical resistance of the filter membrane was determined and corrected for resistance of the empty filter and the area as previously described [52].

4.10. Wound Healing Assay

Caco2 cells were seeded on 2-well culture dishes (ibidi, Gräfelfing, Germany, Cat. No. 81176) in culture medium. Confluent cells were kept on starving medium (culture medium without FCS) overnight. The 2-well insert was removed, the starving medium was replaced with culture medium, and cells were exposed to 2.5 μM MI-2 (Selleckchem, Cat. No. S7429). Time-lapse microscopy was performed using the EVOS M7000 Imaging System.

4.11. MALT1 Knockout Cells

sgRNAs were generated by cloning MALT1 specific oligomers (MALT1 CRISPR/Cas9 KO Plasmid (h2), Santa Cruz, Dallas, TX, USA, Cat. No. sc-400791-KO-2) into the pCAG-SpCas9-GFP-U6-gRNA plasmid backbone vector (addgene, Watertown, MA, USA, Cat. No. 79144). Successful cloning was confirmed by plasmid sequencing. HT-29 and HCT116 cells were transfected with Lipofectamine 2000 transfection reagent (Invitrogen, Cat. No. P/N 52887). GFP-positive cells were FACS sorted (BD, FACSAriaII) and *MALT1* knockout was confirmed by Western blot.

4.12. Gene Expression

Total RNA was isolated from whole colon biopsies, small intestinal organoids, HCT116 and Caco2 cells using the NucleoSpin RNA Mini kit for RNA purification (Macherey-Nagel, Düren, Germany, Cat. No. 740955). cDNA was synthesized using the SCRIPT cDNA Synthesis Kit (Jena Bioscience, Jena, Germany; Cat. No. PCR-511). Real-time PCR analysis was performed using LightCycler 480 SYBR Green I Master (Roche, Basel, Switzerland; Cat. No. 04887352001) and specific primer assays (Table 1).

Table 1. Specific primer assays used for real-time PCR analysis.

Primer Assay	Company, Cat. No.
Mm_Acsl4_1_SG QuantiTect Primer Assay	Qiagen (Hilden, Germany), QT00141673
Mm_Birc5_1_SG QuantiTect Primer Assay	Qiagen, QT00113379
Mm_Cldn4_1_SG QuantiTect Primer Assay	Qiagen, QT00252084
Hs_GAPDH_1_SG QuantiTect Primer Assay	Qiagen, QT00079247
Mouse Gapdh forward (tcaccaccatggagaaggc) Mouse Gapdh reverse (gctaagcagttggtggtgca)	Biomers (Ulm, Germany)

Table 1. *Cont.*

Primer Assay	Company, Cat. No.
Mm_Ifit1_1_SG QuantiTect Primer Assay	Qiagen, QT01161286
Hs_MALT1_1_SG QuantiTect Primer Assay	Qiagen, QT00032718
Mm_Mki67_1_SG QuantiTect Primer Assay	Qiagen, QT00247667
Mm_Nos2_1_SG QuantiTect Primer Assay	Qiagen, QT00100275
Mm_Stat3_1_SG QuantiTect Primer Assay	Qiagen, QT00148750
Mm_Tjp1_1_SG QuantiTect Primer Assay	Qiagen, QT00493899

4.13. Immunoblotting

Whole protein lysates were isolated from colon biopsies, HCT116, Caco2 and HT-29 cells using cell lysis buffer (Cell Signaling, Cat. No. 9803) supplemented with 1 mM PMSF (Cell Signaling, Cat. No. 8553) and centrifuged at 14,000 rpm for 20 min. MiniProtean-TGX gels (4–15% polyacrylamide; Bio-Rad, Hercules, CA, USA) were used for protein separation. Separated proteins were blotted on a PVDF (Bio-Rad, Cat. No. 1704272) or nitrocellulose membrane (Bio-Rad, Cat. No. 1704270). Membranes were incubated with the following primary antibodies: MALT1 (Cell Signaling, Cat. No. 2494), ERK (Cell Signaling, Cat. No. 9102), p100/p52 (Cell Signaling, Cat. No. 4882), claudin-4 (Invitrogen, Cat. No. 36-4800). Anti-rabbit IgG, HRP-linked antibody (Cell Signaling, Cat. No. 7074) was used as a secondary antibody. Western Lightning Plus Chemiluminescent Substrate (PerkinElmer, Waltham, MA, USA, Cat. No. NEL105001EA) was used for detection. Densitometric analysis was performed using the Image Lab Software (Bio-Rad).

4.14. Statistical Analysis

Two groups were compared using the unpaired two-tailed *t*-test and multiple groups were compared using the ANOVA multiple comparison analysis. $p < 0.05$ (NS $p \geq 0.05$; * $p < 0.05$; ** $p < 0.01$; *** $p < 0.001$; **** $p < 0.0001$) was considered as statistically significant. Statistical analysis was performed using GraphPad Prism 8.3.0.

Supplementary Materials: The supporting information can be downloaded at https://www.mdpi.com/article/10.3390/ijms24087402/s1.

Author Contributions: L.W. (Leonie Wittner), M.F.N., M.S. and C.G. designed the research. L.W. (Leonie Wittner), L.W. (Lukas Wagener), J.J.W., I.S. and S.M.K. performed the experiments. S.M.K., E.N., R.J., R.B., R.A., A.A.K., G.S., M.G.-A., J.V.P., C.B., B.S., Z.T., B.W., M.S. supplied material. L.W. (Leonie Wittner), M.F.N. and C.G. analyzed the data and wrote the paper. All authors review and editing. All authors have read and agreed to the published version of the manuscript.

Funding: Support came from the Deutsche Forschungsgemeinschaft (DFG, German Research Foundation)—TRR 241–375876048 (A02, A03, IBDome), FOR 2886–405969122 (A02), TRR 305–429280966 (B08), KFO5024–50553912 (A01, A03, B01, B04, Z01) and DFG GU 1431/5-1. Further support was given by the Interdisciplinary Center for Clinical Research (IZKF) of the University Erlangen-Nürnberg (Jochen-Kalden funding program N5, ELAN P119).

Institutional Review Board Statement: All studies with human material were approved by the ethics committee of the University Hospital of Erlangen (# 49_20B, 159_15 B), or the ethics committee of Charité—Universitätsmedizin Berlin (no. EA4/015/13). Experimental protocols were approved by the Institutional Animal Care and Use Committee of the Regierung von Unterfranken.

Informed Consent Statement: Informed consent was obtained from all subjects involved in the study.

Data Availability Statement: The RNA-seq datasets used in this study have been deposited in the Array Express service of the Molecular Biology Laboratory–European Bioinformatics Institute under the accession IDs E-MTAB-9850 (DSS time course) [53] and E-MTAB-10824 (wound healing time course) [35].

Acknowledgments: We acknowledge the help provided by Elena Percivalle and Jennifer Redlingshöfer for technical aspects, animal husbandry, and experimentation during this work.

Conflicts of Interest: Authors declare no conflict of interest.

References

1. Du, L.; Ha, C. Epidemiology and Pathogenesis of Ulcerative Colitis. *Gastroenterol. Clin. North Am.* **2020**, *49*, 643–654. [CrossRef] [PubMed]
2. Ungaro, R.; Mehandru, S.; Allen, P.B.; Peyrin-Biroulet, L.; Colombel, J.-F. Ulcerative Colitis. *Lancet Lond. Engl.* **2017**, *389*, 1756–1770. [CrossRef] [PubMed]
3. Di Tommaso, N.; Gasbarrini, A.; Ponziani, F.R. Intestinal Barrier in Human Health and Disease. *Int. J. Environ. Res. Public. Health* **2021**, *18*, 12836. [CrossRef] [PubMed]
4. Woznicki, J.A.; Saini, N.; Flood, P.; Rajaram, S.; Lee, C.M.; Stamou, P.; Skowyra, A.; Bustamante-Garrido, M.; Regazzoni, K.; Crawford, N.; et al. TNF-α Synergises with IFN-γ to Induce Caspase-8-JAK1/2-STAT1-Dependent Death of Intestinal Epithelial Cells. *Cell Death Dis.* **2021**, *12*, 864. [CrossRef]
5. Wang, R.; Li, H.; Wu, J.; Cai, Z.-Y.; Li, B.; Ni, H.; Qiu, X.; Chen, H.; Liu, W.; Yang, Z.-H.; et al. Gut Stem Cell Necroptosis by Genome Instability Triggers Bowel Inflammation. *Nature* **2020**, *580*, 386–390. [CrossRef]
6. Xu, M.; Tao, J.; Yang, Y.; Tan, S.; Liu, H.; Jiang, J.; Zheng, F.; Wu, B. Ferroptosis Involves in Intestinal Epithelial Cell Death in Ulcerative Colitis. *Cell Death Dis.* **2020**, *11*, 86. [CrossRef]
7. Günther, C.; Martini, E.; Wittkopf, N.; Amann, K.; Weigmann, B.; Neumann, H.; Waldner, M.J.; Hedrick, S.M.; Tenzer, S.; Neurath, M.F.; et al. Caspase-8 Regulates TNF-α-Induced Epithelial Necroptosis and Terminal Ileitis. *Nature* **2011**, *477*, 335–339. [CrossRef] [PubMed]
8. Günther, C.; Ruder, B.; Stolzer, I.; Dorner, H.; He, G.-W.; Chiriac, M.T.; Aden, K.; Strigli, A.; Bittel, M.; Zeissig, S.; et al. Interferon Lambda Promotes Paneth Cell Death via STAT1 Signaling in Mice and Is Increased in Inflamed Ileal Tissues of Patients with Crohn's Disease. *Gastroenterology* **2019**, *157*, 1310–1322.e13. [CrossRef] [PubMed]
9. Egan, L.J.; de Lecea, A.; Lehrman, E.D.; Myhre, G.M.; Eckmann, L.; Kagnoff, M.F. Nuclear Factor-Kappa B Activation Promotes Restitution of Wounded Intestinal Epithelial Monolayers. *Am. J. Physiol. Cell Physiol.* **2003**, *285*, C1028–C1035. [CrossRef]
10. Steinbrecher, K.A.; Harmel-Laws, E.; Sitcheran, R.; Baldwin, A.S. Loss of Epithelial RelA Results in Deregulated Intestinal Proliferative/Apoptotic Homeostasis and Susceptibility to Inflammation. *J. Immunol. Baltim. Md 1950* **2008**, *180*, 2588–2599. [CrossRef]
11. Nenci, A.; Becker, C.; Wullaert, A.; Gareus, R.; van Loo, G.; Danese, S.; Huth, M.; Nikolaev, A.; Neufert, C.; Madison, B.; et al. Epithelial NEMO Links Innate Immunity to Chronic Intestinal Inflammation. *Nature* **2007**, *446*, 557–561. [CrossRef]
12. Demeyer, A.; Skordos, I.; Driege, Y.; Kreike, M.; Hochepied, T.; Baens, M.; Staal, J.; Beyaert, R. MALT1 Proteolytic Activity Suppresses Autoimmunity in a T Cell Intrinsic Manner. *Front. Immunol.* **2019**, *10*, 1898. [CrossRef] [PubMed]
13. Xia, X.; Cao, G.; Sun, G.; Zhu, L.; Tian, Y.; Song, Y.; Guo, C.; Wang, X.; Zhong, J.; Zhou, W.; et al. GLS1-Mediated Glutaminolysis Unbridled by MALT1 Protease Promotes Psoriasis Pathogenesis. *J. Clin. Investig.* **2020**, *130*, 5180–5196. [CrossRef] [PubMed]
14. Sonoda, M.; Ishimura, M.; Eguchi, K.; Yada, Y.; Lenhartová, N.; Shiraishi, A.; Tanaka, T.; Sakai, Y.; Ohga, S. Progressive B Cell Depletion in Human MALT1 Deficiency. *Clin. Exp. Immunol.* **2021**, *206*, 237–247. [CrossRef] [PubMed]
15. Gross, O.; Grupp, C.; Steinberg, C.; Zimmermann, S.; Strasser, D.; Hannesschläger, N.; Reindl, W.; Jonsson, H.; Huo, H.; Littman, D.R.; et al. Multiple ITAM-Coupled NK-Cell Receptors Engage the Bcl10/Malt1 Complex via Carma1 for NF-KappaB and MAPK Activation to Selectively Control Cytokine Production. *Blood* **2008**, *112*, 2421–2428. [CrossRef] [PubMed]
16. Liu, X.; Yue, C.; Shi, L.; Liu, G.; Cao, Q.; Shan, Q.; Wang, Y.; Chen, X.; Li, H.; Wang, J.; et al. MALT1 Is a Potential Therapeutic Target in Glioblastoma and Plays a Crucial Role in EGFR-Induced NF-KB Activation. *J. Cell. Mol. Med.* **2020**, *24*, 7550–7562. [CrossRef]
17. Lee, J.-Y.L.; Ekambaram, P.; Carleton, N.M.; Hu, D.; Klei, L.R.; Cai, Z.; Myers, M.I.; Hubel, N.E.; Covic, L.; Agnihotri, S.; et al. MALT1 Is a Targetable Driver of Epithelial-to-Mesenchymal Transition in Claudin-Low, Triple-Negative Breast Cancer. *Mol. Cancer Res. MCR* **2022**, *20*, 373–386. [CrossRef]
18. Martinez-Climent, J.A. The Origin and Targeting of Mucosa-Associated Lymphoid Tissue Lymphomas. *Curr. Opin. Hematol.* **2014**, *21*, 309–319. [CrossRef]
19. Baumjohann, D.; Heissmeyer, V. Posttranscriptional Gene Regulation of T Follicular Helper Cells by RNA-Binding Proteins and MicroRNAs. *Front. Immunol.* **2018**, *9*, 1794. [CrossRef]
20. Bell, P.A.; Scheuermann, S.; Renner, F.; Pan, C.L.; Lu, H.Y.; Turvey, S.E.; Bornancin, F.; Régnier, C.H.; Overall, C.M. Integrating Knowledge of Protein Sequence with Protein Function for the Prediction and Validation of New MALT1 Substrates. *Comput. Struct. Biotechnol. J.* **2022**, *20*, 4717–4732. [CrossRef]
21. Juilland, M.; Thome, M. Holding All the CARDs: How MALT1 Controls CARMA/CARD-Dependent Signaling. *Front. Immunol.* **2018**, *9*, 1927. [CrossRef] [PubMed]
22. Yin, H.; Karayel, O.; Chao, Y.-Y.; Seeholzer, T.; Hamp, I.; Plettenburg, O.; Gehring, T.; Zielinski, C.; Mann, M.; Krappmann, D. A20 and ABIN-1 Cooperate in Balancing CBM Complex-Triggered NF-κB Signaling in Activated T Cells. *Cell. Mol. Life Sci. CMLS* **2022**, *79*, 112. [CrossRef] [PubMed]

23. Yu, Z.; Li, X.; Yang, M.; Huang, J.; Fang, Q.; Jia, J.; Li, Z.; Gu, Y.; Chen, T.; Cao, X. TRIM41 Is Required to Innate Antiviral Response by Polyubiquitinating BCL10 and Recruiting NEMO. *Signal Transduct. Target. Ther.* **2021**, *6*, 90. [CrossRef] [PubMed]
24. Lu, H.Y.; Sharma, M.; Sharma, A.A.; Lacson, A.; Szpurko, A.; Luider, J.; Dharmani-Khan, P.; Shameli, A.; Bell, P.A.; Guilcher, G.M.T.; et al. Mechanistic Understanding of the Combined Immunodeficiency in Complete Human CARD11 Deficiency. *J. Allergy Clin. Immunol.* **2021**, *148*, 1559–1574.e13. [CrossRef] [PubMed]
25. Martin, K.; Touil, R.; Kolb, Y.; Cvijetic, G.; Murakami, K.; Israel, L.; Duraes, F.; Buffet, D.; Glück, A.; Niwa, S.; et al. Malt1 Protease Deficiency in Mice Disrupts Immune Homeostasis at Environmental Barriers and Drives Systemic T Cell-Mediated Autoimmunity. *J. Immunol. Baltim. Md 1950* **2019**, *203*, 2791–2806. [CrossRef]
26. Gewies, A.; Gorka, O.; Bergmann, H.; Pechloff, K.; Petermann, F.; Jeltsch, K.M.; Rudelius, M.; Kriegsmann, M.; Weichert, W.; Horsch, M.; et al. Uncoupling Malt1 Threshold Function from Paracaspase Activity Results in Destructive Autoimmune Inflammation. *Cell Rep.* **2014**, *9*, 1292–1305. [CrossRef]
27. Lee, K.W.; Kim, M.; Lee, C.H. Treatment of Dextran Sulfate Sodium-Induced Colitis with Mucosa-Associated Lymphoid Tissue Lymphoma Translocation 1 Inhibitor MI-2 Is Associated with Restoration of Gut Immune Function and the Microbiota. *Infect. Immun.* **2018**, *86*, e00091-18. [CrossRef]
28. Haberman, Y.; Karns, R.; Dexheimer, P.J.; Schirmer, M.; Somekh, J.; Jurickova, I.; Braun, T.; Novak, E.; Bauman, L.; Collins, M.H.; et al. Ulcerative Colitis Mucosal Transcriptomes Reveal Mitochondriopathy and Personalized Mechanisms Underlying Disease Severity and Treatment Response. *Nat. Commun.* **2019**, *10*, 38. [CrossRef]
29. Sokol, H.; Conway, K.L.; Zhang, M.; Choi, M.; Morin, B.; Cao, Z.; Villablanca, E.J.; Li, C.; Wijmenga, C.; Yun, S.H.; et al. Card9 Mediates Intestinal Epithelial Cell Restitution, T-Helper 17 Responses, and Control of Bacterial Infection in Mice. *Gastroenterology* **2013**, *145*, 591–601.e3. [CrossRef]
30. Fontan, L.; Yang, C.; Kabaleeswaran, V.; Volpon, L.; Osborne, M.J.; Beltran, E.; Garcia, M.; Cerchietti, L.; Shaknovich, R.; Yang, S.N.; et al. MALT1 Small Molecule Inhibitors Specifically Suppress ABC-DLBCL In Vitro and In Vivo. *Cancer Cell* **2012**, *22*, 812–824. [CrossRef]
31. Friedmann Angeli, J.P.; Schneider, M.; Proneth, B.; Tyurina, Y.Y.; Tyurin, V.A.; Hammond, V.J.; Herbach, N.; Aichler, M.; Walch, A.; Eggenhofer, E.; et al. Inactivation of the Ferroptosis Regulator Gpx4 Triggers Acute Renal Failure in Mice. *Nat. Cell Biol.* **2014**, *16*, 1180–1191. [CrossRef] [PubMed]
32. Barbara, G.; Barbaro, M.R.; Fuschi, D.; Palombo, M.; Falangone, F.; Cremon, C.; Marasco, G.; Stanghellini, V. Inflammatory and Microbiota-Related Regulation of the Intestinal Epithelial Barrier. *Front. Nutr.* **2021**, *8*, 718356. [CrossRef] [PubMed]
33. Bornancin, F.; Renner, F.; Touil, R.; Sic, H.; Kolb, Y.; Touil-Allaoui, I.; Rush, J.S.; Smith, P.A.; Bigaud, M.; Junker-Walker, U.; et al. Deficiency of MALT1 Paracaspase Activity Results in Unbalanced Regulatory and Effector T and B Cell Responses Leading to Multiorgan Inflammation. *J. Immunol. Baltim. Md 1950* **2015**, *194*, 3723–3734. [CrossRef] [PubMed]
34. Monajemi, M.; Pang, Y.C.F.; Bjornson, S.; Menzies, S.C.; van Rooijen, N.; Sly, L.M. Malt1 Blocks IL-1β Production by Macrophages In Vitro and Limits Dextran Sodium Sulfate-Induced Intestinal Inflammation In Vivo. *J. Leukoc. Biol.* **2018**, *104*, 557–572. [CrossRef]
35. Leppkes, M.; Lindemann, A.; Gößwein, S.; Paulus, S.; Roth, D.; Hartung, H.; Liebing, E.; Zundler, S.; Gonzalez-Acera, M.; Patankar, J.V.; et al. Neutrophils Prevent Rectal Bleeding in Ulcerative Colitis by Peptidyl-Arginine Diminase-4-Dependent Immunothrombosis. *Gut* **2022**, *71*, 2414–2429. [CrossRef]
36. Kuo, W.-T.; Zuo, L.; Odenwald, M.A.; Madha, S.; Singh, G.; Gurniak, C.B.; Abraham, C.; Turner, J.R. The Tight Junction Protein ZO-1 Is Dispensable for Barrier Function but Critical for Effective Mucosal Repair. *Gastroenterology* **2021**, *161*, 1924–1939. [CrossRef]
37. Zhang, H.-L.; Hu, B.-X.; Li, Z.-L.; Du, T.; Shan, J.-L.; Ye, Z.-P.; Peng, X.-D.; Li, X.; Huang, Y.; Zhu, X.-Y.; et al. PKCβII Phosphorylates ACSL4 to Amplify Lipid Peroxidation to Induce Ferroptosis. *Nat. Cell Biol.* **2022**, *24*, 88–98. [CrossRef]
38. Pickert, G.; Neufert, C.; Leppkes, M.; Zheng, Y.; Wittkopf, N.; Warntjen, M.; Lehr, H.-A.; Hirth, S.; Weigmann, B.; Wirtz, S.; et al. STAT3 Links IL-22 Signaling in Intestinal Epithelial Cells to Mucosal Wound Healing. *J. Exp. Med.* **2009**, *206*, 1465–1472. [CrossRef]
39. Shojaei-Ghahrizjani, F.; Rahmati, S.; Mirzaei, S.A.; Banitalebi-Dehkordi, M. Does Survivin Overexpression Enhance the Efficiency of Fibroblast Cell-Based Wound Therapy? *Mol. Biol. Rep.* **2020**, *47*, 5851–5864. [CrossRef]
40. Martini, E.; Wittkopf, N.; Günther, C.; Leppkes, M.; Okada, H.; Watson, A.J.; Podstawa, E.; Backert, I.; Amann, K.; Neurath, M.F.; et al. Loss of Survivin in Intestinal Epithelial Progenitor Cells Leads to Mitotic Catastrophe and Breakdown of Gut Immune Homeostasis. *Cell Rep.* **2016**, *14*, 1062–1073. [CrossRef]
41. Galoczova, M.; Coates, P.; Vojtesek, B. STAT3, Stem Cells, Cancer Stem Cells and P63. *Cell. Mol. Biol. Lett.* **2018**, *23*, 12. [CrossRef] [PubMed]
42. Boal Carvalho, P.; Cotter, J. Mucosal Healing in Ulcerative Colitis: A Comprehensive Review. *Drugs* **2017**, *77*, 159–173. [CrossRef] [PubMed]
43. Sommer, K.; Wiendl, M.; Müller, T.M.; Heidbreder, K.; Voskens, C.; Neurath, M.F.; Zundler, S. Intestinal Mucosal Wound Healing and Barrier Integrity in IBD-Crosstalk and Trafficking of Cellular Players. *Front. Med.* **2021**, *8*, 643973. [CrossRef] [PubMed]
44. Vancamelbeke, M.; Vanuytsel, T.; Farré, R.; Verstockt, S.; Ferrante, M.; Van Assche, G.; Rutgeerts, P.; Schuit, F.; Vermeire, S.; Arijs, I.; et al. Genetic and Transcriptomic Bases of Intestinal Epithelial Barrier Dysfunction in Inflammatory Bowel Disease. *Inflamm. Bowel Dis.* **2017**, *23*, 1718–1729. [CrossRef]

45. Cui, D.-J.; Chen, C.; Yuan, W.-Q.; Yang, Y.-H.; Han, L. Integrative Analysis of Ferroptosis-Related Genes in Ulcerative Colitis. *J. Int. Med. Res.* **2021**, *49*, 3000605211042975. [CrossRef]
46. Arkteg, C.B.; Goll, R.; Gundersen, M.D.; Anderssen, E.; Fenton, C.; Florholmen, J. Mucosal Gene Transcription of Ulcerative Colitis in Endoscopic Remission. *Scand. J. Gastroenterol.* **2020**, *55*, 139–147. [CrossRef]
47. Demeyer, A.; Van Nuffel, E.; Baudelet, G.; Driege, Y.; Kreike, M.; Muyllaert, D.; Staal, J.; Beyaert, R. MALT1-Deficient Mice Develop Atopic-Like Dermatitis Upon Aging. *Front. Immunol.* **2019**, *10*, 2330. [CrossRef]
48. Madison, B.B.; Dunbar, L.; Qiao, X.T.; Braunstein, K.; Braunstein, E.; Gumucio, D.L. Cis Elements of the Villin Gene Control Expression in Restricted Domains of the Vertical (Crypt) and Horizontal (Duodenum, Cecum) Axes of the Intestine. *J. Biol. Chem.* **2002**, *277*, 33275–33283. [CrossRef]
49. el Marjou, F.; Janssen, K.-P.; Chang, B.H.-J.; Li, M.; Hindie, V.; Chan, L.; Louvard, D.; Chambon, P.; Metzger, D.; Robine, S. Tissue-Specific and Inducible Cre-Mediated Recombination in the Gut Epithelium. *Genes. N. Y. N 2000* **2004**, *39*, 186–193. [CrossRef]
50. Becker, C.; Fantini, M.C.; Wirtz, S.; Nikolaev, A.; Kiesslich, R.; Lehr, H.A.; Galle, P.R.; Neurath, M.F. In Vivo Imaging of Colitis and Colon Cancer Development in Mice Using High Resolution Chromoendoscopy. *Gut* **2005**, *54*, 950–954. [CrossRef]
51. Sato, T.; Vries, R.G.; Snippert, H.J.; van de Wetering, M.; Barker, N.; Stange, D.E.; van Es, J.H.; Abo, A.; Kujala, P.; Peters, P.J.; et al. Single Lgr5 Stem Cells Build Crypt-Villus Structures in Vitro without a Mesenchymal Niche. *Nature* **2009**, *459*, 262–265. [CrossRef] [PubMed]
52. Kreusel, K.M.; Fromm, M.; Schulzke, J.D.; Hegel, U. Cl- Secretion in Epithelial Monolayers of Mucus-Forming Human Colon Cells (HT-29/B6). *Am. J. Physiol.* **1991**, *261*, C574–C582. [CrossRef] [PubMed]
53. Patankar, J.V.; Müller, T.M.; Kantham, S.; Acera, M.G.; Mascia, F.; Scheibe, K.; Mahapatro, M.; Heichler, C.; Yu, Y.; Li, W.; et al. E-Type Prostanoid Receptor 4 Drives Resolution of Intestinal Inflammation by Blocking Epithelial Necroptosis. *Nat. Cell Biol.* **2021**, *23*, 796–807. [CrossRef] [PubMed]

Disclaimer/Publisher's Note: The statements, opinions and data contained in all publications are solely those of the individual author(s) and contributor(s) and not of MDPI and/or the editor(s). MDPI and/or the editor(s) disclaim responsibility for any injury to people or property resulting from any ideas, methods, instructions or products referred to in the content.

Review

Role of Muscarinic Acetylcholine Receptors in Intestinal Epithelial Homeostasis: Insights for the Treatment of Inflammatory Bowel Disease

Junsuke Uwada [1,*], Hitomi Nakazawa [1], Ikunobu Muramatsu [1,2,3], Takayoshi Masuoka [1] and Takashi Yazawa [4,*]

1. Department of Pharmacology, School of Medicine, Kanazawa Medical University, Uchinada 920-0293, Japan
2. Division of Genomic Science and Microbiology, School of Medicine, University of Fukui, Eiheiji 910-1193, Japan
3. Kimura Hospital, Awara, Fukui 919-0634, Japan
4. Department of Biochemistry, Asahikawa Medical University, Asahikawa 078-8510, Japan

* Correspondence: uwada@kanazawa-med.ac.jp (J.U.); yazawa@asahihikawa-med.ac.jp (T.Y.); Tel.: +81-166-68-2342 (T.Y.)

Abstract: Inflammatory bowel disease (IBD), which includes Crohn's disease and ulcerative colitis, is an intestinal disorder that causes prolonged inflammation of the gastrointestinal tract. Currently, the etiology of IBD is not fully understood and treatments are insufficient to completely cure the disease. In addition to absorbing essential nutrients, intestinal epithelial cells prevent the entry of foreign antigens (micro-organisms and undigested food) through mucus secretion and epithelial barrier formation. Disruption of the intestinal epithelial homeostasis exacerbates inflammation. Thus, the maintenance and reinforcement of epithelial function may have therapeutic benefits in the treatment of IBD. Muscarinic acetylcholine receptors (mAChRs) are G protein-coupled receptors for acetylcholine that are expressed in intestinal epithelial cells. Recent studies have revealed the role of mAChRs in the maintenance of intestinal epithelial homeostasis. The importance of non-neuronal acetylcholine in mAChR activation in epithelial cells has also been recognized. This review aimed to summarize recent advances in research on mAChRs for intestinal epithelial homeostasis and the involvement of non-neuronal acetylcholine systems, and highlight their potential as targets for IBD therapy.

Keywords: inflammatory bowel disease; epithelial barrier; homeostasis; acetylcholine; muscarinic receptor; non-neuronal acetylcholine

1. Introduction

The intestinal lumen is exposed to various substances via food intake and other sources. Furthermore, a wide variety of bacteria reside in the intestinal lumen and form the gut microbiota. The intestinal epithelial cells separate the inner lamina propria from the luminal environment. Intestinal epithelial cells not only absorb essential nutrients but also form a barrier that blocks the invasion of unwanted antigens and bacteria. Disturbances in homeostasis and barrier function of the intestinal epithelium can result in the entry of bacteria and other antigens, thereby triggering an inflammatory response. Patients with inflammatory bowel disease (IBD), including Crohn's disease and ulcerative colitis, often have impaired intestinal barrier function and exacerbated inflammation [1,2]. Current treatments for IBD generally aim to suppress inflammatory responses. In contrast, the maintenance or regeneration of the epithelial barrier results in removal of the cause of inflammation, which could be a viable strategy for the treatment of IBD. Therefore, the mechanisms that maintain the homeostasis of intestinal epithelial function should be clarified.

Gut function is governed by the autonomic nervous system. The parasympathetic nervous system, through its neurotransmitter, acetylcholine (ACh), activates muscarinic acetylcholine receptors (mAChRs) in intestinal smooth muscle cells to promote intestinal motility [3]. According to previous reports, mAChRs also exist in intestinal epithelial cells and regulate chloride (Cl$^-$) secretion, which is important for mucosal hydration [4,5]. ACh also acts on nicotinic acetylcholine receptors (nAChRs). nAChRs exert anti-inflammatory effects in the gut. For example, stimulation of the vagus nerve activates α7-nAChRs expressed on macrophages in the spleen and gut, which suppress the release of pro-inflammatory cytokines, such as tumor necrosis factor-α (TNF-α) [6]. Therefore, nicotinic ACh signaling is a potential therapeutic target for IBD. On the other hand, in recent years, numerous reports have been published on the role of mAChRs in the maintenance of intestinal epithelial homeostasis. However, some of these reports contradict the function of mAChRs and the receptor subtypes involved. This review aimed to summarize the muscarinic receptor subtypes expressed in the intestinal epithelium and the role of mAChRs in intestinal epithelial homeostasis, with a focus on maintenance of the mucus layer, protection and regeneration of barrier function, and differentiation and proliferation of stem cells. In addition to the parasympathetic nerves, several other cell types secrete ACh to activate mAChRs in epithelial cells. As the mode of ACh synthesis and secretion by epithelial cells has been elucidated in recent years, reports on non-neuronal ACh systems were also reviewed. Finally, we discussed the potential of mAChRs as pharmacological targets for the treatment of IBD by protecting and improving intestinal epithelial function.

2. mAChRs in the Intestinal Epithelium

Muscarinic acetylcholine receptors (mAChRs) belong to the G protein-coupled receptor (GPCR) family and receive ACh as an endogenous ligand. In mammals, mAChRs consist of five subtypes (M_1–M_5). The M_1, M_3, and M_5 subtypes couple to $G\alpha_{q/11}$ proteins, which can activate phospholipase Cβ, leading to the production of diacylglycerol and inositol 1,4,5-trisphosphate, which activates protein kinase C (PKC) and mobilizes intracellular Ca^{2+}, respectively. In contrast, the M_2 and M_4 receptors signal via $G\alpha_{i/o}$ proteins to inhibit adenylyl cyclase activity and downregulate cyclic AMP production. mAChRs have been actively studied for a long time as they play a role in the regulation of motility in intestinal smooth muscle cells and the secretion of anions, such as chloride, in intestinal epithelial cells. The intestinal epithelium comprises aligned enterocytes/colonocytes, goblet cells, and Paneth cells. These cells differentiate from a common origin, the few leucine-rich repeat-containing G protein-coupled receptor 5 (Lgr5)-positive stem cells in the crypt base.

The expression of mAChR subtypes in these cells has been examined using immunohistochemistry, in situ hybridization, quantitative PCR, and pharmacological assays. In a previous review, Hirota et al. summarized the mAChR subtypes in the gut [7]. Here, we provide an update based on a recent study that evaluated mAChR subtypes with a focus on the intestinal epithelium (Table 1).

Table 1. mAChR subtypes in intestinal epithelial cells.

	Tissues	Region/Cell Types	Subtypes	Methods	Ref.
mouse	small intestine	villi	M_1, M_2, M_3, M_4 (M_5-)	qPCR	[8]
		crypts	M_1, M_3, M_4 (M_2-, M_5-)	qPCR	[8]
		epithelial cells	M_1, M_2, M_3, M_4, M_5	IHC	[9]
			M_1, M_3 (M_2-, M_4-, M_5-)	qPCR	[10]
			M_1, M_2, M_3, M_4, M_5	qPCR, IHC	[11]
		goblet cells	M_3, M_4, (M_1-, M_2-, M_5-)	qPCR, microarray	[12]
		Paneth cells	M_2	IHC	[11]
			M_3	IHC	[10]
		stem cells (crypt base)	M_1 (M_2-, M_3-, M_4-, M_5-)	qPCR	[13]
			M_1, M_3	qPCR	[8]
			M_3	IHC	[10]
		endocrine cells	M_3	IHC	[10]
	colon	crypts	M_1 (80%), M_3 (20%)	pharmacological	[14]
			M_1	qPCR	[15]
		goblet cell	M_3, M_4, (M_1-, M_2-, M_5-)	qPCR, microarray	[12]
rat	small intestine	stem cell	M_3, M_5	IHC	[16]
human	colon	epithelial cells	M_1	ISH	[17]
			M_3 (M_1-)	IHC	[18]
	cell line (colon)	HT-29/B6 cells	M_3 (M_1-)	pharmacological, qPCR	[19]
	cell line (colon)	T84 cells	M_3 (65%), M_1 (35%)	pharmacological	[20]

qPCR—quantitative PCR; IHC—immunohistochemistry; ISH—in situ hybridization. "-" indicates that they were not detected in the subtypes.

The mAChR subtypes that are mainly expressed in colonocytes are M_1 and M_3. In intestinal epithelial cells, mAChRs, especially the M_3 subtype, act to promote Cl⁻ secretion [7]. Muscarinic toxin 7 (MT7) is a peptide antagonist derived from snake venom that is highly specific to the M_1 subtype [21]. Experiments on the pharmacological binding of MT7 to colonic crypts have revealed that it consists of approximately 80% M_1 and 20% M_3 receptors. Functionally, M_3 receptors promote Cl⁻ secretion, whereas M_1 receptors may act in an inhibitory manner [14]. The human colonocyte cell-derived cell line, T84, which is often used as a model for intestinal epithelial cells, expresses both M_1 and M_3 [20], although the M_3 subtype is responsible for Cl⁻ secretion [22]. However, as mAChR-stimulated ion secretion is maintained in M_3 receptor-knockout (KO) mice, other subtypes, such as M_1 receptors, may play compensatory roles [15,23]. Thus, both M_1 and M_3, expressed in colonocytes, couple to $G\alpha_{q/11}$ proteins; however, their functions may be partially different.

Other epithelial cell types, such as Paneth cells, goblet cells, and stem cells, express mAChRs. Estimating the major mAChR subtype that is functional on the cell surface is a difficult task in pharmacological binding experiments owing to the relatively small population of these cells in the tissue. Therefore, studies evaluating the functional impact of cell-specific receptor KO mice or subtype-selective ligands are particularly important. In addition to the epithelial cells mentioned here, immune cells in the submucosal region express mAChRs, suggesting that ACh stimulation may indirectly affect epithelial cells via mAChRs on these immune cells. The relationship between mAChR subtypes expressed in these cells and their functions in epithelial homeostasis are described below.

3. Role of mAChRs in Mucus Layer Maintenance

Mucus and antimicrobial peptides (AMPs) on the surface of the epithelium prevent the invasion of macromolecules and bacteria before they reach the intestinal epithelium. Defects in the mucosal layer would facilitate bacterial infections and trigger inflammatory responses. Abnormalities in the mucosal barrier are frequently observed in patients with IBD [24]. Thus, improvement in mucus secretion and AMPs might be beneficial for IBD treatment.

Goblet cells, which reside in the intestinal crypts and villi, secrete mucus. ACh from the enteric nerve acts on mAChRs in goblet cells to induce mucus release [25,26]. The mAChR subtypes that are critical for the maintenance of the mucus layer have not been determined.

In other tissues, the M_3 subtype primarily mediates secretion in response to cholinergic stimulation. For example, in the conjunctival goblet cells, genetic disruption of the M_3 subtype has been demonstrated to significantly reduce tear secretion [27]. Recent studies have suggested that the M_1 subtype is primarily responsible for mucus secretion in the gut [28]. The expression of M_1 in intestinal goblet cells was supported by a single-cell RNA-seq study [29]. The secretion of mucus from goblet cells is classified into compound exocytosis, in which multiple vesicles fuse in an intracellular Ca^{2+}-dependent manner, and primary exocytosis, in which vesicles fuse individually. Mucus release by ACh stimulation is the former mechanism, and the process might be triggered by intracellular Ca^{2+} elevation by $G\alpha_{q/11}$-coupled mAChR subtypes, such as M_1 and M_3 [30,31]. Furthermore, a study of M_3 subtype KO mice revealed that M_3 is important for the maintenance of goblet cells and the expression of Muc2, the main factor of mucus [32]. In contrast, Knoop et al. showed that M_4 receptors are abundantly expressed with M_3 receptors in goblet cells [12]. This research revealed that the M_4 subtype plays an important role in immune tolerance in the small intestine through a mechanism called goblet cell-associated antigen passages (GAPs), which deliver luminal antigens to antigen-presenting cells in the lamina propria. In contrast, in the colonic mucosa, M_3 receptors are involved in the induction of GAPs [28]. Thus, mAChR in goblet cells regulates the prevention of antigen entry by mucus secretion and the uptake and transport of antigens by GAPs.

Antimicrobial peptides are secreted from Paneth cells in the crypts of the small intestine. As AMPs prevent bacterial infections and control intestinal bacterial composites, their abnormalities are associated with pathologies, such as IBD [33]. Paneth cell secretion is affected by cholinergic stimuli as well as the bacterial milieu [34,35]. Stimulation of mAChRs in Paneth cells increases intracellular Ca^{2+} concentrations, which may induce the exocytosis of AMP-containing vesicles [36,37]. In *Caenorhabditis elegans*, cholinergic neurons induce Wnt expression in the intestinal epithelium via mAChR, leading to the upregulation of AMPs, such as C-type lectins and lysozymes [38]. Therefore, mAChRs may not only act on the secretion, but also on gene expression of AMPs.

Overall, mAChRs contribute to intestinal epithelial homeostasis by preventing the entry of macromolecules and bacteria into the epithelium via the release of mucus and AMPs.

4. Role of mAChRs in the Epithelial Barrier against Inflammatory Cytokines

Immune cells in the lamina propria are activated in response to bacterial and antigenic penetration. In the intestinal mucosa of IBD patients, the secretion of pro-inflammatory cytokines, such as TNF-α or interferon γ (IFNγ), is elevated [39–41]. These cytokines are known to increase the membrane permeability of intestinal epithelial cells and disrupt barrier functions [42,43]. Reducing the effects of these pro-inflammatory cytokines on the intestinal epithelium would be beneficial, as revealed by the efficacy of TNF-α-neutralizing antibodies in the treatment of IBD [44].

In rat colonic epithelium, the TNF-α/IFNγ-induced increase in paracellular permeability was prevented by prestimulation with a muscarinic agonist [19]. Nuclear factor κB (NF-κB) is a main signaling mediator of TNF-α and is involved in the dysregulation of intestinal epithelial integrity [45–47]. In HT-29/B6 cells, a human colorectal adenocarcinoma-derived cell line that can be used to study intestinal epithelial barrier function [48], TNF-α decreased barrier function and increased the expression of inflammatory cytokine (IL-8) in association with an increase in NF-κB signaling, both of which were suppressed by mAChR stimulation [19]. This attenuation of TNF-α effects is due to the shedding of the TNF-α receptors (TNFRs). Ectodomain shedding of TNFRs leads to the downregulation of TNF-α effects by reducing the density of cell surface TNFRs and neutralizing TNF-α with the cleaved, soluble form of TNFRs (sTNFRs) [49,50]. As HT-29/B6 cells predominantly express the M_3 subtype, the action of TNF-α might be suppressed via this mAChR subtype. Tumor necrosis factor-α converting enzyme (TACE/ADAM-17) is a metalloprotease that can act on the shedding of TNFRs [51]. One upstream signaling molecule involved in TACE activation is p38 MAPK [52]. Based on further studies, the M_3 subtype induces the reduction of TNF-α action by activating p38 MAPK following $G\alpha_{q/11}$ protein-mediated Ca^{2+} responses, particularly store-operated calcium entry (SOCE) [53,54]. Activation of TACE by the M_3 subtype also induces epidermal growth factor receptor (EGFR) transactivation [54], which may contribute to the optimal regulation of ion secretion [55] and intestinal epithelial homeostasis [56].

Stimulation of mAChRs confers resistance to interleukin-1β (IL-1β)-induced barrier dysfunction [57]. Treatment with IL-1β enhances the expression of chemokines (CXCL-1, CXCL-10, IL-8, and CCL-7) and myosin light-chain kinase (MLCK) through NF-κB signaling. Stimulation of mAChRs was not found to suppress the activation of NF-κB by IL-1β; therefore, the expression of these cytokines or MLCK was not suppressed. In contrast, mAChR stimulation markedly inhibited MLCK-mediated phosphorylation of the myosin light chain (MLC) by IL-1β; however, the mechanism is unclear. Activation of MLCK leads to barrier disruption through endocytosis of tight junction factors, including occludin [58,59]. In fact, IL-1β reduced the amount of occludin localized to the tight junction, which was inhibited by mAChR stimulation. Thus, mAChR may inhibit IL-1β-induced impairment of barrier function via the suppression of MLC phosphorylation by MLCK [57].

Dextran sulfate sodium (DSS)-induced colitis is widely used as a model of human ulcerative colitis [60]. The administration of DSS damages intestinal epithelial cells, resulting in the infiltration of macrophages and the release of pro-inflammatory cytokines, such as TNF-α and IL-1β, in response to invading bacteria. Neutralizing antibodies against TNF-α were found to improve mucosal integrity in the DSS-induced colitis model [61]. Notably, DSS-induced colitis was more severe in M_3 KO mice [23]. Recently, McN-A-343 was reported to exhibit anti-inflammatory effects in acetic acid-treated mice, another experimental model of ulcerative colitis [62]. McN-A-343 is widely used as an M1 selective agonist owing to its relatively high efficacy against the M1 subtype; however, it also acts on other mAChR subtypes [63]. Therefore, mAChRs, especially the M_1 and M_3 subtypes, may reduce the action of pro-inflammatory cytokines, such as TNF-α and IL-1β, released by the activated innate immune system and prevent the disruption of the intestinal epithelial barrier.

Hosic and colleagues established a primary culture system of human small intestinal epithelial cells, rather than immortalized cell lines, to determine the effects of TNF-α on barrier function [64]. In their study, neither nicotinic nor muscarinic stimulation improved TNF-α-induced barrier disruption. Therefore, it may be necessary to reconsider the role of mAChRs in epithelial cells by comparing the expressed mAChR subtypes and responsiveness between this primary culture system, cell lines, and in vivo.

5. Role of mAChRs in Epithelial Barrier Repair

As disruption of epithelial barrier function allows continued macromolecular and bacterial invasion, repair of the barrier function is important to prevent further inflammatory responses. In a porcine colonocyte culture system, stimulation with carbachol or oxotremorine increased transepithelial resistance during the establishment of epithelial barrier function [65]. This effect was inhibited by co-treatment with atropine, suggesting that muscarinic stimulation facilitates epithelial barrier formation, and mAChRs may play a role in the regeneration of the damaged epithelial barrier. Colonocyte-derived ACh was also detected, and the administration of atropine without muscarinic agonists suppressed the establishment of barrier function. Therefore, the autocrine/paracrine action of colonocyte-derived non-neuronal ACh may be involved in barrier formation [65].

Studies using T84 cells derived from human colonocytes expressing the M_1 and M_3 subtypes have reported that M_1 receptor-mediated extracellular signal-regulated kinase 1/2 (ERK1/2) activation and focal adhesion kinase (FAK) activation contribute to recovery from ethanol-induced epithelial injury [20]. FAK activity is important for epithelial barrier maintenance and repair through the regulation of tight junction complex redistribution [66]. Activation of ERK1/2 also facilitates intestinal barrier function via expression of the tight junction factors [67,68]. The importance of the M_1 subtype, rather than M_3, for ERK1/2 activation has been demonstrated using rodent colonic mucosal fragments [14]. Khan et al. showed that the expression of the M_1 subtype was reduced by IFNγ-induced barrier perturbation in T84 cells [20]. This observation suggests that inflammatory cytokines inhibit barrier restoration by suppressing M_1 receptor levels. Tyrosine kinase inhibitors used as anticancer drugs have been demonstrated to reduce the barrier function of T84 cell monolayers, whereas cholinergic stimulation with carbachol delays barrier function impairment through ERK1/2 activation [69]. Thus, signaling through ERK1/2 and FAK may contribute to mAChR-induced epithelial barrier maintenance or repair. These kinases are involved in cell proliferation and migration as well. Therefore, the activation of these kinases by mAChRs is expected to participate in the replenishment of epithelial cells from stem and progenitor cells, and the maintenance of epithelial cell homeostasis, as described below.

Although mAChRs are important for maintaining barrier function against injury or restoring impaired barrier function, they may not be essential for constitutive epithelial barrier function, at least in the colon. This notion is because genetic ablation of M_1, M_3 or M_1/M_3 showed no significant difference in intestinal epithelial permeability [32,70]. However, in the small intestine, the constitutive barrier function is partially impaired in M_3 KO mice [70]. Therefore, the role of mAChRs in barrier function may differ in the small and large intestine.

6. Role of mAChRs in Epithelial Cell Regeneration

The differentiation and proliferation of stem and progenitor cells are essential for the maintenance of intestinal epithelial cells, which undergo rapid turnover and replenishment of epithelial cells after injury. Released ACh from enteric cholinergic neurons upregulates mucosal growth in a scopolamine-sensitive manner, suggesting that mAChRs may facilitate these processes [16,71]. The stem cells responsible for intestinal epithelium regeneration are Lgr5-positive cells located at the bottom of the crypts. Several studies have revealed the mAChR subtypes expressed in Lgr5-positive stem cells. Greig et al. detected only the M_1 subtype in jejunal and ileal crypt-based samples using RT-PCR [13]. In contrast, immunohistochemical studies have suggested the expression of the M_3 and M_5 subtypes [10,16]. Importantly, scopolamine treatment inhibited the differentiation and proliferation of Lgr5-positive cells, and caused their disappearance from the crypt base of the small intestine [10]. In addition, administration of the M_1-selective agonist McN-A-343 promoted cell proliferation and increased intestinal mucosal growth in mice [13]. Therefore, mAChRs may contribute to the maintenance of stem cell function in the intestinal epithelium.

Conversely, some reports have revealed the negative effects of mAChRs on intestinal stem cell function. Treatment with the mAChR agonist inhibited organoid proliferation and differentiation in crypt-villus organoid cultures of the small intestine [8,9], while treatment with atropine alone promoted them. Such findings indicate that mAChRs inhibit the differentiation and proliferation of stem and progenitor cells by receiving non-neuronal ACh secreted by the intestinal epithelial cells themselves [9]. In addition, M_3 KO mice displayed an increase in crypt size and the facilitation of cell proliferation and migration [72]. The increased villus height has been observed in conventional mAChR knockout mice, especially in M_2, M_3, and M_5 receptor-KO mice [73].

Taken together, stimulation with M_3 and M_5 receptors may have inhibitory effects on differentiation and proliferation, whereas the M_1 receptors contribute to epithelial cell regeneration and maintenance by maintaining and promoting the function of Lgr5-positive stem and progenitor cells. This proposal is intriguing as the M_1, M_3, and M_5 subtypes are coupled to the same $G\alpha_{q/11}$ protein. One possibility is that one of the M_1 or M_3/M_5 subtypes is expressed not on Lgr5-positive stem cells, but on cells that form a stem cell niche near the stem cells, and indirectly regulates stem cell function. Alternatively, this phenomenon may be related to prior findings that the activities of ERK1/2 and FAK, which contribute to cell proliferation and migration in intestinal epithelial cells, are selectively induced by the M_1 receptor rather than by the M_3 receptor [14,20]. In fact, ERK1/2 inhibitors have been reported to suppress cell proliferation by inhibiting enhanced ERK1/2 activity in the intestinal organoids of M_3 KO mice [72]. It is unclear why such a difference exists between M_1- and M_3-mediated signaling. In experiments performed with varying amounts of the $G\alpha_{q/11}$ protein in the intestinal epithelial cell line, $G\alpha_{q/11}$ signaling was suggested to act in a growth-suppressive manner and may be responsible for physiological effects, such as secretion and absorption in terminally differentiated intestinal epithelial cells [74]. Thus, the M_1 receptor may activate ERK1/2 in a $G\alpha_{q/11}$ protein-independent pathway. On the other hand, deletion of $G\alpha_{q/11}$ in intestinal epithelial cells impairs proper differentiation, particularly into Paneth cells, suggesting that the effects of M_1/M_3-mediated $G\alpha_{q/11}$ signaling on differentiation regulation require further studies [75].

Overall, an mAChR subtype-specific balance regulation may exist between the promotion and inhibition of proliferation and differentiation for intestinal epithelial regeneration.

7. Involvement of mAChRs in Epithelial Barrier Impairment

As described above, mAChRs in the intestinal epithelial cells contribute to epithelial homeostasis through various mechanisms. However, several studies have reported that mAChRs may reduce epithelial barrier function. For example, experiments on rat ileal segments have revealed that carbachol treatment enhances transport from the mucosa to the plasma membrane via endocytosis and the paracellular pathway [76]. Furthermore, electrical stimulation of the vagus nerve led to permeability of the jejunal epithelium through the activation of mAChRs [26]. Notably, the passage of bacteria increased when the small intestinal epithelium, stimulated with mAChRs via the intraperitoneal administration of pilocarpine, was examined in the Ussing chamber [77]. This study also revealed a pilocarpine-induced decrease in mucus secretion. In the mouse ileum, the M_3 subtype increased the barrier permeability of macromolecules [78]. In contrast, mAChR activation in primary cultured intestinal epithelial cells or colonic cell lines, such as Caco-2 and T84 cells, was not found to exacerbate epithelial barrier function [57,64,65,79].

The presence of various cell types in the intestinal tissue could explain this difference. In addition to the epithelium, the tissue used in the Ussing chamber also contains immune and nervous system cells in the submucosal layer. Stress has been demonstrated to increase intestinal epithelial permeability via the activation of mAChRs by cholinergic neurons. Corticotropin-releasing factor (CRF) and the activation of mast cells play important roles in this process [80,81]. Wallon et al. demonstrated the presence of eosinophils expressing muscarinic M_2 and M_3 receptors in the subepithelial regions. The release of CRF by eosinophils via the activation of M_3 receptors reduces intestinal epithelial barrier function by activating neighboring mast cells [79]. This research also found increased levels of activated and degranulated eosinophils in patients with ulcerative colitis, suggesting a link between mAChR stimulation-mediated eosinophil activation and the exacerbation of inflammation. In addition, activation of M_3 receptors on macrophages leads to their differentiation into classically activated phenotypes, thereby facilitating inflammatory responses [32].

These studies indicate that the activation of mAChRs in a tissue-wide or subtype-unselective manner may have deleterious effects on intestinal epithelial barrier function. Therefore, local or subtype-specific activation of mAChRs is important for epithelial homeostasis.

8. Non-Neuronal Acetylcholine

Multiple sources of ACh—including ACh released from parasympathetic or enteric cholinergic nerves, and non-neuronal ACh released from intestinal epithelial cells and T cells—act on intestinal epithelial cells and their surrounding cells. Acetylcholine from parasympathetic and enteric neurons act on macrophage $\alpha7$ nicotinic receptors to suppress pro-inflammatory cytokine release and stimulate mucus secretion from goblet cells via mAChR activation [26,82]. Neuronal ACh may also act on cryptic basal stem and progenitor cells, promoting intestinal mucosal tissue growth [16,71].

The importance of ACh released from non-neuronal cells in several tissues has been gradually recognized [83]. As ACh is an unstable substance that is easily degraded by acetylcholinesterase (AChE), ACh from nerve endings may be insufficient to activate receptors on epithelial cells. It has therefore been suggested that ACh released by epithelial cells may act in an autocrine/paracrine manner. Indeed, non-neuronal ACh has been demonstrated to be involved in epithelial barrier formation and the regulation of mucosal growth [9,65].

Choline acetyltransferase (ChAT) is responsible for ACh synthesis from choline. Transgenic mice expressing fluorescent proteins under the control of the ChAT promoter showed that ChAT-positive cells exist as scattered solitary cells in the epithelium of the small intestine and colon [84]. These tuft cells expressing ChAT were not found to express the vesicular ACh transporter (vAChT), except in the proximal colon, suggesting that ACh was released in a vesicle-independent manner. Consistently, vesamicol, an inhibitor of vAChT, was not found to inhibit non-neuronal ACh secretion in the colonic epithelium [85]. The polyspecific organic cation transporter OCTN1 has a variant (amino acid substitution L503F) associated with Crohn's disease [86]. Interestingly, OCTN1 can transport ACh, and its transport function has been demonstrated to be reduced in the L503F variant [87]. Therefore, OCTN1 is one of the possible candidates responsible for the release of non-neuronal ACh in intestinal epithelial cells. As tuft cells do not express a high-affinity choline transporter (CHT1), they may provide choline for ACh synthesis via a different mechanism from cholinergic neurons [84]. The choline transporter-like (CTL) family consists of five members, of which CTL4 has been reported to contribute to choline uptake associated with ACh synthesis and secretion [88]. The expression of both CTL4 and ChAT increased when an inflammatory response was induced in the mouse ileum by lipopolysaccharide (LPS) treatment [89]. Therefore, inflammation may increase non-neuronal ACh production in the intestinal epithelium. However, in a previous study, ChAT expression was decreased in the intestinal epithelium in specimens from patients with Crohn's disease and ulcerative colitis [57].

CD4+ T cells that infiltrate the gut express ChAT and synthesize ACh. ChAT-positive T cells participate in host defense against bacterial infections [90]. In addition, T cell-derived ACh has been reported to contribute to the expression of AMPs, including lysozymes and defensin A [91]. In DSS colitis models, ChAT-positive T cells exacerbate the acute immune response but support the later resolution of intestinal inflammation [92].

As described above, neuronal and non-neuronal ACh systems differ in certain factors involved in the choline uptake and ACh release mechanisms. Therefore, neuronal and non-neuronal ACh levels may be pharmacologically distinguished and regulated by targeting these differences.

9. mAChRs as a Potential Therapeutic Target for IBD

As summarized in Figure 1, the activation of mAChRs in intestinal epithelial cells is effective in the maintenance of homeostasis. However, as each mAChR subtype is expressed in different cell types and plays different roles, the outcome may vary depending on the subtype activated. For example, M_1 receptors have been demonstrated to be responsible for epithelial barrier regeneration and mucus secretion, while M_3 receptors are involved in the protection against inflammatory cytokines. The activation of M_3 receptors expressed on eosinophils and macrophages may indirectly threaten epithelial barrier function. In addition, the migration and invasion of colon cancer cells are stimulated by the activation of M_3 receptors [93], whose expression is increased in cancer cells [94]. In this context, the activation of M_3 receptors may adversely affect intestinal epithelial homeostasis. Therefore, it is important to determine the effects of subtype-selective agonists and positive allosteric modulators (PAMs) on intestinal epithelial cell homeostasis and their impact on IBD treatment. In particular, M_1 receptor-selective agonists and PAMs are being actively developed as potential therapeutic agents for schizophrenia and Alzheimer's disease [95,96]. Exploring the potential of these drugs in the treatment of IBD is an interesting challenge. Gastrointestinal disorders, such as diarrhea, are major adverse effects of muscarinic stimulation. This effect is mainly due to the M_3 subtype in smooth muscle, despite reports of the involvement of the M_1 and M_2 subtypes [97,98]. Therefore, the stimulation of epithelial cell-specific muscarinic receptors, such as in drug delivery systems, is desirable for safe treatment.

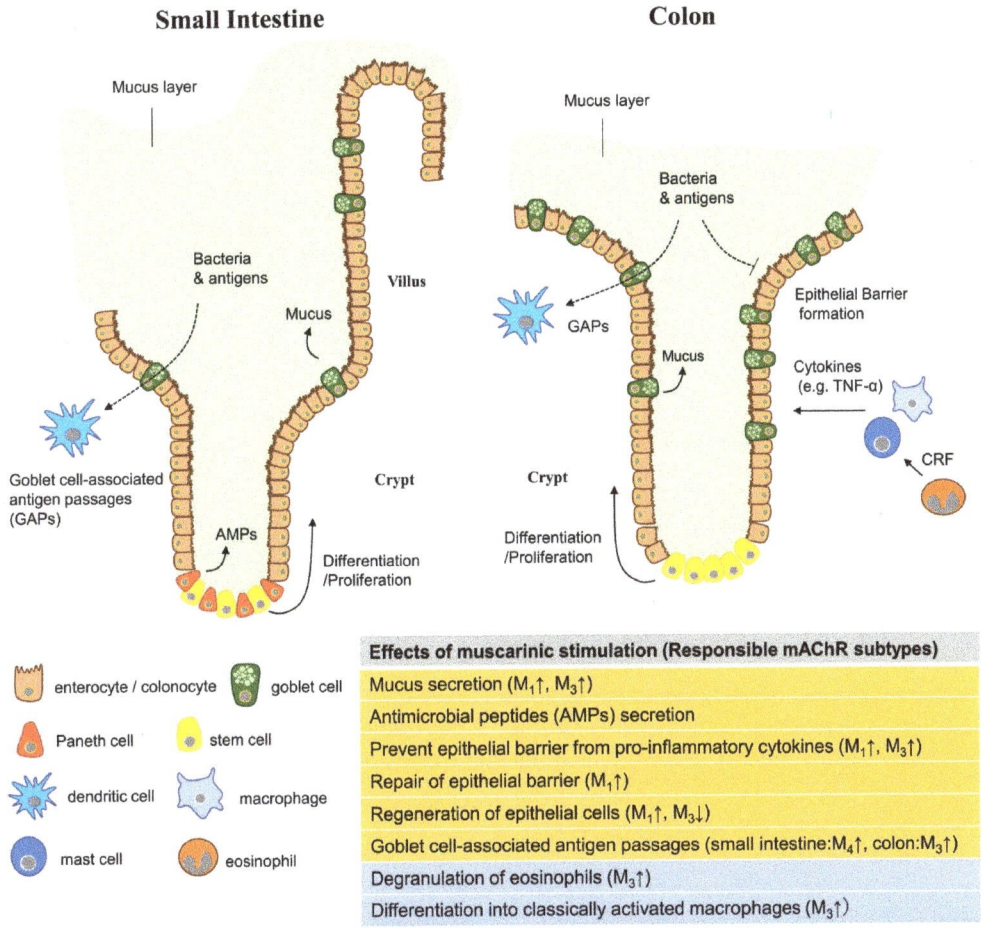

Figure 1. Mucosal defense system and muscarinic receptor action in intestinal epithelial tissue. The intestinal epithelium of the small intestine (left panel) and colon (right panel) are shown. Intestinal epithelial cells are composed of enterocytes/colonocytes, goblet cells, Paneth cells, and stem cells that are responsible for the formation of the epithelial barrier, secretion of mucus and antimicrobial peptides (AMPs), and replenishment of epithelial cells through differentiation and proliferation, respectively. Various immune cells reside or infiltrate the submucosal layer and are responsible for the immune response against invading bacteria. These cells express mAChRs that modulate the function of each cell. The table below summarizes the effects of mAChRs on each of these functions. The effects on epithelial cells are highlighted in orange while those on other cells are highlighted in blue. The up and down arrows marked to the right of the mAChR subtypes indicate that activating each subtype enhances or inhibits that response, respectively.

High AChE activity has been observed in the intestinal epithelium [89,99]. Therefore, AChE inhibitors may be effective at maintaining intestinal epithelial homeostasis by increasing ACh stability near the intestinal epithelial cells and enhancing ACh signaling. In fact, the inhibition of cholinesterase by paraoxon has been demonstrated to promote the degranulation of goblet and Paneth cells, which promotes defense against orally administered *Salmonella* [100]. The acetylcholinesterase inhibitor, pyridostigmine, was also found to attenuate the pathology of DSS-induced colitis [101].

The promotion of ACh synthesis and release also enhances ACh signaling. Brain orexins stimulate the vagal cholinergic pathway, which prevents LPS-induced colonic epithelial permeation in an mAChR-dependent manner [102]. As ACh-producing tuft cells express chemoreceptors and respond to bitter substances, ACh release may be regulated by dietary components [84]. Moreover, the short-chain fatty acid generated by intestinal bacteria, propionate, induces the secretion of non-neuronal ACh in the colon [103,104]. Therefore, prebiotics or probiotics may contribute to the upregulation of non-neuronal ACh in the colonic epithelium. Importantly, the effect of propionate is expected to be specific to intestinal epithelial cells, whereas AChE inhibitors are expected to enhance ACh in both neuronal and non-neuronal cells. Owing to its local action, ACh is thought to exert different effects depending on the localization of the released cells. However, the effects of epithelial cell-derived non-neuronal ACh on intestinal epithelial homeostasis and IBD are not fully understood. Therefore, the facilitative effect of propionate-mediated non-neuronal ACh release on intestinal epithelial homeostasis is an interesting subject for basic research and clinical applications.

10. Conclusions

In summary, mAChRs are involved in various functions related to intestinal epithelial homeostasis, in addition to the previously known intestinal contractions and secretions. However, the subtypes of mAChRs that function on different cell types in the intestinal epithelium and surrounding cell populations, including immune cells, are not fully understood. In addition, the cholinergic system that delivers ACh to the mAChRs in each cell is unclear. As a result, the complete mechanism of action of the mAChRs in the intestinal epithelium remains elusive. Although not discussed in detail in this review, nicotinic receptors are also important targets of ACh, and their involvement in the intestinal inflammatory response is a topic of intense research. Therefore, a comprehensive understanding of the ACh network throughout the intestinal tissue, including the relationship between muscarinic and nicotinic receptors, would highlight a new strategy for IBD treatment that contributes to intestinal epithelial homeostasis.

Author Contributions: Conceptualization, J.U. and T.Y.; writing—original draft preparation, J.U.; writing—review and editing, J.U., H.N., I.M., T.M. and T.Y.; All authors have read and agreed to the published version of the manuscript.

Funding: This research was funded in part by JSPS grant number 19K09794 (T.Y.), 22K07358 (H.N.) and 22K06637 (J.U.) (Grant-in-Aid for Scientific Research (C)) granted by Japan Society for the Promotion of Science, the Smoking Research Foundation of Japan (2021G008 to T.M. and 2020G006 to T.Y.), Kobayashi Foundation (no.181 to T.Y.), Akiyama Life Science Foundation (J.U. and 141-032 to T.Y.) and the Grant of National Center for Child Health and Development (2021-A1 to T.Y.).

Institutional Review Board Statement: Not applicable.

Informed Consent Statement: Not applicable.

Data Availability Statement: No new data were created or analyzed in this study. Data sharing is not applicable to this article.

Acknowledgments: The authors thank to Keiko Ikeda for the efficient secretarial assistance.

Conflicts of Interest: The authors declare no conflict of interest.

References

1. Irvine, E.J.; Marshall, J.K. Increased intestinal permeability precedes the onset of Crohn's disease in a subject with familial risk. *Gastroenterology* **2000**, *119*, 1740–1744. [CrossRef] [PubMed]
2. Michielan, A.; D'Inca, R. Intestinal Permeability in Inflammatory Bowel Disease: Pathogenesis, Clinical Evaluation, and Therapy of Leaky Gut. *Mediat. Inflamm.* **2015**, *2015*, 628157. [CrossRef] [PubMed]
3. Tanahashi, Y.; Komori, S.; Matsuyama, H.; Kitazawa, T.; Unno, T. Functions of Muscarinic Receptor Subtypes in Gastrointestinal Smooth Muscle: A Review of Studies with Receptor-Knockout Mice. *Int. J. Mol. Sci.* **2021**, *22*, 926. [CrossRef] [PubMed]
4. Khan, M.R.; Islam, M.T.; Yazawa, T.; Hayashi, H.; Suzuki, Y.; Uwada, J.; Anisuzzaman, A.S.; Taniguchi, T. Muscarinic cholinoceptor-mediated activation of JNK negatively regulates intestinal secretion in mice. *J. Pharmacol. Sci.* **2015**, *127*, 150–153. [CrossRef]
5. Keely, S.J.; Barrett, K.E. Regulation of chloride secretion. Novel pathways and messengers. *Ann. N. Y. Acad. Sci.* **2000**, *915*, 67–76. [CrossRef]
6. Serafini, M.A.; Paz, A.H.; Nunes, N.S. Cholinergic immunomodulation in inflammatory bowel diseases. *Brain Behav. Immun. Health* **2022**, *19*, 100401. [CrossRef] [PubMed]
7. Hirota, C.L.; McKay, D.M. Cholinergic regulation of epithelial ion transport in the mammalian intestine. *Br. J. Pharmacol.* **2006**, *149*, 463–479. [CrossRef]
8. Davis, E.A.; Zhou, W.; Dailey, M.J. Evidence for a direct effect of the autonomic nervous system on intestinal epithelial stem cell proliferation. *Physiol. Rep.* **2018**, *6*, e13745. [CrossRef] [PubMed]
9. Takahashi, T.; Ohnishi, H.; Sugiura, Y.; Honda, K.; Suematsu, M.; Kawasaki, T.; Deguchi, T.; Fujii, T.; Orihashi, K.; Hippo, Y.; et al. Non-neuronal acetylcholine acts as an endogenous regulator of proliferation and differentiation of Lgr5-positive stem cells in mice. *FEBS J.* **2014**, *281*, 4672–4690. [CrossRef] [PubMed]
10. Middelhoff, M.; Nienhuser, H.; Valenti, G.; Maurer, H.C.; Hayakawa, Y.; Takahashi, R.; Kim, W.; Jiang, Z.; Malagola, E.; Cuti, K.; et al. Prox1-positive cells monitor and sustain the murine intestinal epithelial cholinergic niche. *Nat. Commun.* **2020**, *11*, 111. [CrossRef]
11. Muise, E.D.; Gandotra, N.; Tackett, J.J.; Bamdad, M.C.; Cowles, R.A. Distribution of muscarinic acetylcholine receptor subtypes in the murine small intestine. *Life Sci.* **2017**, *169*, 6–10. [CrossRef] [PubMed]
12. Knoop, K.A.; McDonald, K.G.; McCrate, S.; McDole, J.R.; Newberry, R.D. Microbial sensing by goblet cells controls immune surveillance of luminal antigens in the colon. *Mucosal Immunol.* **2015**, *8*, 198–210. [CrossRef] [PubMed]
13. Greig, C.J.; Armenia, S.J.; Cowles, R.A. The M1 muscarinic acetylcholine receptor in the crypt stem cell compartment mediates intestinal mucosal growth. *Exp. Biol. Med.* **2020**, *245*, 1194–1199. [CrossRef]
14. Khan, M.R.; Anisuzzaman, A.S.; Semba, S.; Ma, Y.; Uwada, J.; Hayashi, H.; Suzuki, Y.; Takano, T.; Ikeuchi, H.; Uchino, M.; et al. M1 is a major subtype of muscarinic acetylcholine receptors on mouse colonic epithelial cells. *J. Gastroenterol.* **2013**, *48*, 885–896. [CrossRef]
15. Haberberger, R.; Schultheiss, G.; Diener, M. Epithelial muscarinic M1 receptors contribute to carbachol-induced ion secretion in mouse colon. *Eur. J. Pharmacol.* **2006**, *530*, 229–233. [CrossRef]
16. Lundgren, O.; Jodal, M.; Jansson, M.; Ryberg, A.T.; Svensson, L. Intestinal epithelial stem/progenitor cells are controlled by mucosal afferent nerves. *PLoS ONE* **2011**, *6*, e16295. [CrossRef] [PubMed]
17. Tsukimi, Y.; Pustovit, R.V.; Harrington, A.M.; Garcia-Caraballo, S.; Brierley, S.M.; Di Natale, M.; Molero, J.C.; Furness, J.B. Effects and sites of action of a M1 receptor positive allosteric modulator on colonic motility in rats and dogs compared with 5-HT(4) agonism and cholinesterase inhibition. *Neurogastroenterol. Motil.* **2020**, *32*, e13866. [CrossRef] [PubMed]
18. Harrington, A.M.; Peck, C.J.; Liu, L.; Burcher, E.; Hutson, J.M.; Southwell, B.R. Localization of muscarinic receptors M1R, M2R and M3R in the human colon. *Neurogastroenterol. Motil.* **2010**, *22*, e262–e263. [CrossRef]
19. Khan, M.R.; Uwada, J.; Yazawa, T.; Islam, M.T.; Krug, S.M.; Fromm, M.; Karaki, S.; Suzuki, Y.; Kuwahara, A.; Yoshiki, H.; et al. Activation of muscarinic cholinoceptor ameliorates tumor necrosis factor-alpha-induced barrier dysfunction in intestinal epithelial cells. *FEBS Lett.* **2015**, *589*, 3640–3647. [CrossRef]
20. Khan, R.I.; Yazawa, T.; Anisuzzaman, A.S.; Semba, S.; Ma, Y.; Uwada, J.; Hayashi, H.; Suzuki, Y.; Ikeuchi, H.; Uchino, M.; et al. Activation of focal adhesion kinase via M1 muscarinic acetylcholine receptor is required in restitution of intestinal barrier function after epithelial injury. *Biochim. Biophys. Acta* **2014**, *1842*, 635–645. [CrossRef]
21. Onali, P.; Adem, A.; Karlsson, E.; Olianas, M.C. The pharmacological action of MT-7. *Life Sci.* **2005**, *76*, 1547–1552. [CrossRef] [PubMed]
22. Dickinson, K.E.; Frizzell, R.A.; Sekar, M.C. Activation of T84 cell chloride channels by carbachol involves a phosphoinositide-coupled muscarinic M3 receptor. *Eur. J. Pharmacol.* **1992**, *225*, 291–298. [CrossRef] [PubMed]
23. Hirota, C.L.; McKay, D.M. M3 muscarinic receptor-deficient mice retain bethanechol-mediated intestinal ion transport and are more sensitive to colitis. *Can. J. Physiol. Pharmacol.* **2006**, *84*, 1153–1161. [CrossRef]
24. Sun, J.; Shen, X.; Li, Y.; Guo, Z.; Zhu, W.; Zuo, L.; Zhao, J.; Gu, L.; Gong, J.; Li, J. Therapeutic Potential to Modify the Mucus Barrier in Inflammatory Bowel Disease. *Nutrients* **2016**, *8*, 44. [CrossRef] [PubMed]
25. Specian, R.D.; Neutra, M.R. Mechanism of rapid mucus secretion in goblet cells stimulated by acetylcholine. *J. Cell Biol.* **1980**, *85*, 626–640. [CrossRef]
26. Greenwood, B.; Mantle, M. Mucin and protein release in the rabbit jejunum: Effects of bethanechol and vagal nerve stimulation. *Gastroenterology* **1992**, *103*, 496–505. [CrossRef]

27. Musayeva, A.; Jiang, S.; Ruan, Y.; Zadeh, J.K.; Chronopoulos, P.; Pfeiffer, N.; Muller, W.E.G.; Ackermann, M.; Xia, N.; Li, H.; et al. Aged Mice Devoid of the M(3) Muscarinic Acetylcholine Receptor Develop Mild Dry Eye Disease. *Int. J. Mol. Sci.* **2021**, *22*, 6133. [CrossRef]
28. Gustafsson, J.K.; Davis, J.E.; Rappai, T.; McDonald, K.G.; Kulkarni, D.H.; Knoop, K.A.; Hogan, S.P.; Fitzpatrick, J.A.; Lencer, W.I.; Newberry, R.D. Intestinal goblet cells sample and deliver lumenal antigens by regulated endocytic uptake and transcytosis. *Elife* **2021**, *10*, e67292. [CrossRef]
29. Haber, A.L.; Biton, M.; Rogel, N.; Herbst, R.H.; Shekhar, K.; Smillie, C.; Burgin, G.; Delorey, T.M.; Howitt, M.R.; Katz, Y.; et al. A single-cell survey of the small intestinal epithelium. *Nature* **2017**, *551*, 333–339. [CrossRef]
30. Phillips, T.E.; Phillips, T.H.; Neutra, M.R. Regulation of intestinal goblet cell secretion. III. Isolated intestinal epithelium. *Am. J. Physiol.* **1984**, *247*, G674-81. [CrossRef]
31. Epple, H.J.; Kreusel, K.M.; Hanski, C.; Schulzke, J.D.; Riecken, E.O.; Fromm, M. Differential stimulation of intestinal mucin secretion by cholera toxin and carbachol. *Pflugers Arch.* **1997**, *433*, 638–647. [CrossRef] [PubMed]
32. McLean, L.P.; Smith, A.; Cheung, L.; Sun, R.; Grinchuk, V.; Vanuytsel, T.; Desai, N.; Urban, J.F., Jr.; Zhao, A.; Raufman, J.P.; et al. Type 3 Muscarinic Receptors Contribute to Clearance of Citrobacter rodentium. *Inflamm. Bowel Dis.* **2015**, *21*, 1860–1871. [CrossRef] [PubMed]
33. Gubatan, J.; Holman, D.R.; Puntasecca, C.J.; Polevoi, D.; Rubin, S.J.; Rogalla, S. Antimicrobial peptides and the gut microbiome in inflammatory bowel disease. *World J. Gastroenterol.* **2021**, *27*, 7402–7422. [CrossRef] [PubMed]
34. Satoh, Y. Atropine inhibits the degranulation of Paneth cells in ex-germ-free mice. *Cell Tissue Res.* **1988**, *253*, 397–402. [CrossRef] [PubMed]
35. Qu, X.D.; Lloyd, K.C.; Walsh, J.H.; Lehrer, R.I. Secretion of type II phospholipase A2 and cryptdin by rat small intestinal Paneth cells. *Infect. Immun.* **1996**, *64*, 5161–5165. [CrossRef] [PubMed]
36. Satoh, Y.; Ishikawa, K.; Oomori, Y.; Takeda, S.; Ono, K. Bethanechol and a G-protein activator, NaF/AlCl3, induce secretory response in Paneth cells of mouse intestine. *Cell Tissue Res.* **1992**, *269*, 213–220. [CrossRef] [PubMed]
37. Satoh, Y.; Habara, Y.; Ono, K.; Kanno, T. Carbamylcholine- and catecholamine-induced intracellular calcium dynamics of epithelial cells in mouse ileal crypts. *Gastroenterology* **1995**, *108*, 1345–1356. [CrossRef]
38. Labed, S.A.; Wani, K.A.; Jagadeesan, S.; Hakkim, A.; Najibi, M.; Irazoqui, J.E. Intestinal Epithelial Wnt Signaling Mediates Acetylcholine-Triggered Host Defense against Infection. *Immunity* **2018**, *48*, 963–978.e3. [CrossRef]
39. Dionne, S.; Hiscott, J.; D'Agata, I.; Duhaime, A.; Seidman, E.G. Quantitative PCR analysis of TNF-alpha and IL-1 beta mRNA levels in pediatric IBD mucosal biopsies. *Dig. Dis. Sci.* **1997**, *42*, 1557–1566. [CrossRef]
40. Matsuda, R.; Koide, T.; Tokoro, C.; Yamamoto, T.; Godai, T.; Morohashi, T.; Fujita, Y.; Takahashi, D.; Kawana, I.; Suzuki, S.; et al. Quantitive cytokine mRNA expression profiles in the colonic mucosa of patients with steroid naive ulcerative colitis during active and quiescent disease. *Inflamm. Bowel Dis.* **2009**, *15*, 328–334. [CrossRef]
41. Verma, R.; Verma, N.; Paul, J. Expression of inflammatory genes in the colon of ulcerative colitis patients varies with activity both at the mRNA and protein level. *Eur. Cytokine Netw.* **2013**, *24*, 130–138. [CrossRef] [PubMed]
42. Amasheh, M.; Grotjohann, I.; Amasheh, S.; Fromm, A.; Soderholm, J.D.; Zeitz, M.; Fromm, M.; Schulzke, J.D. Regulation of mucosal structure and barrier function in rat colon exposed to tumor necrosis factor alpha and interferon gamma in vitro: A novel model for studying the pathomechanisms of inflammatory bowel disease cytokines. *Scand. J. Gastroenterol.* **2009**, *44*, 1226–1235. [CrossRef] [PubMed]
43. McKay, D.M.; Singh, P.K. Superantigen activation of immune cells evokes epithelial (T84) transport and barrier abnormalities via IFN-gamma and TNF alpha: Inhibition of increased permeability, but not diminished secretory responses by TGF-beta2. *J. Immunol.* **1997**, *159*, 2382–2390. [CrossRef]
44. Billmeier, U.; Dieterich, W.; Neurath, M.F.; Atreya, R. Molecular mechanism of action of anti-tumor necrosis factor antibodies in inflammatory bowel diseases. *World J. Gastroenterol.* **2016**, *22*, 9300–9313. [CrossRef] [PubMed]
45. Al-Sadi, R.; Guo, S.; Ye, D.; Rawat, M.; Ma, T.Y. TNF-alpha Modulation of Intestinal Tight Junction Permeability Is Mediated by NIK/IKK-alpha Axis Activation of the Canonical NF-kappaB Pathway. *Am. J. Pathol.* **2016**, *186*, 1151–1165. [CrossRef]
46. Vereecke, L.; Sze, M.; Mc Guire, C.; Rogiers, B.; Chu, Y.; Schmidt-Supprian, M.; Pasparakis, M.; Beyaert, R.; van Loo, G. Enterocyte-specific A20 deficiency sensitizes to tumor necrosis factor-induced toxicity and experimental colitis. *J. Exp. Med.* **2010**, *207*, 1513–1523. [CrossRef]
47. Vlantis, K.; Wullaert, A.; Sasaki, Y.; Schmidt-Supprian, M.; Rajewsky, K.; Roskams, T.; Pasparakis, M. Constitutive IKK2 activation in intestinal epithelial cells induces intestinal tumors in mice. *J. Clin. Investig.* **2011**, *121*, 2781–2793. [CrossRef] [PubMed]
48. Krug, S.M.; Fromm, M.; Gunzel, D. Two-path impedance spectroscopy for measuring paracellular and transcellular epithelial resistance. *Biophys. J.* **2009**, *97*, 2202–2211. [CrossRef] [PubMed]
49. Wang, J.; Al-Lamki, R.S.; Zhang, H.; Kirkiles-Smith, N.; Gaeta, M.L.; Thiru, S.; Pober, J.S.; Bradley, J.R. Histamine antagonizes tumor necrosis factor (TNF) signaling by stimulating TNF receptor shedding from the cell surface and Golgi storage pool. *J. Biol. Chem.* **2003**, *278*, 21751–21760. [CrossRef]
50. Van Zee, K.J.; Kohno, T.; Fischer, E.; Rock, C.S.; Moldawer, L.L.; Lowry, S.F. Tumor necrosis factor soluble receptors circulate during experimental and clinical inflammation and can protect against excessive tumor necrosis factor alpha in vitro and in vivo. *Proc. Natl. Acad. Sci. USA* **1992**, *89*, 4845–4849. [CrossRef]

51. Peschon, J.J.; Slack, J.L.; Reddy, P.; Stocking, K.L.; Sunnarborg, S.W.; Lee, D.C.; Russell, W.E.; Castner, B.J.; Johnson, R.S.; Fitzner, J.N.; et al. An essential role for ectodomain shedding in mammalian development. *Science* **1998**, *282*, 1281–1284. [CrossRef] [PubMed]
52. Xu, P.; Derynck, R. Direct activation of TACE-mediated ectodomain shedding by p38 MAP kinase regulates EGF receptor-dependent cell proliferation. *Mol. Cell* **2010**, *37*, 551–566. [CrossRef] [PubMed]
53. Uwada, J.; Yazawa, T.; Nakazawa, H.; Mikami, D.; Krug, S.M.; Fromm, M.; Sada, K.; Muramatsu, I.; Taniguchi, T. Store-operated calcium entry (SOCE) contributes to phosphorylation of p38 MAPK and suppression of TNF-alpha signalling in the intestinal epithelial cells. *Cell. Signal.* **2019**, *63*, 109358. [CrossRef]
54. Uwada, J.; Yazawa, T.; Islam, M.T.; Khan, M.R.I.; Krug, S.M.; Fromm, M.; Karaki, S.I.; Suzuki, Y.; Kuwahara, A.; Yoshiki, H.; et al. Activation of muscarinic receptors prevents TNF-alpha-mediated intestinal epithelial barrier disruption through p38 MAPK. *Cell. Signal.* **2017**, *35*, 188–196. [CrossRef]
55. McCole, D.F.; Keely, S.J.; Coffey, R.J.; Barrett, K.E. Transactivation of the epidermal growth factor receptor in colonic epithelial cells by carbachol requires extracellular release of transforming growth factor-alpha. *J. Biol. Chem.* **2002**, *277*, 42603–42612. [CrossRef] [PubMed]
56. Chalaris, A.; Adam, N.; Sina, C.; Rosenstiel, P.; Lehmann-Koch, J.; Schirmacher, P.; Hartmann, D.; Cichy, J.; Gavrilova, O.; Schreiber, S.; et al. Critical role of the disintegrin metalloprotease ADAM17 for intestinal inflammation and regeneration in mice. *J. Exp. Med.* **2010**, *207*, 1617–1624. [CrossRef] [PubMed]
57. Dhawan, S.; Hiemstra, I.H.; Verseijden, C.; Hilbers, F.W.; Te Velde, A.A.; Willemsen, L.E.; Stap, J.; den Haan, J.M.; de Jonge, W.J. Cholinergic receptor activation on epithelia protects against cytokine-induced barrier dysfunction. *Acta Physiol.* **2015**, *213*, 846–859. [CrossRef]
58. Ma, T.Y.; Hoa, N.T.; Tran, D.D.; Bui, V.; Pedram, A.; Mills, S.; Merryfield, M. Cytochalasin B modulation of Caco-2 tight junction barrier: Role of myosin light chain kinase. *Am. J. Physiol. Gastrointest Liver Physiol.* **2000**, *279*, G875–G885. [CrossRef]
59. He, W.Q.; Wang, J.; Sheng, J.Y.; Zha, J.M.; Graham, W.V.; Turner, J.R. Contributions of Myosin Light Chain Kinase to Regulation of Epithelial Paracellular Permeability and Mucosal Homeostasis. *Int. J. Mol. Sci.* **2020**, *21*, 993. [CrossRef]
60. Chassaing, B.; Aitken, J.D.; Malleshappa, M.; Vijay-Kumar, M. Dextran sulfate sodium (DSS)-induced colitis in mice. *Curr. Protoc. Immunol.* **2014**, *104*, 15.25.1–15.25.14. [CrossRef]
61. Lenzen, H.; Qian, J.; Manns, M.P.; Seidler, U.; Jorns, A. Restoration of mucosal integrity and epithelial transport function by concomitant anti-TNFalpha treatment in chronic DSS-induced colitis. *J. Mol. Med.* **2018**, *96*, 831–843. [CrossRef]
62. Magalhaes, D.A.; Batista, J.A.; Sousa, S.G.; Ferreira, J.D.S.; da Rocha Rodrigues, L.; Pereira, C.M.C.; do Nascimento Lima, J.V.; de Albuquerque, I.F.; Bezerra, N.; Monteiro, C.; et al. McN-A-343, a muscarinic agonist, reduces inflammation and oxidative stress in an experimental model of ulcerative colitis. *Life Sci.* **2021**, *272*, 119194. [CrossRef] [PubMed]
63. Mitchelson, F.J. The pharmacology of McN-A-343. *Pharmacol. Ther.* **2012**, *135*, 216–245. [CrossRef] [PubMed]
64. Hosic, S.; Lake, W.; Stas, E.; Koppes, R.; Breault, D.T.; Murthy, S.K.; Koppes, A.N. Cholinergic Activation of Primary Human Derived Intestinal Epithelium Does Not Ameliorate TNF-alpha Induced Injury. *Cell Mol. Bioeng.* **2020**, *13*, 487–505. [CrossRef] [PubMed]
65. Lesko, S.; Wessler, I.; Gabel, G.; Petto, C.; Pfannkuche, H. Cholinergic modulation of epithelial integrity in the proximal colon of pigs. *Cells Tissues Organs* **2013**, *197*, 411–420. [CrossRef] [PubMed]
66. Ma, Y.; Semba, S.; Khan, R.I.; Bochimoto, H.; Watanabe, T.; Fujiya, M.; Kohgo, Y.; Liu, Y.; Taniguchi, T. Focal adhesion kinase regulates intestinal epithelial barrier function via redistribution of tight junction. *Biochim. Biophys. Acta* **2013**, *1832*, 151–159. [CrossRef]
67. Howe, K.L.; Reardon, C.; Wang, A.; Nazli, A.; McKay, D.M. Transforming growth factor-beta regulation of epithelial tight junction proteins enhances barrier function and blocks enterohemorrhagic Escherichia coli O157:H7-induced increased permeability. *Am. J. Pathol.* **2005**, *167*, 1587–1597. [CrossRef] [PubMed]
68. Ewaschuk, J.B.; Diaz, H.; Meddings, L.; Diederichs, B.; Dmytrash, A.; Backer, J.; Looijer-van Langen, M.; Madsen, K.L. Secreted bioactive factors from Bifidobacterium infantis enhance epithelial cell barrier function. *Am. J. Physiol. Gastrointest Liver Physiol.* **2008**, *295*, G1025–G1034. [CrossRef] [PubMed]
69. Kim, Y.; Quach, A.; Das, S.; Barrett, K.E. Potentiation of calcium-activated chloride secretion and barrier dysfunction may underlie EGF receptor tyrosine kinase inhibitor-induced diarrhea. *Physiol. Rep.* **2020**, *8*, e14490. [CrossRef] [PubMed]
70. McLean, L.P.; Smith, A.; Cheung, L.; Urban, J.F., Jr.; Sun, R.; Grinchuk, V.; Desai, N.; Zhao, A.; Raufman, J.P.; Shea-Donohue, T. Type 3 muscarinic receptors contribute to intestinal mucosal homeostasis and clearance of Nippostrongylus brasiliensis through induction of TH2 cytokines. *Am. J. Physiol. Gastrointest Liver Physiol.* **2016**, *311*, G130–G141. [CrossRef]
71. Gross, E.R.; Gershon, M.D.; Margolis, K.G.; Gertsberg, Z.V.; Li, Z.; Cowles, R.A. Neuronal serotonin regulates growth of the intestinal mucosa in mice. *Gastroenterology* **2012**, *143*, 408–417.e2. [CrossRef] [PubMed]
72. Takahashi, T.; Shiraishi, A.; Murata, J.; Matsubara, S.; Nakaoka, S.; Kirimoto, S.; Osawa, M. Muscarinic receptor M3 contributes to intestinal stem cell maintenance via EphB/ephrin-B signaling. *Life Sci. Alliance* **2021**, *4*, e202000962. [CrossRef]
73. Greig, C.J.; Cowles, R.A. Muscarinic acetylcholine receptors participate in small intestinal mucosal homeostasis. *J. Pediatr. Surg.* **2017**, *52*, 1031–1034. [CrossRef] [PubMed]
74. Mashima, H.; Watanabe, N.; Sekine, M.; Matsumoto, S.; Asano, T.; Yuhashi, K.; Sagihara, N.; Urayoshi, S.; Uehara, T.; Fujiwara, J.; et al. The role of Galpha(q)/Galpha(11) signaling in intestinal epithelial cells. *Biochem. Biophys. Rep.* **2018**, *13*, 93–98. [PubMed]

75. Watanabe, N.; Mashima, H.; Miura, K.; Goto, T.; Yoshida, M.; Goto, A.; Ohnishi, H. Requirement of Galpha(q)/Galpha(11) Signaling in the Preservation of Mouse Intestinal Epithelial Homeostasis. *Cell Mol. Gastroenterol. Hepatol.* **2016**, *2*, 767–782.e6. [PubMed]
76. Bijlsma, P.B.; Kiliaan, A.J.; Scholten, G.; Heyman, M.; Groot, J.A.; Taminiau, J.A. Carbachol, but not forskolin, increases mucosal-to-serosal transport of intact protein in rat ileum in vitro. *Am. J. Physiol.* **1996**, *271*, G147-55. [CrossRef]
77. Albanese, C.T.; Cardona, M.; Smith, S.D.; Watkins, S.; Kurkchubasche, A.G.; Ulman, I.; Simmons, R.L.; Rowe, M.I. Role of intestinal mucus in transepithelial passage of bacteria across the intact ileum in vitro. *Surgery* **1994**, *116*, 76–82.
78. Cameron, H.L.; Perdue, M.H. Muscarinic acetylcholine receptor activation increases transcellular transport of macromolecules across mouse and human intestinal epithelium in vitro. *Neurogastroenterol. Motil.* **2007**, *19*, 47–56.
79. Wallon, C.; Persborn, M.; Jonsson, M.; Wang, A.; Phan, V.; Lampinen, M.; Vicario, M.; Santos, J.; Sherman, P.M.; Carlson, M.; et al. Eosinophils express muscarinic receptors and corticotropin-releasing factor to disrupt the mucosal barrier in ulcerative colitis. *Gastroenterology* **2011**, *140*, 1597–1607.
80. Keita, A.V.; Soderholm, J.D.; Ericson, A.C. Stress-induced barrier disruption of rat follicle-associated epithelium involves corticotropin-releasing hormone, acetylcholine, substance P. and mast cells. *Neurogastroenterol. Motil.* **2010**, *22*, 770–778, e221-2. [CrossRef]
81. Gareau, M.G.; Jury, J.; Perdue, M.H. Neonatal maternal separation of rat pups results in abnormal cholinergic regulation of epithelial permeability. *Am. J. Physiol. Gastrointest Liver Physiol.* **2007**, *293*, G198-203. [CrossRef]
82. Wang, H.; Yu, M.; Ochani, M.; Amella, C.A.; Tanovic, M.; Susarla, S.; Li, J.H.; Wang, H.; Yang, H.; Ulloa, L.; et al. Nicotinic acetylcholine receptor alpha7 subunit is an essential regulator of inflammation. *Nature* **2003**, *421*, 384–388. [CrossRef] [PubMed]
83. Beckmann, J.; Lips, K.S. The non-neuronal cholinergic system in health and disease. *Pharmacology* **2013**, *92*, 286–302. [CrossRef]
84. Schutz, B.; Jurastow, I.; Bader, S.; Ringer, C.; von Engelhardt, J.; Chubanov, V.; Gudermann, T.; Diener, M.; Kummer, W.; Krasteva-Christ, G.; et al. Chemical coding and chemosensory properties of cholinergic brush cells in the mouse gastrointestinal and biliary tract. *Front. Physiol.* **2015**, *6*, 87.
85. Bader, S.; Klein, J.; Diener, M. Choline acetyltransferase and organic cation transporters are responsible for synthesis and propionate-induced release of acetylcholine in colon epithelium. *Eur. J. Pharmacol.* **2014**, *733*, 23–33. [CrossRef]
86. Peltekova, V.D.; Wintle, R.F.; Rubin, L.A.; Amos, C.I.; Huang, Q.; Gu, X.; Newman, B.; Van Oene, M.; Cescon, D.; Greenberg, G.; et al. Functional variants of OCTN cation transporter genes are associated with Crohn disease. *Nat. Genet.* **2004**, *36*, 471–475. [CrossRef] [PubMed]
87. Pochini, L.; Scalise, M.; Galluccio, M.; Pani, G.; Siminovitch, K.A.; Indiveri, C. The human OCTN1 (SLC22A4) reconstituted in liposomes catalyzes acetylcholine transport which is defective in the mutant L503F associated to the Crohn's disease. *Biochim. Biophys. Acta* **2012**, *1818*, 559–565. [CrossRef]
88. Song, P.; Rekow, S.S.; Singleton, C.A.; Sekhon, H.S.; Dissen, G.A.; Zhou, M.; Campling, B.; Lindstrom, J.; Spindel, E.R. Choline transporter-like protein 4 (CTL4) links to non-neuronal acetylcholine synthesis. *J. Neurochem.* **2013**, *126*, 451–461. [CrossRef] [PubMed]
89. Yajima, M.; Kimura, S.; Karaki, S.; Nio-Kobayashi, J.; Tsuruta, T.; Kuwahara, A.; Yajima, T.; Iwanaga, T. Non-neuronal, but atropine-sensitive ileal contractile responses to short-chain fatty acids: Age-dependent desensitization and restoration under inflammatory conditions in mice. *Physiol. Rep.* **2016**, *4*, e12579. [CrossRef]
90. Ramirez, V.T.; Godinez, D.R.; Brust-Mascher, I.; Nonnecke, E.B.; Castillo, P.A.; Gardner, M.B.; Tu, D.; Sladek, J.A.; Miller, E.N.; Lebrilla, C.B.; et al. T-cell derived acetylcholine aids host defenses during enteric bacterial infection with Citrobacter rodentium. *PLoS Pathog.* **2019**, *15*, e1007719. [CrossRef]
91. Dhawan, S.; De Palma, G.; Willemze, R.A.; Hilbers, F.W.; Verseijden, C.; Luyer, M.D.; Nuding, S.; Wehkamp, J.; Souwer, Y.; de Jong, E.C.; et al. Acetylcholine-producing T cells in the intestine regulate antimicrobial peptide expression and microbial diversity. *Am. J. Physiol. Gastrointest Liver Physiol.* **2016**, *311*, G920–G933. [CrossRef] [PubMed]
92. Willemze, R.A.; Brinkman, D.J.; Welting, O.; van Hamersveld, P.H.P.; Verseijden, C.; Luyer, M.D.; Wildenberg, M.E.; Seppen, J.; de Jonge, W.J. Acetylcholine-producing T cells augment innate immune-driven colitis but are redundant in T cell-driven colitis. *Am. J. Physiol. Gastrointest Liver Physiol.* **2019**, *317*, G557–G568. [CrossRef]
93. Belo, A.; Cheng, K.; Chahdi, A.; Shant, J.; Xie, G.; Khurana, S.; Raufman, J.P. Muscarinic receptor agonists stimulate human colon cancer cell migration and invasion. *Am. J. Physiol. Gastrointest Liver Physiol.* **2011**, *300*, G749–G760. [CrossRef]
94. Cheng, K.; Shang, A.C.; Drachenberg, C.B.; Zhan, M.; Raufman, J.P. Differential expression of M3 muscarinic receptors in progressive colon neoplasia and metastasis. *Oncotarget* **2017**, *8*, 21106–21114. [CrossRef] [PubMed]
95. Dwomoh, L.; Tejeda, G.S.; Tobin, A.B. Targeting the M1 muscarinic acetylcholine receptor in Alzheimer's disease. *Neuronal Signal.* **2022**, *6*, NS20210004. [CrossRef]
96. Nguyen, H.T.M.; van der Westhuizen, E.T.; Langmead, C.J.; Tobin, A.B.; Sexton, P.M.; Christopoulos, A.; Valant, C. Opportunities and challenges for the development of M(1) muscarinic receptor positive allosteric modulators in the treatment for neurocognitive deficits. *Br. J. Pharmacol.* **2022**, in press. [CrossRef] [PubMed]
97. Kurimoto, E.; Matsuda, S.; Shimizu, Y.; Sako, Y.; Mandai, T.; Sugimoto, T.; Sakamoto, H.; Kimura, H. An Approach to Discovering Novel Muscarinic M(1) Receptor Positive Allosteric Modulators with Potent Cognitive Improvement and Minimized Gastrointestinal Dysfunction. *J. Pharmacol. Exp. Ther.* **2018**, *364*, 28–37. [CrossRef] [PubMed]

98. Matsui, M.; Motomura, D.; Fujikawa, T.; Jiang, J.; Takahashi, S.; Manabe, T.; Taketo, M.M. Mice lacking M2 and M3 muscarinic acetylcholine receptors are devoid of cholinergic smooth muscle contractions but still viable. *J. Neurosci.* **2002**, *22*, 10627–10632. [CrossRef]
99. Bader, S.; Diener, M. Novel aspects of cholinergic regulation of colonic ion transport. *Pharmacol. Res. Perspect.* **2015**, *3*, e00139. [CrossRef]
100. Al-Barazie, R.M.; Bashir, G.H.; Qureshi, M.M.; Mohamed, Y.A.; Al-Sbiei, A.; Tariq, S.; Lammers, W.J.; Al-Ramadi, B.K.; Fernandez-Cabezudo, M.J. Cholinergic Activation Enhances Resistance to Oral Salmonella Infection by Modulating Innate Immune Defense Mechanisms at the Intestinal Barrier. *Front. Immunol.* **2018**, *9*, 551. [CrossRef]
101. Singh, S.P.; Chand, H.S.; Banerjee, S.; Agarwal, H.; Raizada, V.; Roy, S.; Sopori, M. Acetylcholinesterase Inhibitor Pyridostigmine Bromide Attenuates Gut Pathology and Bacterial Dysbiosis in a Murine Model of Ulcerative Colitis. *Dig. Dis. Sci.* **2020**, *65*, 141–149. [CrossRef] [PubMed]
102. Okumura, T.; Nozu, T.; Ishioh, M.; Igarashi, S.; Kumei, S.; Ohhira, M. Brain orexin improves intestinal barrier function via the vagal cholinergic pathway. *Neurosci. Lett.* **2020**, *714*, 134592. [CrossRef] [PubMed]
103. Yajima, T.; Inoue, R.; Yajima, M.; Tsuruta, T.; Karaki, S.; Hira, T.; Kuwahara, A. The G-protein on cholesterol-rich membrane microdomains mediates mucosal sensing of short-chain fatty acid and secretory response in rat colon. *Acta Physiol.* **2011**, *203*, 381–389. [CrossRef] [PubMed]
104. Yajima, T.; Inoue, R.; Matsumoto, M.; Yajima, M. Non-neuronal release of ACh plays a key role in secretory response to luminal propionate in rat colon. *J. Physiol.* **2011**, *589*, 953–962. [CrossRef] [PubMed]

Disclaimer/Publisher's Note: The statements, opinions and data contained in all publications are solely those of the individual author(s) and contributor(s) and not of MDPI and/or the editor(s). MDPI and/or the editor(s) disclaim responsibility for any injury to people or property resulting from any ideas, methods, instructions or products referred to in the content.

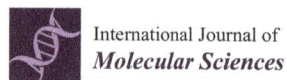

Review

Contribution of Blood Vessel Activation, Remodeling and Barrier Function to Inflammatory Bowel Diseases

Nathalie Britzen-Laurent [1,2,*], Carl Weidinger [3] and Michael Stürzl [2,4]

1. Division of Surgical Research, Department of Surgery, Translational Research Center, Universitätsklinikum Erlangen, Friedrich-Alexander-Universität Erlangen-Nürnberg (FAU), 91054 Erlangen, Germany
2. Comprehensive Cancer Center Erlangen-EMN (CCC ER-EMN), 91054 Erlangen, Germany
3. Department of Gastroenterology, Infectious Diseases and Rheumatology, Charité-Universitätsmedizin Berlin, Campus Benjamin Franklin, 12203 Berlin, Germany
4. Division of Molecular and Experimental Surgery, Translational Research Center, Universitätsklinikum Erlangen, Friedrich-Alexander-Universität Erlangen-Nürnberg (FAU), 91054 Erlangen, Germany
* Correspondence: nathalie.britzen-laurent@uk-erlangen.de

Abstract: Inflammatory bowel diseases (IBDs) consist of a group of chronic inflammatory disorders with a complex etiology, which represent a clinical challenge due to their often therapy-refractory nature. In IBD, inflammation of the intestinal mucosa is characterized by strong and sustained leukocyte infiltration, resulting in the loss of epithelial barrier function and subsequent tissue destruction. This is accompanied by the activation and the massive remodeling of mucosal micro-vessels. The role of the gut vasculature in the induction and perpetuation of mucosal inflammation is receiving increasing recognition. While the vascular barrier is considered to offer protection against bacterial translocation and sepsis after the breakdown of the epithelial barrier, endothelium activation and angiogenesis are thought to promote inflammation. The present review examines the respective pathological contributions of the different phenotypical changes observed in the microvascular endothelium during IBD, and provides an overview of potential vessel-specific targeted therapy options for the treatment of IBD.

Keywords: inflammatory bowel diseases (IBDs); vasculature; angiogenesis; gut vascular barrier; vessel permeability

1. Introduction

Inflammatory bowel diseases (IBD) are a group of intestinal chronic inflammatory disorders characterized by cyclic flares of destructive inflammation that comprise two major forms, Crohn's disease (CD) and ulcerative colitis (UC) [1]. Although inflammation in UC is restricted to the colon and only extends to the mucosal layers, transmural inflammation can be observed in CD, which can manifest at any site of the gut. The etiology of IBD is thought to be multifactorial and to involve the patient's genetics and immune response, the intestinal microbiome, and environmental factors [2]. IBD is considered to result from an inappropriate immune response to the intestinal microflora and environmental triggers in genetically susceptible individuals [1]. The resulting inflammation induces tissue damage and, notably, a disruption of the epithelial barrier, leading to the perturbation of the intestinal microenvironment and the relationship between the mucosal surface and the commensal microbiota. This disequilibrium not only affects the maintenance, function, and repair of the epithelial barrier, it also results in the perturbation of the commensal microbiota composition, leading to dysbiosis [3,4].

The intestinal microvasculature lies in close vicinity to the epithelial layer and represents a second barrier to the penetration and dissemination of commensals and microbial products. In IBD, the microvascular endothelium is strongly affected by inflammation [5]. Endothelial cells (ECs) of the gut microvasculature are activated to allow leukocyte recruitment and infiltration, whereas the vascular barrier function is compromised and local bursts of angiogenesis are observed. Despite its well-defined function in inflammation, the contribution of the endothelium to the development and maintenance of IBD has been rather overlooked, in particular as a potential therapeutic target. In the present review, we summarize the respective contributions of blood vessel activation, remodeling, and barrier function to the pathogenesis of IBD, and discuss the status and perspectives of vessel-directed therapies.

2. The Intestinal Vasculature in Homeostasis

The intestine is vascularized by arterioles from the submucosa, which divide into capillary networks in the mucosa and muscle layers, with the mucosal layers receiving 80% of the total blood flow [6]. The anatomy of the mucosal vasculature differs between the small and large intestine (colon) due to their different tissue architectures. In the small intestine, the epithelium builds villi and crypts. Each villus contains a single arteriole going to the tip, forming a tuft-like network of capillaries which are located directly under the epithelial monolayer, and the blood is collected into a single central venule. The crypts are infused with a capillary network which drains into the venule as well. In contrast to the small intestine, the colon epithelium does not have villi. The arterioles and their capillary branches are arranged along the colonic crypts, developing into a capillary honeycomb-like network around the crypts that is in very close proximity to the epithelial layer (1 μm) [6,7]. Intestinal post-capillary veins are devoid of smooth-muscle cells and represent the most reactive segment of the microvasculature [8]. The intestinal microcirculation regulates oxygen and nutrient exchange, tissue fluid homeostasis, and leucocyte abundance [9–11].

Under physiological conditions, the single layer of ECs lining the vessel lumen provides an anti-adhesive and selectively permeable exchange barrier. In the past few years, the general opinion about the role of the intestinal microvasculature has evolved, and it is now viewed as an integral component of the intestinal barrier [12]. The intestinal barrier is tightly regulated to allow the absorption of essential nutrients, electrolytes, and water from the intestinal lumen into the circulation, while preventing the entry of microbiota through different layers of protection. The first barrier is formed by a tight epithelial monolayer covered by a thick layer of mucus produced by specialized enterocytes, the goblet cells. In addition, another population, the Paneth cells, secretes antimicrobial peptides. This intestinal epithelial barrier prevents the penetration of microbes or microbe-derived molecules into the tissue. A second barrier, the gut vascular barrier (GVB), has been identified in humans and mice, and provides a second layer of protection, which blocks microbial dissemination into the systemic circulation (Figure 1) [12–14].

In contrast to the blood–brain barrier (BBB), which has a size exclusion threshold of 500 Da, the GVB is permeable to molecules as large as 4 kDa, allowing the passage of nutrients and antigens for tolerance induction [14]. Spadoni et al. demonstrated that endothelial cells in the intestine are closely associated with pericytes and enteric glial cells to form what they termed gut–vascular units (Figure 1) [13]. Enteric glial cells seem to be crucial for the development and maintenance of the GVB, as it has been shown that transgenic mice lacking enteric glial cells feature increased epithelial permeability and microvascular disturbances, resulting in the uncontrolled spread of bacteria into the blood circulation and the subsequent death of the affected animals (Table 1) [15,16]. Interestingly, the interplay of the GVB with the commensal microbiota was found to increase angiogenesis, endothelial coverage, and the formation of the enteric glial cell network in the lamina propria using human ECs and murine models [17–20], suggesting that the microbiota supports the formation and maintenance of the GVB.

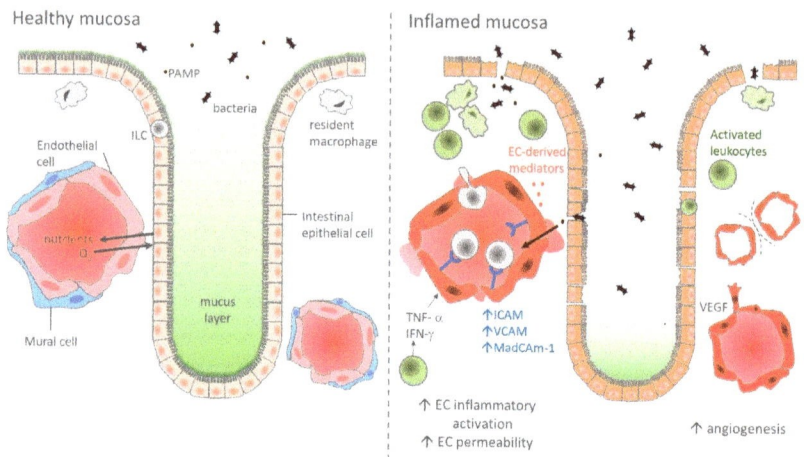

Figure 1. In the healthy intestine (depicted here, the colon mucosa), the mucosal microvasculature participates in homeostasis by regulating the absorption of essential nutrients, electrolytes, and water, while building a second barrier towards luminal microbes. During IBD, inflammation activates the intestinal microvasculature through release of cytokines and growth factors, leading to adhesion molecule expression, leukocyte extravasation, vascular hyperpermeability, and an increase in both sprouting and intussusceptive angiogenesis.

Table 1. Different mesenteric vascular cell subtypes in homeostasis and in IBD.

Cell Type	In Homeostasis	In IBD
HIMECs	Tolerance to bacterial products from the gut microbiota Constitutive iNOS expression	Leukocyte hyperadhesion Angiogenesis ↑ αvβ3 integrin expression ↑ vessel permeability ↓ iNOS and eNOS expression ↓ protein C system activation ↑ secretion of inflammatory mediators
HEVs	Recruitment and trafficking of lymphocytes from blood to lymph nodes and secondary lymphoid organs	↑ density ↑ leukocyte binding Formation of extrafollicular HEVs
Lymphatic ECs	Absorption of fatty acids Immune regulation	↑ density ↓ contractile activity Lymphangitis
Mural cells	Development and maintenance of the GVB	↓ vessel coverage ↑ MMP expression
Enteric glial cells	Part of gut–vascular units Development and maintenance of the GVB	Sensing of bacterial translocation Closure of the PVB

Abbreviations: ECs: endothelial cells; HIMECs: human intestinal microvascular ECs; HEVs: high endothelial venules; TJs: tight junctions; GVB: gut–vascular barrier; PVB: plexus–vascular barrier; ↑: increase; ↓: decrease.

Within the gut–vascular units, endothelial cells form tight cell–cell contacts, which are enhanced through interaction with enteric glial cells and pericytes. Adherens junctions (AJs) and tight junctions (TJs) found in human and mouse intestinal microvascular ECs regulate paracellular trafficking of molecules and leukocytes and express different classes of transporters (such as ATP-binding cassette transporters and sugar transporters) [12]. TJs control permeability for ions and small molecules (<800 Da), whereas AJs are primarily responsible for the maintenance of vascular barrier function and control its permeability for molecules of high molecular weight [21]. In intestinal ECs, AJs are composed of vascular endothelial cadherin (VE-cadherin), α- and β-catenin, and p120, all of which are expressed homogenously throughout the intestines and the vascular beds. The building of VE-cadherin adhesions is considered to be the primary event during vascular development [13,21]. It precedes TJ formation and is required for TJ maintenance. Disruption of AJs leads to disassembly of TJs [13,21]. Although numerous TJs can be found in small arterioles, the level of TJs is reduced in capillaries and post-capillary veins. As a result, AJs are predominantly found in capillaries and post-capillary venules [21]. In intestinal ECs, TJs are formed by occludin, zonula occludens-1 (ZO-1), cingulin, junctional adhesion molecule-A (JAM-A), and claudins [13,22]. The expression of endothelial claudins has been extensively studied in the mouse intestine and varies between gut areas and cell types. While claudin-1 is expressed at similar levels in ECs throughout the intestines, the channel-forming claudins-7, -12, and -15 are exclusively expressed in the colon [22]. Outside of the BBB and the blood–retinal barrier, where a high expression of claudin-5 prevents the passage of small molecules, claudin-5 exhibits diminishing expression along the arteriovenous axis [23]. In the gut, claudin-5 expression is restricted to lymphatic ECs, high endothelial venules (HEVs), and certain capillary ECs [13,24]. These different patterns of expression are thought to be responsible for variations in permeability and to reflect the site-specific physiological function of the GVB. In humans, claudins working as channels show a higher expression in the colon, where they regulate solute paracellular transport, compared to the small intestine or the BBB [25,26].

Kalucka et al. performed a single-cell transcriptome analysis of murine ECs across 11 tissues, revealing heterogeneity between tissues and vascular beds [24]. Overall, they found that colon and small-intestine ECs are characterized by the high expression of genes involved in vascular barrier integrity and maintenance. In addition, two specific EC-fractions were found in the intestine. First, a subset of capillary ECs was described, which display an elevated expression of genes involved in the uptake and metabolism of glycerol and fatty acids. Cells in this cluster were notably characterized by a high expression of aquaglyceroporin 7 (*Aqp7*), a pore-forming transmembrane protein involved in glycerol transport across cell membranes, and were therefore termed Aqp7+ capillary ECs. Second, a subset of intestinal venous ECs showing enriched expression of HEV markers (*Madcam1*, *Lrg1*, *Ackr1*) was identified. HEVs represent a specialized subtype of post-capillary venules mediating the recruiting and trafficking of lymphocytes from blood to lymph nodes and secondary lymphoid organs, which take their name from the cuboidal appearance of their endothelial cells (Table 1).

The investigation of isolated human intestinal mucosa-derived endothelial cells (HIMECs) has revealed unique functional features when compared to human umbilical veins (HUVECs) (Table 1). For instance, exposure to lipopolysaccharide (LPS) induces a transient increase in the presence of adhesion molecules in HIMECs, compared to a long-lasting increase in the presence of adhesion molecules in HUVECs [27]. This reflects the relative tolerance of intestinal microvascular cells to bacterial products from the gut microbiota. In addition, HIMECs produce different cytokines, including IL-3 and IL-6, as HUVECs upon activation with inflammatory cytokines [28]. Furthermore, HIMECs constitutively express the (otherwise) inducible nitric oxide synthase (iNOS) in addition to endothelial NOS (eNOS) [29]. Under physiological conditions, endothelial-derived NO maintains the anti-adhesive state of the endothelium by limiting leukocyte and platelet adhesion, and regulates vasodilatation [29,30].

Overall, in the state of homeostasis, intestinal ECs are involved in barrier function maintenance, nutrient uptake, and immune tolerance.

3. The Intestinal Vasculature in IBD

The intestinal microvasculature plays a crucial role during inflammation by regulating tissue recruitment of inflammatory cells and wound healing. However, uncontrolled inflammation induces a sustained EC activation (Figure 1), causing an increase in leakiness (edema), adhesiveness (leukocyte recruitment), pro-coagulant activity (thrombus), and angiogenesis (immature vessels) [5,31]. As a result, inflammation is enhanced, ultimately leading to sustained tissue and vessel damage.

The histopathological analysis of inflamed human and murine intestinal tissues has revealed massive changes in the blood microvasculature, including vasodilatation, vaso-congestion, edema, flares of angiogenesis, microvascular occlusions, and abnormal vessel architecture characterized by tortuous vessels of varying diameter (Figure 2) [32–34]. These profound alterations have been considered to be an early event since they precede the development of mucosal ulceration, and to significantly enhance inflammation in IBD [32]. Hence, the intestinal microvasculature can be seen both as a regulating factor and as a target of inflammation. In the following, we examine the respective contributions of intestinal vascular changes to IBD pathogenesis (Figure 2).

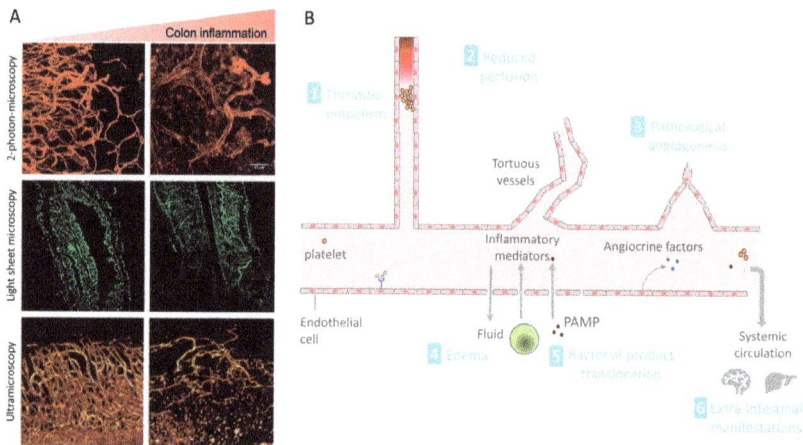

Figure 2. (**A**) The colonic microvascular architecture is massively remodeled in the presence of inflammation. The vessel structure was analyzed in mouse colon samples in the absence (left) or presence (right) of colitis. Vessels were visualized via the staining of CD31 (2-photon microscopy) or via lectin-staining (light sheet microscopy and ultramicroscopy). (**B**). Vascular changes and dysfunction observed in IBD participate in the initiation and perpetuation of mucosal inflammation and extra-cellular manifestations. PAMP: pathogen-associated molecular pattern.

3.1. Endothelial Cell Activation and Leukocyte Recruitment

The recruitment of circulating leukocytes into tissues is an early and central event during inflammation. It starts with the activation of the microvascular endothelium by inflammatory mediators, including cytokines such as IFN-γ, IL-1β, and TNF-α (Table 2). The activated endothelium regulates the leukocyte extravasation cascade in a tightly coordinated sequence, including tethering and rolling, activation, adhesion, spreading, and the transmigration of leukocytes [35]. Activated ECs are characterized by an elevation in the level of cell adhesion molecules (CAMs), the production of chemokines, and the expression of costimulatory molecules, which further amplify the recruitment and activation of leukocytes (Figure 1). Leukocyte hyper-adhesion has been observed in the intestinal ECs of patients with IBD. For instance, Binion et al. described a significant increase in leukocyte binding in HIMECs isolated from inflamed regions of IBD patients compared to

HIMECs that were obtained from non-inflamed intestinal sites or from the guts of control subjects [36].

Table 2. Vessel-directed effects of key inflammatory cytokines involved in the pathogenesis of IBD.

Cytokines	Effect
IFN-γ	EC activation, ↑ CAM expression (notably MadCAM-1) ↑ vascular permeability Disassembly of VE-cadherin junctions, ↓ VE-cadherin expression ↓ EC proliferation and migration, ↓ angiogenesis ↓ vascular coverage, ↓ PDGF-B ↑ TLR3 expression ↑ CX3CL1 (fractalkine)
TNF-α	EC activation, ↑ CAM expression (notably MadCAM-1) ↑ vascular permeability, ↑ Phosphorylation of VE-cadherin, ↑ monolayer tension ↓ TJ protein expression in EC ↑ circulating levels, ↑ vascular dysfunction ↓ EC proliferation and migration, ↓ angiogenesis ↑ CX3CL1 (fractalkine)
IL-1β	EC activation, ↑ CAM expression (notably MadCAM-1) ↑ CX3CL1 (fractalkine)

Abbreviations: ↑: increase; ↓: decrease.

At the molecular level, the MAPK pathway has been shown to play an important role in the upregulation of CAMs and the production of chemokines by activated HIMECs, as well as lymphocyte extravasation [37]. In the inflamed mucosa of IBD patients, increased levels of phosphorylated MAPK have been detected in the microvasculature [37].

Among the various CAMs expressed in activated ECs, P- and E-selectins are glycoproteins involved in the rolling and recruitment of leukocytes. Although P-selectin is constitutively available as a pool that can be mobilized upon activation, E-selectin expression is induced in response to inflammatory stimuli. A notable increase in P-selectin levels has been observed in the colons of UC patients compared to controls, whereas serum levels of the decoy soluble P-selectin were decreased [37–39].

An important class of adhesion molecules expressed in ECs is the immunoglobin CAM superfamily, which includes intracellular cell adhesion molecule 1 (ICAM-1), vascular cell adhesion molecule 1 (VCAM-1), platelet endothelial cell adhesion molecule (PECAM-1, also known as CD31), as well as the gut-specific mucosal addressin cell adhesion molecule 1 (MadCAM-1). Upon EC activation, ICAM-1 is recruited from the EC junctions to the apical surface [27]. The microvascular expression of ICAM-1 is increased in IBD patients, and ICAM-1 has been shown to be crucial to T-cell recruitment in the T-cell transfer murine colitis model [40]. ICAM-1 is constitutively expressed in HIMECs and can be upregulated by inflammatory cytokines and vascular endothelial growth factor-A (VEGF-A) [27,41,42]. VCAM-1, which mediates adhesion to lymphocytes expressing integrin α4β1 or α4β7, is also inducible in HIMECs, notably by VEGF-A. The expression of VCAM-1 in the mucosal vasculature is increased in patients with IBD and murine colitis models, where its expression correlates with disease severity [43,44]. PECAM-1/CD31 is also inducible by inflammatory cytokines and is involved in leukocyte rolling and firm adhesion during IBD [45]. A large amount of attention has been paid to MadCAM-1, a gut-specific homing molecule mediating the recruitment of T and B cells expressing integrin α4β7 [46]. High MadCAM-1 expression has been observed in the inflamed intestinal endothelium during IBD [36]. In HIMECs, MadCAM-1 expression can be induced by inflammatory cytokines (IFN-γ, IL-1β, TNF-α) [47,48]. Interestingly, the expression of MadCAM-1 in HIMECs is inversely correlated to cellular density, suggesting that high MadCAM-1 expression might be a marker of proliferating vessels [47,48]. Recently, MadCAM-1 has been found to be critical for the recruitment of antibody-producing B cells into the intestinal mucosa in the IL-10-knockout colitis model [49].

3.2. Pathological Angiogenesis in IBD

Angiogenesis is a hallmark of chronic inflammation [50]. In human IBD and in several murine models of colitis, the microvascular density is increased and directly correlates with disease severity (Figures 1 and 2) [51–53]. Angiogenic ECs exhibit increased proliferation and migration, as well as a unique cell-surface molecular pattern. For instance, the integrins $\alpha v \beta 3$ and $\alpha v \beta 5$ are specifically expressed at the surface of ECs from newly formed vessels, and an increased expression of $\alpha v \beta 3$ has been observed in the inflamed mucosa of IBD patients [51]. The blockade of $\alpha v \beta 3$ was found to reduce disease activity in the IL-10 knock-out colitis model, suggesting that angiogenesis contributes to IBD pathogenesis [54]. The angiogenic expansion of the vascular bed is assumed to physically increase blood supply through the increased endothelial surface, and therefore to enhance the leukocyte supply to the tissue. However, the newly formed vessels in the context of chronic inflammation show an immature phenotype in mouse and human tissues [34,55,56]. They are leaky, have less or no coverage by pericytes, and are hypoperfused and often hyperthrombic [32–34]. Stenoses are also frequently observed [32]. Hence, pathological angiogenesis appears to contribute to the intense vascular remodeling observed in IBD.

The fact that mucosal extracts of IBD patients could induce dose-dependent HIMEC migration in vitro supported the presence of a pro-angiogenic microenvironment in the inflamed gut mucosa [57]. Two main mechanisms of angiogenesis have been proposed to occur during IBD, namely, extension from existing vessels (sprouting) and vessel splitting (intussusception). Angiogenesis through the recruitment of endothelial progenitor cells seems less likely to occur during colitis since the number of bone-marrow-derived endothelial progenitor cells is reduced in UC [58–60].

The induction of sprouting angiogenesis during IBD has been partly attributed to inflammation-related hypoxia, with hypoxia-inducible factor-1 and -2 transcriptionally activating the expression of vascular endothelial growth factor A (VEGF-A), the major angiogenic growth factor (AGF) [61]. In agreement with this hypothesis, the human inflamed intestinal epithelium was found to represent an important source of VEGF-A, which is also produced by leukocytes [62–65]. Furthermore, increased expression of VEGF and other AGFs including basic fibroblast growth factor (bFGF) and platelet-derived growth factor (PDGF) has been detected in mucosal extracts and in the serum of IBD patients as compared to controls (Table 3) [51,53,66–70], although this increase was more evident for UC than for CD, especially for VEGF [61,71–73]. However, experimental colitis models have provided conflicting results regarding the contribution of sprouting angiogenesis to disease activity. The inhibition of angiogenesis via the neutralization of VEGF-A improved the course of intestinal inflammation in mice [34,64,74,75] and modestly in rats [76]. In contrast, the knock-out of placental growth factor, a VEGF homolog, also caused decreased angiogenesis, but lead to an aggravation of colonic injury in the mouse dextran sodium sulfate (DSS)-induced colitis model [77]. These results are reflected in the responses of cancer patients treated with anti-angiogenic treatment. Rare adverse effects of bevacizumab, a humanized monoclonal antibody against VEGF, include intestinal perforation, gastrointestinal bleeding, and ulcerative colitis [78–80]. However, anti-VEGF therapy is well tolerated by most patients with quiescent and moderately active IBD [81]. The frequency of inflammatory side effects is higher when the PDFG pathway is involved. For instance, an exaggeration of UC has been observed during treatment with the angiogenic inhibitors sunitinib and sorafenib, which target both the VEGF and PDGF pathways [82–84].

Table 3. Pathogenic effects of vascular factors in IBD.

Factor	Effect on the Intestinal Vasculature
Angiogenic growth factors	
VEGF	Expression increased in IBD ↑ sprouting angiogenesis ↑ EC proliferation and migration ↑ ICAM-1 and VCAM-1 expression ↑ recruitment of VEGFR- expressing immune cells ↑ vascular permeability, disassembly of VE-cadherin junctions ↓ vascular coverage ↑ wound healing
bFGF	Expression increased in IBD ↑ sprouting angiogenesis
PDGF	Expression increased in IBD ↑ sprouting angiogenesis ↑ vascular coverage Protective effect in UC
Nitric oxide (NO)	Decreased constitutive expression of eNOS and iNOS in intestinal EC during IBD ↓ CAM expression ↓ ROS production ↑ intestinal endothelial barrier function ↑ vasodilatation Potentiates VEGF-mediated effects
Coagulation factors	Increased platelet activation and thrombi in IBD ↓ thrombomodulin expression in IBD ↓ protein C receptor expression in IBD Impaired protein C activation in activated intestinal EC
Toll-like receptors (TLR)	Tolerance to endotoxin in intestinal EC Expression of TLR3 and TLR5 by intestinal EC, protective against colitis in mice ↑ endothelial barrier function
Angiocrine factors	↑ CX3CL1 (fractalkine) → ↑ adhesion and activation of CX3CR1+ leukocytes ↑ CL25 → recruitment of CCR9+ immune cells → protective effect ↑ NO ↑ CXCL10 → epithelial cell survival

Abbreviations: ↑: increase; ↓: decrease.

Several reasons might explain the contradictory effects of angiogenesis in IBD. Firstly, while angiogenic and inflammatory vessels can synchronously co-exist in the inflamed mucosa during mouse colitis [32], the two phenotypes are mutually exclusive in a single EC. In particular, inflammatory cytokines (ICs) such as IFN-γ, TNF-α, and IL1-β can inhibit AGF-induced proliferation and the migration of human ECs in vitro (Table 2) [85–87]. In addition to ICs, several anti-angiogenic factors are upregulated during intestinal inflammation, including the chemokine CXCL-10, thrombospondin, angiostatin—a cleaved fragment of plasminogen, and endostatin—a cleaved fragment of collagen XVIII [63,88–92]. Hence, the balance between angiogenic and inflammatory-associated angiostatic stimuli might explain the relative contribution of angiogenesis to IBD pathogenesis.

Secondly, there is a strong interplay between angiogenesis, inflammatory vessel activation, and barrier function during inflammation. For instance, human and murine VEGF-A stimulates angiogenesis and increases vessel permeability, while reducing vessel coverage [41,42,93]. In murine colitis models, the permeability marker CD146/MUC18 was shown to induce angiogenesis, lymphangiogenesis, and leukocyte recruitment [94–96].

In a similar manner, mice that are deficient in CD40 or CD40L display both a decrease in leukocyte and platelet recruitment and impaired angiogenesis in the gut [97–99].

Thirdly, the importance of intussusceptive angiogenesis during IBD might have been underestimated. The vessel splitting that is characteristic of intussusceptive angiogenesis occurs through intraluminal endothelial cell rearrangements rather than endothelial cell proliferation [100]. These are triggered by increased blow flow and are regulated by the nitric oxide (NO), endoglin, and ephrinB2/EphB4 signaling pathways [101–105]. Intussusceptive angiogenesis has been observed in murine colitis [100,106,107], where it was induced through mechanical forces and changes in the intraluminal blood flow, and was regulated by MT1-MMP [100,106]. EC-specific knockout of MT1-MMP ameliorated dextran sulfate (DSS)-induced colitis in mice [107]. The predominance of intussusceptive angiogenesis compared to sprouting angiogenesis during colitis might explain the relative success of classical anti-angiogenic approaches in animal models of IBD.

Finally, angiogenesis not only sustains inflammation, it also plays an essential role during mucosal healing. For instance, VEGF-A is involved in UC healing and angiogenesis via the recruitment of cells expressing vascular endothelial growth factor receptor 1 (VEGFR1), including monocytes, Tregs, and bone-marrow derived stem cells, to ulcerated tissues [108]. Furthermore, the expression of the Wnt pathway member adenomatous polyposis coli (APC) in murine intestinal ECs has been shown to mediate mucosal repair following colonic inflammation through angiogenesis [109]. Hence, treatment with angiogenesis inhibitors might result in wound healing complications. Despite the activation of angiogenic signals, impaired mucosal healing is observed and represents a major issue in IBD, notably in UC. Pathological angiogenesis or an increase in anti-angiogenic signals such as endostatin and angiostatin might explain why mucosal lesions are slow to repair in UC [91]. In addition, the decrease in the number of bone-marrow-derived endothelial progenitor cells (BMD-EPC) observed in UC, whether it is due to a decreased release from the bone marrow and/or impaired homing in colonic lesions, participates in mucosal healing impairment [59,60]. In addition, there is crosstalk between VEGF and transforming growth factor-beta (TGF-β), which is essential for wound healing, tissue repair, and the resolution of inflammation. A dysregulation of the TGF-β pathway, as seen in case of the impairment of endoglin, the endothelial-specific co-receptor for TGF-β, caused the levels of VEGF to spike in the acute DSS colitis model [110,111]. This resulted in enhanced and chronic intestinal inflammation, characterized by higher angiogenesis and MAdCAM-1 vascular expression [110,111]. Hence, both the therapeutic inhibition of angiogenesis and the presence of exacerbated or pathological angiogenesis seem to impair wound healing in IBD and experimental colitis models.

Another example of the interplay between vascular remodeling and inflammation in IBD is given by HEVs (Table 1). Subsequently to the ectopic formation of tertiary lymphoid organs observed in the inflamed gut mucosa, the density of HEVs has been found to increase in the mucosa of IBD patients [112,113]. However, HEVs not only regulate the lymph drainage of antigen-presenting cells, they also regulate the homing of T-cells. Extrafollicular HEV formation has been observed in the intestinal mucosa of IBD patients during active inflammation, where it correlates with T-cell infiltration and disease activity [113,114]. Human intestinal HEVs express high levels of MadCAM-1, and in UC, the O-glycosylation of MadCAM1 is increased, which induces a higher binding to L-selectin, expressed on leukocytes [112,115]. Taken together, pathological angiogenesis in IBD seems to both potentiate inflammation and impair mucosal healing.

3.3. The Gut–Vascular Barrier in IBD

During IBD, the epithelial barrier is compromised, as shown by an increased permeability and mucosal damage such as erosions or ulcers [116,117]. In consequence, the passage of antigens, bacteria, and bacterial products into the submucosa is increased [117]. This further enhances the local inflammation, resulting in the release of large amounts of inflammatory mediators from—but not restricted to—immune cells, which can in turn affect the gut–vascular barrier [118].

IBD is associated with increased gut vascular permeability (Figure 1), which is indicative of a loss of intestinal vascular barrier function, and results in edema and tissue damage [33,34,69,119–121]. For instance, human CD146 (MUC18), a cell junction molecule constitutively expressed in ECs, and its soluble form (sCD146), which is considered a marker for vascular permeability, are upregulated in intestinal ECs and serum of IBD patients, respectively [96,122]. Endothelial damage and increased colonic vascular permeability have been observed early during the development of experimental ulcerative colitis in rats and mice [123]. Post-capillary venules, the most reactive part of the vascular tree, were also shown to be the major site of vascular leakage [124]. The increased vascular permeability of inflamed post-capillary venules has been attributed to endothelial cell-cell contact disruption, to the contraction of activated ECs, to EC death and detachment, and/or to plasma protein extravasation at the site of leukocyte transendothelial migration [125,126]. A variety of inflammation mediators found in IBD can induce vascular permeability, including histamine, serotonin, substance P, bradykinin, and ICs, notably IFN-γ and TNF-α (Table 2) [121]. In addition, the reduction of anti-inflammatory cytokines such as IL-10 can further amplify intestinal vascular permeability induced by IFN-γ in experimental colitis [121]. Vascular permeability is also increased during angiogenesis, notably through a direct effect of VEGF [127–129]. Intussusceptive angiogenesis has also been associated with an enhanced permeability, likely because it induces holes in the vascular layer. In particular, endothelial cell-specific MT1-MMP knockout mice, which are characterized by a lower intussusceptive angiogenesis, also display a reduced vessel permeability during DSS-induced colitis [107].

In a study comparing the respective effects of IFN-γ and VEGF on disease development, both endothelial-specific knockout of the IFN-γ receptor (IFNγR) and VEGF blockade inhibited DSS-induced colitis in mice [34]. In agreement with the angiostatic properties of IFN-γ and the pro-angiogenic effect of VEGF, angiogenesis was increased in the case of IFNγR knockout, whereas it was decreased after VEGF blockade as compared to controls. Both approaches, however, led to a strong decrease in vascular permeability [34,74]. These results suggested that the induction of vascular permeability by VEGF might contribute more to colitis pathogenesis than the mere induction of angiogenesis. Several reports further support the promoting role of GVB disruption in IBD. Vascular permeability is associated with disease activity in UC and CD [34]. The inhibition of vascular permeability with the RTK inhibitor imatinib restores VE-cadherin junctions, increases vascular coverage, and inhibits DSS-induced colitis [34]. Fibrinogen, which is upregulated in UC and mouse colitis, was shown to promote DSS-induced colitis by enhancing vascular permeability [130]. Moreover, transient receptor potential vanilloid 4 (TRPV4) channels were found to enhance DSS-induced colonic inflammation in mice through an increase in vascular permeability [131]. Taken together, these studies have established the pathogenic contribution of vascular barrier breakdown to IBD.

3.3.1. VE-Cadherin and Vascular Barrier Regulation in IBD

VE-cadherin, the major component of endothelial adherens junctions and the master regulator of vascular barrier function, is regarded as the primary target during inflammation-induced vascular permeability [132–134]. In IBD patients, membrane VE-cadherin expression is significantly reduced in blood vessels found in inflamed areas compared to uninvolved intestinal tissues [34]. Several mechanisms of VE-cadherin junction disruption have been described. Inflammation-induced proteases such as matrix metalloproteinases (MMPs) or elastase, which are produced by leukocytes, smooth muscle cells, and ECs, can promote vascular permeability through the degradation of VE-cadherin AJs and TJs [5,34,135–138]. In IBD, vascular smooth muscle cells and pericytes express MMP-1 and MMP-9 [137], and MMP-9 serum levels are increased [139–141]. This is supported by the fact that MMP9 deficiency was found to attenuate intestinal injury in animal colitis models [142–144]. In addition, MMP-catalyzed VE-cadherin cleavage results in the generation of soluble VE-cadherin, which itself can further destabilize the vascular barrier by impairing the binding of VE-cadherin molecules, as shown in human rheumatoid arthritis, systemic inflammation, and sepsis [145–147].

The vascular hyperpermeability induced by VEGF and inflammatory cytokines also involves the direct disassembly of VE-cadherin junctions. Binding of VEGF to VEGFR2 at the surface of human ECs activates the Src kinase, resulting in VE-cadherin phosphorylation and internalization, which occurs via clathrin-dependent endocytosis and is mediated by neuropilin and Rac [127,129,147–150]. In a similar manner, TNF-α was shown to increase tyrosine phosphorylation of VE-cadherin and to open the paracellular pathway in the human lung endothelium through the activation of the Fyn kinase [138]. The effect of IFN-γ on the disruption of the VE-cadherin junction was found to be even stronger and longer lasting than the effect of VEGF in human ECs and mouse intestinal endothelial cells (MIECs) [33,34,151]. However, the molecular mechanism by which IFN-γ dismantles VE-cadherin junctions remains to be elucidated.

VE-cadherin disruption can also result from EC contraction, since the VE-cadherin complex and the actin cytoskeleton are functionally connected [134,152,153]. For instance, treatment of ECs with TNF-α was found to induce an almost immediate rise in mechanical substrate traction force and internal monolayer tension [154]. VEGF also induces actin reorganization and the migration of endothelial cells via the serine/threonine kinase Akt [155]. A similar disruption of actin has been observed in human ECs following exposure to IFN-γ, and might explain, at least partially, the IFN-γ-induced destabilization of VE-cadherin [156]. Such a mechanism was also observed during experimental colitis, where fibrinogen was shown to induce vascular permeability through activation of AKT and depolymerization of actin microfilaments [130].

Downregulation of AJ and TJ adhesion molecule expression has also been observed upon exposure to ICs and VEGF. For instance, VE-cadherin expression decreases in MIECs after treatment with IFN-γ [34]. Using an in-vitro intestinal endothelial barrier model composed of rat intestinal microvascular endothelial cells, Liu et al. found that TNF-α decreases the expression of TJ proteins, including ZO-1, occludin, and claudin-1, while increasing the expression of pore-forming claudin-2 [157]. Nevertheless, several reports showed no difference in the TJ-associated protein expression of zonula occludens-1 (ZO-1) in MIECs or intestinal endothelial cells during DSS-induced colitis [34,158]. In this model, ZO-1 was notably only reduced in epithelial cells but not in ECs [158], supporting the predominant role of VE-cadherin junctions in the regulation of the GVB.

3.3.2. Vessel Coverage and Permeability

During intestinal inflammation, vessel coverage with adventitial support cells, the so-called mural cells (pericytes and smooth muscle cells), is reduced in mouse models of colitis [159,160]. Mural cell recruitment is regulated by the PDGF-B-PDGFR-β pathway. PDGF-B is secreted by sprouting ECs and signals through PDGFR-β at the surface of mural cells [159]. This induces the proliferation and migration of mural cells. PDGF-B/PDGFR-β knockout models in mice showed reduced mural cell coverage and increased vessel permeability [159,161,162]. In the DSS colitis model, vessel coverage has been found to promote the stabilization of the vascular barrier, decreasing vessel permeability and inflammation [163,164]. Endothelial IFN-γ receptor knockout leads to increased vessel coverage during DSS-induced colitis in mice [33,34]. This could be attributed to the fact that IFN-γ inhibits PDGF-like protein release and decreases the PDGF-B chain mRNA level in HUVECs [165]. Similarly, excess VEGF-A disrupts pericyte recruitment and VEGF blockade was found to increase vessel coverage in the DSS-colitis model [34,166].

3.4. Microvascular Dysfunction in IBD

In IBD, the mucosal vasculature displays pathological traits, including tortuous structures, edema, arteriolar dilatation, hypercoagulation, and vascular damage (Figure 2) [32].

These vascular defects are multifactorial. For instance, chronic high levels of angiogenic factors and inflammatory cytokines can alter microvascular structure and function [167]. More precisely, structural changes in vessels have been shown to result from pathological angiogenesis and inflammation-driven GVB dysfunction, including the loss of mural cell coverage and an immature phenotype [167]. Another example is edema formation, which results both from increased afferent blood flow (hyperemia) due to arteriolar dilatation and from hyperpermeability. The imbalances in vascular function observed during IBD lead to complex and sometimes contradictory effects. In IBD patients, for instance, hyperemia has been observed in submucosal arterioles enlarged by increased afferent blood flow, whereas decreased perfusion was found in the intestinal mucosa [168].

3.4.1. The Role of Nitric Oxide in Vascular Dysfunction during IBD

Among the numerous mediators involved in microvascular function, nitric oxide (NO) has attracted a large amount of interest due to its broad range of functions. Under physiological conditions, NO counteracts leukocyte and platelet adhesion to ECs, regulates vasodilatation and endothelial permeability, and acts as radical scavenger [30]. As mentioned above, HIMECs express both the endogenous endothelial and the inducible form of NO-synthase (eNOS and iNOS), indicating the high tolerance of the gut microvasculature towards inflammatory activation [29]. The resulting high NO levels can, for instance, inhibit the expression of endothelial CAMs and MMPs induced by ICs (Table 3). During IBD, the production of NO by ECs is reduced due to the loss of iNOS and eNOS in HIMECs, and leukocyte adhesion is increased [169,170]. Furthermore, an upregulation of arginase expression and activity has been observed in inflamed HIMECs. Arginase competes with NOS for L-arginine, and therefore can limit NO production due to reduced substrate availability [170]. The decreased production of NO in ECs during IBD results in a loss of NO-mediated vasodilatation and an increase in ROS production in the microvessels of affected intestinal areas [171,172]. In parallel, NO also plays a role in VEGF-driven angiogenesis, as well as in intussusceptive angiogenesis [107], hence contributing both to the perpetuation of inflammation and to wound healing. Finally, NO has been shown to regulate endothelial barrier function in human, murine, and bovine ECs, notably by promoting VEGF-induced permeability through targeting of the VE-cadherin/β-catenin and Rho pathways [173,174]. However, NO can also protect ECs from hypoxia-induced barrier dysfunction [175]. In line with these contradictory results, the deficiency of eNOS and iNOS has been associated with either a better or a more severe course of disease in mouse models of colitis [176–179]. These differences might be attributed to the different roles played by NO in different cell compartments. The expression of eNOS by intestinal endothelial cells has been shown to specifically maintain mucosal integrity and prevent bacterial translocation in an TNBS-colitis model in mice [179]. Overall, the impairment of NO production during IBD increases the inflammatory activation of ECs and impairs vasodilatation, which might ultimately lead to pathological vasoconstriction, reduced mucosal perfusion, impaired wound healing, and the maintenance of chronic inflammation.

3.4.2. Coagulation

In mucosal tissues from patients with IBD or murine colitis models, the presence of thrombi due to increased platelet activation and binding to the EC surface has been observed [57]. This, in turn, can result in ischemic inflammation in the intestinal microvasculature, further enhancing tissue damage. In the DSS-colitis model and in IBD patient samples, accumulation of platelets in mucosal venules is linked to an increased leukocyte binding and disease activity [57,180,181]. The increase in thrombus formation associated with IBD has been attributed to several factors (Table 3). At the endothelial level, the activation of ECs through ICs and the decrease in NO levels upregulate the surface expression of adhesion molecules. Activated platelets found in the general circulation and in the intestinal mucosa of IBD patients can activate ECs, notably through the expression of P-selectin or CD40L, as well as the release of the soluble form of CD40L (sCD40L) [182,183]. In turn,

P-selectin and CD40L/sCD40L activate HIMECs, resulting in increased adhesion molecule expression, the secretion of cytokines such as IL-8, and increased binding to leukocytes, as well as to platelets themselves [97,183]. Increased coagulation has also been attributed to a reduced expression of thrombomodulin and protein C receptor (PCR) in the mucosal microvasculature of IBD patients and in colitic mice [184–187]. Protein C activation is also impaired in HIMECs under inflammatory conditions. This dampening of the PC system is correlated with increased adhesiveness of ECs, thereby promoting leukocyte recruitment and inflammation.

3.5. Regulatory Role of the Vasculature during Mucosal Inflammation

3.5.1. Vasculature and Innate Immunity

Following the rupture of the gut–epithelial barrier, mucosal microvascular ECs are exposed to bacteria and bacterial products. ECs can then launch an innate immune reaction through the engagement of toll-like receptors (TLRs) via pathogen-associated molecular patterns (PAMPs). Gut microvascular ECs exhibit a particular TLR response pattern compared to ECs from other origins (Table 3). For instance, tolerance to lipopolysaccharide (LPS), an activator of TLR4, has been observed in HIMECs but not in HUVECs after repeated exposure [188]. TLR3 and TLR5 are expressed at the surfaces of intestinal ECs. TLR3 is involved in the anti-viral response and is constitutively expressed in HIMECs, where it can be further upregulated by IFN-γ [189]. TLR5, a receptor for flagellin, was shown to play an important role in the EC innate immune response [190,191]. Activation of TLR3 and TLR5 in HIMECs induces the upregulation of inflammatory mediators and ICAM-1, leading to leukocyte recruitment [189,192]. TLRs expressed by intestinal ECs serve as a second barrier in the case of epithelial barrier breakdown. In particular, flagellin has been described as a dominant antigen in CD [193–195]. In agreement with this protective function of the GVB, TLR3 and TLR5 expression on ECs is protective against colitis in mice [196,197]. Taken together, the propensity of HIMECs to develop endotoxin tolerance might prevent an excessive immune reaction from occurring in the case of luminal bacterial penetration into the mucosa, while the response to viruses and flagellin remains intact, protecting against systemic propagation.

3.5.2. Paracrine Effects of the Inflamed Vasculature

ECs are highly reactive and can themselves express and secrete inflammatory mediators upon activation [192,198,199]. Those factors can either further promote or dampen inflammation through local or systemic effects (Table 3). For example, CX3CL1 (fractalkine), a chemokine that is upregulated in ECs via the MAPK pathway upon stimulation by TNF-α, IL-1, LPS, and IFN-γ, is highly upregulated in the mucosal endothelia of IBD patients [200,201]. CX3CL1 released from ECs stimulates the adhesion and transmigration of leukocytes expressing the CX3CR1 receptor. Higher levels of circulating and infiltrating CX3CL1$^+$ T cells have been observed during IBD [202]. Under inflammatory conditions, HIMECs are also able to express monocyte chemotactic protein 1 (MCP-1) [199]. In addition, intestinal vessels might exert angiocrine activity on epithelial cells during IBD through the release of TIMP1 and CXCL10, the latter being able to increase crypt survival [199].

Vascular ECs also secrete the C-C chemokine ligands 5 (CCL5) and 25 (CCL25) during inflammation [5]. CCL25 leads to the recruitment of immune cells expressing CCR9 [203]. Both CCR9 and CCL25 are upregulated during DSS-induced colitis, in which the CCL25-CCR9 axis exerts a protective anti-colitic effect in the intestinal mucosa by balancing different dendritic cell subsets [203]. Furthermore, during experimental colitis, NO of endothelial origin protects the intestinal mucosa of mice against inflammation by increasing the number of goblet cells and mucin production, thereby preventing luminal bacteria translocation [179].

3.6. Role of the Mesenteric Lymphatic Vasculature in IBD

Intestinal lymphatic vessels are involved in the removal of excess interstitial fluids, immune regulation, and the absorption of fatty acids by lacteal lymphatic endothelial cells [204]. During inflammation, lymphatic endothelial cells participate in the regulation of the adaptive inflammatory response and promote the resolution of inflammation through the clearance of immune cells and mediators [204]. Lymphangiogenesis is frequently observed during inflammation [205]. An increase in lymphatic vessel density has been observed in UC and CD throughout the mucosa, including in non-inflamed areas [206–208]. This development of the lymphatic system is thought to be a reaction to the inflammation and edema in the mucosa, aiming to dampen tissue damage by draining immune cells and excess fluid. However, similarly to blood vessels, lymph vessels show abnormal architectures and are often dysfunctional [209,210]. In CD, granulomatous structures characteristic of chronic lymphangitis have been observed in mesenteric lymph nodes and lymphatic vessels of the intestinal mucosa, and these correlate with disease activity [57,209,211]. In addition, lymphangiectasia, lymphadenopathy, and lymphatic vessel obstruction occurring during IBD compromise lymph drainage and leukocyte trafficking. This ultimately leads to edema, lymph leakage, and the deposition of adipose tissue into the mucosa, further fostering inflammation [211–213]. These observations are supported by the fact that a notable reduction in lymphatic contractile activity has been observed during murine experimental colitis, both locally and systematically [209,210,214]. Taken together, the lymphangiogenesis observed in IBD cannot resolve inflammation due the dysfunctionality of the newly formed lymphatics. The normalization of lymphatic function might represent an additional therapeutic approach in IBD.

3.7. Vascular Function and Extra-Intestinal Manifestations of IBD

More than one third of patients with CD and UC are affected by extraintestinal manifestations in addition to intestinal inflammation (Figure 2). The most common manifestations include thromboembolisms; hepatobiliary disorders; arthropathies; and cutaneous, pulmonary, and ocular manifestations, as well as neurological and psychosocial disturbances [14,215,216]. For example, major depressive disorder and multiple sclerosis are well-described IBD comorbidities [216–218]. Some of these extraintestinal manifestations correlate with flares of intestinal inflammation but others occur independently [215]. It remains unclear why only a fraction of patients with IBD present extra-intestinal manifestations.

3.7.1. Systemic Vascular Barrier Dysfunction in IBD

The GVB has been shown to lie at the heart of the gut–liver–brain axis. Increased GVB leakiness and dysfunction has been observed in patients during *Salmonella* infection, diet-induced nonalcoholic steatohepatitis, and metastatic colorectal cancer, leading to an impaired gut–liver axis connection [13,219,220]. The breakdown of the GVB in IBD may induce widespread low-grade vascular inflammation through the uncontrolled release of microbial products or pro-inflammatory factors into the systemic circulation, which might then compromise the vascular barrier at distant organs and result in extra-intestinal manifestations [12]. A strong link between the GVB and the blood–brain barrier (BBB) has been established in IBD. Manifestations of anxiety and depression have been reported in up to 40% of patients with active IBD (14), together with deterioration in cognitive functions [216–218,221–224]. Similar observations have been made in DSS-colitis models where mice displayed increased anxiety- and depression-like behaviors and alterations of the limbic system [158,225–227]. Carloni et al. have recently shown that after DSS challenge, there is a persistent increase in intestinal vascular permeability in treated mice, even after recovery [158]. They also observed an increased absolute number and percentage of innate immune cells in the liver and the brain, suggesting that acute intestinal inflammation quickly spreads to other organs, including the brain [158]. Interestingly, vascular permeability induced by DSS treatment was only increased transiently in the brain due to the closure of the vascular barrier in the brain choroid plexus (PVB), which was then released after discontinuation of the application of DSS. In a transgenic mouse model of the inducible closure of the PVB, animals exhibited anxiety-like behavior and a deficit in short-term memory, suggesting that PVB closure may correlate with cognitive and mental disturbances [158]. These observations are further supported by the fact that a disruption of the BBB has been observed during TNBS-induced colitis in mice [228].

The translocation of bacteria into the bloodstream during IBD-related intestinal inflammation has been proposed to contribute to extra-intestinal effects. Indeed, patients with IBD have an elevated risk of sepsis [229,230]. Nevertheless, sepsis represents a rare complication of IBD, mainly occurring after surgery [230]. In DSS-induced colitis, mice treated with the glucocorticoid budesonide, bacterial translocation to the liver, and endotoxemia have been observed following massive intestinal barrier disruption [231]. However, these effects were not observed in the transfer colitis model, or in DSS-treated mice which did not receive budesonide. Together, these data suggest that the translocation of bacteria and bacterial products is limited during IBD and experimental colitis [231].

Bacterial products, on the contrary, have been frequently detected in the circulation of patients with IBD. Bacterial DNA can be found in the blood for up to 50% of IBD patients [232], and bacterial DNA translocation represents an independent risk factor of relapse at 6 months in CD patients [233]. The presence of bacterial endotoxin and LPS-binding protein can also be detected in the circulation of IBD patients [234–238]. Higher serum levels of LPS were observed in patients with IBD-associated spondylarthritis compared to IBD alone, indicating that an increased translocation of bacterial products is linked to the development of extra-intestinal manifestations [236]. Recently, Carloni et al. showed that the LPS blood concentration increases only transiently after DSS challenge in mice. The fact that patients with UC have elevated serum concentrations of LPS-binding protein but not of LPS supports the idea of a transient increase [158]. The authors proposed that increased scavenging by circulating inflammatory cells might explain the transient character of the serum LPS spike.

The release of inflammatory mediators by the inflamed intestinal endothelium might also lead to systemic low-grade inflammation, resulting in vascular activation and/or barrier dysfunction at distant organs. Increased levels of circulating inflammatory cytokines (IL-6, TNF-α ...), for instance, can be found in IBD patients and animals with colitis [158]. There is indeed increasing evidence that circulating pro-inflammatory mediators in IBD patients may contribute to the progression of several central nervous system (CNS) disorders [158,239–241].

3.7.2. Endothelial Damage and Systemic Vascular Inflammation

During IBD, local endothelial dysfunction, which can spread into systemic vascular barrier defects, might also promote generalized vascular inflammation. There is evidence linking IBD with atherosclerosis, coronary dysfunction, and an increased risk of cardiovascular (CV) morbidity and mortality [242–248]. Furthermore, IBD patients have an elevated risk of vasculitis, which is linked to more frequent headaches and extraintestinal symptoms [249,250]. Antibodies to endothelial cells reflect vascular injury and have been detected in the serum of patients with vasculitis. Anti-endothelial cell antibody levels are elevated in UC and CD patients compared with healthy controls [251]. In addition, increased anti-EC antibody levels were found to correlate with circulating levels of Von Willebrand factor, a marker of vascular inflammation and injury, indicating the occurrence of vasculitis during IBD. Some association between anti-endothelial cell antibody levels and disease activity has been found in both UC and CD [252,253].

Increasing evidence links intestinal microbiota dysbiosis, vascular aging, and cardiovascular diseases (the "gut–heart axis"). The passage of bacterial products into the bloodstream has been associated with increased arterial stiffness, atherosclerosis, hypertension, and cardiovascular risk in human individuals [254]. For instance, the reduction of short chain fatty acids and the increased production of trimethylamine-N-oxide, which are associated with gut dysbiosis, increase cardiovascular risk. In addition, the transmigration of LPS into the bloodstream activates vascular inflammation [254].

3.7.3. Coagulation and Thrombosis in IBD

The local increase of pro-coagulant and pro-thrombotic events in the microvasculature of inflamed intestinal tissues is associated with systemic subclinical thrombosis in patients with IBD. Markers of coagulation are elevated in the serum of IBD patients, and increased extra-intestinal thrombus formation is enhanced in the DSS-colitis model [184,255]. Thrombosis represents a significant comorbidity, and thromboembolitic events have been estimated to account for up to 25% of IBD-related deaths [256]. The risk of venous thromboembolism is particularly increased in patients with IBD during a flare up or in the presence of chronically active inflammation [257–263]. In comparison, the overall risk of arterial disease is only modestly increased [260].

3.8. Targeting the Vasculature in IBD Therapy

The role of the microvasculature in the pathogenesis and perpetuation of IBD is receiving increasing recognition, and it represents an attractive therapy target.

Interestingly, several anti-inflammatory drugs used in the clinical management of IBD also ameliorate vascular dysfunction, suggesting that their efficacy depends in part on their endothelium-directed effects. For instance, mesalazine (5-aminosylicyclic acid), a medication used to treat mildly to moderately severe forms of IBD, has been shown to inhibit platelet activation [264]. In addition, the anti-TNF-α neutralizing antibody infliximab, which blocks TNF-induced inflammation and has been successfully used in IBD therapy, notably improves endothelial dysfunction in CD by enhancing agonist-induced vasodilatation, by reducing thrombus formation through inhibition of the CD40/CD40L/sCD40L pathway, and by inhibiting TNF-α-induced endothelial cell permeability [265–267].

Anti-TNF-α therapy has allowed healthcare professionals to bridge a therapeutic gap for IBD patients who are refractory or intolerant to treatment with classic immunosuppressive agents. However, a significant proportion of patients does not respond to anti-TNF-α therapy. New approaches based on the blockade of T-cell homing have shown promising results. Here, the recruitment of T-cells through the binding of $\alpha 4 \beta 7$ integrins to endothelial MadCAM1 is inhibited [268–270]. The $\alpha 4 \beta 7$-integrin-specific antibody vedolizumab induces long-term remission in CD and UC, and represents a good alternative for patients with refractory disease and colonic inflammation [271–273]. The $\beta 7$-integrin-specific antibody etrolizumab as well as anti-MadCAM1 antibodies are currently being evaluated in clinical trials [269,274,275]. Hence, the specific blockade of the interaction of T-cells with the activated MadCAM1$^+$ endothelium is increasingly being implemented in the clinical routine.

Therapeutic strategies targeting the endothelium represent an interesting way to reduce mucosal inflammation and/or extraintestinal manifestations by normalizing the vascular function. For example, heparin has been administered to IBD patients to prevent venous thromboembolism [276–278]. In addition, treatment with low-molecular-weight heparin has shown therapeutic efficiency in IBD [279,280], which was not only due to the inhibition of microvascular thromboses, but also to immuno-modulating properties (such as the suppression of neutrophil recruitment) and to an increase in mucosal recovery [281,282]. A new therapeutic approach based on the delivery of heparin via nanoparticles (NPs) has provided promising results in the TNBS-induced colitis mouse model [283]. In addition, heparin-coated human serum albumin NPs have been shown to efficiently deliver drugs into the inflamed intestine in a murine model of colitis, opening up new possibilities for combinational treatment [284]. Similarly, the treatment of microvascular lesions with *Panax notoginseng* attenuated inflammation and disease activity in rats with colitis [285]. In another study, the targeting of phosphatidylserine externalized by stressed ECs in capillaries of the mouse colonic mucosa using annexin-V inhibited TNBS-induced colitis [286].

Another promising strategy for vessel-directed therapy of IBD is the inhibition of the loss of GVB function during IBD. The receptor tyrosine kinase imatinib has been shown to inhibit vascular dysfunction and edema in various models [162,287–289]. Treatment with imatinib blocks vessel permeability and alleviates DSS-induced colitis in mice [34]. Imatinib, given in the context of chronic myeloid leukemia, has been reported to induce long-standing remission of CD [290]. Sphingosine 1-phosphate (S1P), a sphingolipid mediator, represents another potential target. S1P signals through high-affinity G protein-coupled receptors S1P1 to 5 to regulate the egress of lymphocytes from lymphoid organs and the maintenance of vascular integrity [291,292], targeting both blood and lymphatic ECs. A dysfunctional S1P signaling axis leads to pathological angiogenesis and increased vascular permeability [293,294]. Several S1P agonists including ozanimod and etrasimod have shown promising results by blocking lymphocyte recruitment and improving barrier function, and are currently being tested in phase 3 clinical trials for UC and CD [293,295,296]. In conclusion, pharmacological normalization of the vasculature could not only prevent vascular co-morbidities in IBD patients, but might also complement the standard anti-inflammatory regimens.

4. Conclusions

The endothelium lies at the heart of the inflammation circle, and the manifold changes it undergoes during activation are regulated by complex mechanisms. These mechanisms can explain in part the refractory character of IBD, but might also represent complementary anti-inflammatory therapy targets. The blockade of leukocyte recruitment by endothelial cells plays an important role in that regard. Vascular damage, hyperpermeability, and the activation of the hyperthrombic state of the inflamed vasculature also represent important contributors to inflammation, whereas the role of angiogenesis appears to be less important than initially thought. In recent years, the intestinal microvascular barrier has been shown to play a decisive role as a second barrier in the gut. The loss of its function has furthermore been found to promote inflammation and has been linked to the development of extra-intestinal manifestations of IBD. Therefore, the intestinal microvascular barrier is now emerging as a promising therapeutic target for the treatment of IBD patients.

Author Contributions: Writing—original draft preparation, N.B.-L.; writing—review and editing, N.B.-L., C.W., M.S.; funding acquisition, N.B.-L., C.W., M.S. All authors have read and agreed to the published version of the manuscript.

Funding: This work has been funded by the Deutsche Forschungsgemeinschaft (DFG, German Research Foundation)—TRR 241-375876048 (A06 to M.S. and N.B.-L.; A09 and B01 to C.W.); TRR305-429280966 (B07 to N.B.-L.); STU 238/10-1-437201724 to M.S.; KFO 257-4-190140969 to M.S.; FOR 2438-2 280163318 to M.S.—as well as by the Interdisciplinary Center for Clinical Research (IZKF) of the Clinical Center Erlangen (ELAN-Fonds project P027 to N.B.-L., Project J19 to N.B.-L., and D34 to M.S.), by the W. Lutz Stiftung, and by the Forschungsstiftung Medizin am Universi-tätsklinikum Erlangen to M.S., by the Deutsche Forschungsgemeinschaft and Frie-drich-Alexander-Universität Erlangen-Nürnberg within the funding programme "Open Access Publication Funding".

Conflicts of Interest: The authors declare no conflict of interest.

References

1. Zhang, Y.Z.; Li, Y.Y. Inflammatory bowel disease: Pathogenesis. *World J. Gastroenterol.* **2014**, *20*, 91–99. [CrossRef]
2. Wallace, K.L.; Zheng, L.B.; Kanazawa, Y.; Shih, D.Q. Immunopathology of inflammatory bowel disease. *World J. Gastroenterol.* **2014**, *20*, 6–21. [CrossRef] [PubMed]
3. Ni, J.; Wu, G.D.; Albenberg, L.; Tomov, V.T. Gut microbiota and IBD: Causation or correlation? *Nat. Rev. Gastroenterol. Hepatol.* **2017**, *14*, 573–584. [CrossRef]
4. Thoo, L.; Noti, M.; Krebs, P. Keep calm: The intestinal barrier at the interface of peace and war. *Cell Death Dis.* **2019**, *10*, 849. [CrossRef]
5. Cromer, W.E.; Mathis, J.M.; Granger, D.N.; Chaitanya, G.V.; Alexander, J.S. Role of the endothelium in inflammatory bowel diseases. *World J. Gastroenterol.* **2011**, *17*, 578–593. [CrossRef] [PubMed]

6. Kvietys, P.R. Integrated Systems Physiology: From Molecule to Function. In *The Gastrointestinal Circulation*; Morgan & Claypool Life Sciences: San Rafael, CA, USA, 2010.
7. Geboes, K.; Geboes, K.P.; Maleux, G. Vascular anatomy of the gastrointestinal tract. *Best Pract. Res. Clin. Gastroenterol.* **2001**, *15*, 1–14. [CrossRef]
8. Arfors, K.E.; Rutili, G.; Svensjö, E. Microvascular transport of macromolecules in normal and inflammatory conditions. *Acta Physiol. Scand. Suppl.* **1979**, *463*, 93–103.
9. Hasibeder, W. Gastrointestinal microcirculation: Still a mystery? *Br. J. Anaesth.* **2010**, *105*, 393–396. [CrossRef]
10. Miller, M.J.; McDole, J.R.; Newberry, R.D. Microanatomy of the intestinal lymphatic system. *Ann. N. Y. Acad. Sci.* **2010**, *1207* (Suppl. 1), E21–E28. [CrossRef]
11. Cifarelli, V.; Eichmann, A. The Intestinal Lymphatic System: Functions and Metabolic Implications. *Cell. Mol. Gastroenterol. Hepatol.* **2019**, *7*, 503–513. [CrossRef] [PubMed]
12. Brescia, P.; Rescigno, M. The gut vascular barrier: A new player in the gut-liver-brain axis. *Trends Mol. Med.* **2021**, *27*, 844–855. [CrossRef]
13. Spadoni, I.; Zagato, E.; Bertocchi, A.; Paolinelli, R.; Hot, E.; Di Sabatino, A.; Caprioli, F.; Bottiglieri, L.; Oldani, A.; Viale, G.; et al. A gut-vascular barrier controls the systemic dissemination of bacteria. *Science* **2015**, *350*, 830–834. [CrossRef] [PubMed]
14. Spadoni, I.; Fornasa, G.; Rescigno, M. Organ-specific protection mediated by cooperation between vascular and epithelial barriers. *Nat. Rev. Immunol.* **2017**, *17*, 761–773. [CrossRef] [PubMed]
15. Bush, T.G.; Savidge, T.C.; Freeman, T.C.; Cox, H.J.; Campbell, E.A.; Mucke, L.; Johnson, M.H.; Sofroniew, M.V. Fulminant jejuno-ileitis following ablation of enteric glia in adult transgenic mice. *Cell* **1998**, *93*, 189–201. [CrossRef]
16. Cornet, A.; Savidge, T.C.; Cabarrocas, J.; Deng, W.L.; Colombel, J.F.; Lassmann, H.; Desreumaux, P.; Liblau, R.S. Enterocolitis induced by autoimmune targeting of enteric glial cells: A possible mechanism in Crohn's disease? *Proc. Natl. Acad. Sci. USA* **2001**, *98*, 13306–13311. [CrossRef]
17. Kabouridis, P.S.; Lasrado, R.; McCallum, S.; Chng, S.H.; Snippert, H.J.; Clevers, H.; Pettersson, S.; Pachnis, V. Microbiota controls the homeostasis of glial cells in the gut lamina propria. *Neuron* **2015**, *85*, 289–295. [CrossRef] [PubMed]
18. Reinhardt, C.; Bergentall, M.; Greiner, T.U.; Schaffner, F.; Ostergren-Lundén, G.; Petersen, L.C.; Ruf, W.; Bäckhed, F. Tissue factor and PAR1 promote microbiota-induced intestinal vascular remodelling. *Nature* **2012**, *483*, 627–631. [CrossRef]
19. Schirbel, A.; Kessler, S.; Rieder, F.; West, G.; Rebert, N.; Asosingh, K.; McDonald, C.; Fiocchi, C. Pro-angiogenic activity of TLRs and NLRs: A novel link between gut microbiota and intestinal angiogenesis. *Gastroenterology* **2013**, *144*, 613–623.e9. [CrossRef]
20. Stappenbeck, T.S.; Hooper, L.V.; Gordon, J.I. Developmental regulation of intestinal angiogenesis by indigenous microbes via Paneth cells. *Proc. Natl. Acad. Sci. USA* **2002**, *99*, 15451–15455. [CrossRef] [PubMed]
21. Komarova, Y.A.; Kruse, K.; Mehta, D.; Malik, A.B. Protein Interactions at Endothelial Junctions and Signaling Mechanisms Regulating Endothelial Permeability. *Circ. Res.* **2017**, *120*, 179–206. [CrossRef]
22. Scalise, A.A.; Kakogiannos, N.; Zanardi, F.; Iannelli, F.; Giannotta, M. The blood–brain and gut–vascular barriers: From the perspective of claudins. *Tissue Barriers* **2021**, *9*, 1926190. [CrossRef]
23. Richards, M.; Nwadozi, E.; Pal, S.; Martinsson, P.; Kaakinen, M.; Gloger, M.; Sjöberg, E.; Koltowska, K.; Betsholtz, C.; Eklund, L.; et al. Claudin5 protects the peripheral endothelial barrier in an organ and vessel-type-specific manner. *eLife* **2022**, *11*, e78517. [CrossRef] [PubMed]
24. Kalucka, J.; de Rooij, L.P.M.H.; Goveia, J.; Rohlenova, K.; Dumas, S.J.; Meta, E.; Conchinha, N.V.; Taverna, F.; Teuwen, L.-A.; Veys, K.; et al. Single—Cell Transcriptome Atlas of Murine Endothelial Cells. *Cell* **2020**, *180*, 764–779.e20. [CrossRef] [PubMed]
25. Günzel, D.; Yu, A.S.L. Claudins and the modulation of tight junction permeability. *Physiol. Rev.* **2013**, *93*, 525–569. [CrossRef]
26. Garcia-Hernandez, V.; Quiros, M.; Nusrat, A. Intestinal epithelial claudins: Expression and regulation in homeostasis and inflammation. *Ann. N. Y. Acad. Sci.* **2017**, *1397*, 66–79. [CrossRef]
27. Haraldsen, G.; Kvale, D.; Lien, B.; Farstad, I.N.; Brandtzaeg, P. Cytokine-regulated expression of E-selectin, intercellular adhesion molecule-1 (ICAM-1), and vascular cell adhesion molecule-1 (VCAM-1) in human microvascular endothelial cells. *J. Immunol.* **1996**, *156*, 2558–2565. [CrossRef] [PubMed]
28. Nilsen, E.M.; Johansen, F.E.; Jahnsen, F.L.; Lundin, K.E.A.; Scholz, T.; Brandtzaeg, P.; Haraldsen, G. Cytokine profiles of cultured microvascular endothelial cells from the human intestine. *Gut* **1998**, *42*, 635–642. [CrossRef]
29. Binion, D.G.; Fu, S.; Ramanujam, K.S.; Chai, Y.C.; Dweik, R.A.; Drazba, J.A.; Wade, J.G.; Ziats, N.P.; Erzurum, S.C.; Wilson, K.T. iNOS expression in human intestinal microvascular endothelial cells inhibits leukocyte adhesion. *Am. J. Physiol.* **1998**, *275*, G592–G603. [CrossRef]
30. Sessa, W.C. Molecular control of blood flow and angiogenesis: Role of nitric oxide. *J. Thromb. Haemost.* **2009**, *7* (Suppl. 1), 35–37. [CrossRef]
31. Pober, J.S.; Sessa, W.C. Evolving functions of endothelial cells in inflammation. *Nat. Rev. Immunol.* **2007**, *7*, 803–815. [CrossRef]
32. Papa, A.; Scaldaferri, F.; Danese, S.; Guglielmo, S.; Roberto, I.; Bonizzi, M.; Mocci, G.; Felice, C.; Ricci, C.; Andrisani, G.; et al. Vascular involvement in inflammatory bowel disease: Pathogenesis and clinical aspects. *Dig. Dis.* **2008**, *26*, 149–155. [CrossRef]
33. Haep, L.; Britzen-Laurent, N.; Weber, T.G.; Naschberger, E.; Schaefer, A.; Kremmer, E.; Foersch, S.; Vieth, M.; Scheuer, W.; Wirtz, S.; et al. Interferon Gamma Counteracts the Angiogenic Switch and Induces Vascular Permeability in Dextran Sulfate Sodium Colitis in Mice. *Inflamm. Bowel Dis.* **2015**, *21*, 2360–2371. [CrossRef]

34. Langer, V.; Vivi, E.; Regensburger, D.; Winkler, T.H.; Waldner, M.J.; Rath, T.; Schmid, B.; Skottke, L.; Lee, S.; Jeon, N.L.; et al. IFN-γ drives inflammatory bowel disease pathogenesis through VE-cadherin-directed vascular barrier disruption. *J. Clin. Investig.* **2019**, *129*, 4691–4707. [CrossRef]
35. Nourshargh, S.; Alon, R. Leukocyte Migration into Inflamed Tissues. *Immunity* **2014**, *41*, 694–707. [CrossRef]
36. Binion, D.G.; West, G.A.; Volk, E.E.; Drazba, J.A.; Ziats, N.P.; Petras, R.E.; Fiocchi, C. Acquired increase in leucocyte binding by intestinal microvascular endothelium in inflammatory bowel disease. *Lancet* **1998**, *352*, 1742–1746. [CrossRef]
37. Scaldaferri, F.; Sans, M.; Vetrano, S.; Correale, C.; Arena, V.; Pagano, N.; Rando, G.; Romeo, F.; Potenza, A.E.; Repici, A.; et al. The role of MAPK in governing lymphocyte adhesion and migration across the microvasculature in inflammatory bowel disease. *Eur. J. Immunol.* **2009**, *39*, 290–300. [CrossRef] [PubMed]
38. Fägerstam, J.P.; Whiss, P.A.; Ström, M.; Andersson, R.G. Expression of platelet P-selectin and detection of soluble P-selectin, NPY and RANTES in patients with inflammatory bowel disease. *Inflamm. Res.* **2000**, *49*, 466–472. [CrossRef] [PubMed]
39. Fägerstam, J.P.; Whiss, P.A. Higher platelet P-selectin in male patients with inflammatory bowel disease compared to healthy males. *World J. Gastroenterol.* **2006**, *12*, 1270–1272. [CrossRef]
40. Ostanin, D.V.; Bao, J.; Koboziev, I.; Gray, L.; Robinson-Jackson, S.A.; Kosloski-Davidson, M.; Price, V.H.; Grisham, M.B. T cell transfer model of chronic colitis: Concepts, considerations, and tricks of the trade. *Am. J. Physiol. Gastrointest. Liver Physiol.* **2009**, *296*, G135–G146. [CrossRef]
41. Zittermann, S.I.; Issekutz, A.C. Endothelial growth factors VEGF and bFGF differentially enhance monocyte and neutrophil recruitment to inflammation. *J. Leukoc. Biol.* **2006**, *80*, 247–257. [CrossRef] [PubMed]
42. Goebel, S.; Huang, M.; Davis, W.C.; Jennings, M.; Siahaan, T.J.; Alexander, J.S.; Kevil, C.G. VEGF-A stimulation of leukocyte adhesion to colonic microvascular endothelium: Implications for inflammatory bowel disease. *Am. J. Physiol. Gastrointest. Liver Physiol.* **2006**, *290*, G648–G654. [CrossRef]
43. Sans, M.; Fuster, D.; Vázquez, A.; Setoain, F.J.; Piera, C.; Piqué, J.M.; Panés, J. 123Iodine-labelled anti-VCAM-1 antibody scintigraphy in the assessment of experimental colitis. *Eur. J. Gastroenterol. Hepatol.* **2001**, *13*, 31–38. [CrossRef]
44. Soriano, A.; Salas, A.; Salas, A.; Sans, M.; Gironella, M.; Elena, M.; Anderson, D.C.; Piqué, J.M.; Panés, J. VCAM-1, but not ICAM-1 or MAdCAM-1, immunoblockade ameliorates DSS-induced colitis in mice. *Lab. Investig.* **2000**, *80*, 1541–1551. [CrossRef] [PubMed]
45. Rijcken, E.; Mennigen, R.B.; Schaefer, S.D.; Laukoetter, M.G.; Anthoni, C.; Spiegel, H.U.; Bruewer, M.; Senninger, N.; Krieglstein, C.F. PECAM-1 (CD 31) mediates transendothelial leukocyte migration in experimental colitis. *Am. J. Physiol. Gastrointest. Liver Physiol.* **2007**, *293*, G446–G452. [CrossRef] [PubMed]
46. Briskin, M.; Winsor-Hines, D.; Shyjan, A.; Cochran, N.; Bloom, S.; Wilson, J.; McEvoy, L.M.; Butcher, E.C.; Kassam, N.; Mackay, C.R.; et al. Human mucosal addressin cell adhesion molecule-1 is preferentially expressed in intestinal tract and associated lymphoid tissue. *Am. J. Pathol.* **1997**, *151*, 97–110.
47. Ogawa, H.; Binion, D.G.; Heidemann, J.; Theriot, M.; Fisher, P.J.; Johnson, N.A.; Otterson, M.F.; Rafiee, P. Mechanisms of MAdCAM-1 gene expression in human intestinal microvascular endothelial cells. *Am. J. Physiol. Cell Physiol.* **2005**, *288*, C272–C281. [CrossRef] [PubMed]
48. Ando, T.; Jordan, P.; Wang, Y.; Itoh, M.; Joh, T.; Sasaki, M.; Elrod, J.W.; Carpenter, A.; Jennings, M.H.; Minagar, A.; et al. MAdCAM-1 expression and regulation in murine colonic endothelial cells in vitro. *Inflamm. Bowel Dis.* **2005**, *11*, 258–264. [CrossRef]
49. Tyler, C.J.; Guzman, M.; Lundborg, L.R.; Yeasmin, S.; Zgajnar, N.; Jedlicka, P.; Bamias, G.; Rivera-Nieves, J. Antibody secreting cells are critically dependent on integrin α4β7/MAdCAM-1 for intestinal recruitment and control of the microbiota during chronic colitis. *Mucosal Immunol.* **2022**, *15*, 109–119. [CrossRef]
50. Jackson, J.R.; Seed, M.P.; Kircher, C.H.; Willoughby, D.A.; Winkler, J.D. The codependence of angiogenesis and chronic inflammation. *FASEB J.* **1997**, *11*, 457–465. [CrossRef]
51. Danese, S.; Sans, M.; de la Motte, C.; Graziani, C.; West, G.; Phillips, M.H.; Pola, R.; Rutella, S.; Willis, J.; Gasbarrini, A.; et al. Angiogenesis as a novel component of inflammatory bowel disease pathogenesis. *Gastroenterology* **2006**, *130*, 2060–2073. [CrossRef]
52. Chidlow, J.H., Jr.; Langston, W.; Greer, J.J.; Ostanin, D.; Abdelbaqi, M.; Houghton, J.; Senthilkumar, A.; Shukla, D.; Mazar, A.P.; Grisham, M.B.; et al. Differential angiogenic regulation of experimental colitis. *Am. J. Pathol.* **2006**, *169*, 2014–2030. [CrossRef] [PubMed]
53. Alkim, C.; Alkim, H.; Koksal, A.R.; Boga, S.; Sen, I. Angiogenesis in Inflammatory Bowel Disease. *Int. J. Inflamm.* **2015**, *2015*, 970890. [CrossRef]
54. Danese, S.; Sans, M.; Spencer, D.M.; Beck, I.; Doñate, F.; Plunkett, M.L.; de la Motte, C.; Redline, R.; Shaw, D.E.; Levine, A.D.; et al. Angiogenesis blockade as a new therapeutic approach to experimental colitis. *Gut* **2007**, *56*, 855–862. [CrossRef] [PubMed]
55. Danese, S. Inflammation and the mucosal microcirculation in inflammatory bowel disease: The ebb and flow. *Curr. Opin. Gastroenterol.* **2007**, *23*, 384–389. [CrossRef]
56. Binion, D.G.; Rafiee, P. Is inflammatory bowel disease a vascular disease? Targeting angiogenesis improves chronic inflammation in inflammatory bowel disease. *Gastroenterology* **2009**, *136*, 400–403. [CrossRef] [PubMed]
57. Danese, S. Role of the vascular and lymphatic endothelium in the pathogenesis of inflammatory bowel disease: 'Brothers in arms'. *Gut* **2011**, *60*, 998–1008. [CrossRef] [PubMed]

58. Dulic-Sills, A.; Blunden, M.J.; Mawdsley, J.; Bastin, A.J.; McAuley, D.; Griffiths, M.; Rampton, D.S.; Yaqoob, M.M.; Macey, M.G.; Agrawal, S.G. New flow cytometric technique for the evaluation of circulating endothelial progenitor cell levels in various disease groups. *J. Immunol. Methods* **2006**, *316*, 107–115. [CrossRef] [PubMed]
59. Garolla, A.; D'Incà, R.; Checchin, D.; Biagioli, A.; De Toni, L.; Nicoletti, V.; Scarpa, M.; Bolzonello, E.; Sturniolo, G.C.; Foresta, C. Reduced endothelial progenitor cell number and function in inflammatory bowel disease: A possible link to the pathogenesis. *Am. J. Gastroenterol.* **2009**, *104*, 2500–2507. [CrossRef]
60. Deng, X.; Szabo, S.; Chen, L.; Paunovic, B.; Khomenko, T.; Tolstanova, G.; Tarnawski, A.S.; Jones, M.K.; Sandor, Z. New cell therapy using bone marrow-derived stem cells/endothelial progenitor cells to accelerate neovascularization in healing of experimental ulcerative colitis. *Curr. Pharm. Des.* **2011**, *17*, 1643–1651. [CrossRef]
61. Giatromanolaki, A.; Sivridis, E.; Maltezos, E.; Papazoglou, D.; Simopoulos, C.; Gatter, K.C.; Harris, A.L.; Koukourakis, M.I. Hypoxia inducible factor 1alpha and 2alpha overexpression in inflammatory bowel disease. *J. Clin. Pathol.* **2003**, *56*, 209–213. [CrossRef]
62. Alkim, C.; Savas, B.; Ensari, A.; Alkim, H.; Dagli, U.; Parlak, E.; Ulker, A.; Sahin, B. Expression of p53, VEGF, microvessel density, and cyclin-D1 in noncancerous tissue of inflammatory bowel disease. *Dig. Dis. Sci.* **2009**, *54*, 1979–1984. [CrossRef] [PubMed]
63. Alkim, C.; Sakiz, D.; Alkim, H.; Livaoglu, A.; Kendir, T.; Demirsoy, H.; Erdem, L.; Akbayir, N.; Sokmen, M. Thrombospondin-1 and VEGF in inflammatory bowel disease. *Libyan J. Med.* **2012**, *7*, 8942. [CrossRef] [PubMed]
64. Scaldaferri, F.; Vetrano, S.; Sans, M.; Arena, V.; Straface, G.; Stigliano, E.; Repici, A.; Sturm, A.; Malesci, A.; Panes, J.; et al. VEGF-A links angiogenesis and inflammation in inflammatory bowel disease pathogenesis. *Gastroenterology* **2009**, *136*, 585–595.e5. [CrossRef]
65. Griga, T.; Gutzeit, A.; Sommerkamp, C.; May, B. Increased production of vascular endothelial growth factor by peripheral blood mononuclear cells in patients with inflammatory bowel disease. *Eur. J. Gastroenterol. Hepatol.* **1999**, *11*, 175–179. [CrossRef] [PubMed]
66. Bousvaros, A.; Leichtner, A.; Zurakowski, D.; Kwon, J.; Law, T.; Keough, K.; Fishman, S. Elevated serum vascular endothelial growth factor in children and young adults with Crohn's disease. *Dig. Dis. Sci.* **1999**, *44*, 424–430. [CrossRef] [PubMed]
67. Pousa, I.D.; Maté, J.; Gisbert, J.P. Angiogenesis in inflammatory bowel disease. *Eur. J. Clin. Investig.* **2008**, *38*, 73–81. [CrossRef] [PubMed]
68. Krzystek-Korpacka, M.; Neubauer, K.; Matusiewicz, M. Platelet-derived growth factor-BB reflects clinical, inflammatory and angiogenic disease activity and oxidative stress in inflammatory bowel disease. *Clin. Biochem.* **2009**, *42*, 1602–1609. [CrossRef] [PubMed]
69. Macé, V.; Ahluwalia, A.; Coron, E.; Le Rhun, M.; Boureille, A.; Bossard, C.; Mosnier, J.F.; Matysiak-Budnik, T.; Tarnawski, A.S. Confocal laser endomicroscopy: A new gold standard for the assessment of mucosal healing in ulcerative colitis. *J. Gastroenterol. Hepatol.* **2015**, *30* (Suppl. 1), 85–92. [CrossRef]
70. Ippolito, C.; Colucci, R.; Segnani, C.; Errede, M.; Girolamo, F.; Virgintino, D.; Dolfi, A.; Tirotta, E.; Buccianti, P.; Di Candio, G.; et al. Fibrotic and Vascular Remodelling of Colonic Wall in Patients with Active Ulcerative Colitis. *J. Crohn's Colitis* **2016**, *10*, 1194–1204. [CrossRef]
71. Kapsoritakis, A.; Sfiridaki, A.; Maltezos, E.; Simopoulos, K.; Giatromanolaki, A.; Sivridis, E.; Koukourakis, M.I. Vascular endothelial growth factor in inflammatory bowel disease. *Int. J. Color. Dis.* **2003**, *18*, 418–422. [CrossRef]
72. Konno, S.; Iizuka, M.; Yukawa, M.; Sasaki, K.; Sato, A.; Horie, Y.; Nanjo, H.; Fukushima, T.; Watanabe, S. Altered expression of angiogenic factors in the VEGF-Ets-1 cascades in inflammatory bowel disease. *J. Gastroenterol.* **2004**, *39*, 931–939. [CrossRef] [PubMed]
73. Magro, F.; Araujo, F.; Pereira, P.; Meireles, E.; Diniz-Ribeiro, M.; Velosom, F.T. Soluble selectins, sICAM, sVCAM, and angiogenic proteins in different activity groups of patients with inflammatory bowel disease. *Dig. Dis. Sci.* **2004**, *49*, 1265–1274. [CrossRef] [PubMed]
74. Tolstanova, G.; Khomenko, T.; Deng, X.; Chen, L.; Tarnawski, A.; Ahluwalia, A.; Szabo, S.; Sandor, Z. Neutralizing anti-vascular endothelial growth factor (VEGF) antibody reduces severity of experimental ulcerative colitis in rats: Direct evidence for the pathogenic role of VEGF. *J. Pharmacol. Exp. Ther.* **2009**, *328*, 749–757. [CrossRef] [PubMed]
75. Cromer, W.E.; Ganta, C.V.; Patel, M.; Traylor, J.; Kevil, C.G.; Alexander, J.S.; Mathis, J.M. VEGF-A isoform modulation in an preclinical TNBS model of ulcerative colitis: Protective effects of a VEGF164b therapy. *J. Transl. Med.* **2013**, *11*, 207. [CrossRef] [PubMed]
76. Ozsoy, Z.; Ozsoy, S.; Gevrek, F.; Demir, E.; Benli, I.; Daldal, E.; Yenidogan, E. Effect of bevacizumab on acetic acid–induced ulcerative colitis in rats. *J. Surg. Res.* **2017**, *216*, 191–200. [CrossRef]
77. Hindryckx, P.; Waeytens, A.; Laukens, D.; Peeters, H.; Van Huysse, J.; Ferdinande, L.; Carmeliet, P.; De Vos, M. Absence of placental growth factor blocks dextran sodium sulfate-induced colonic mucosal angiogenesis, increases mucosal hypoxia and aggravates acute colonic injury. *Lab. Investig.* **2010**, *90*, 566–576. [CrossRef]
78. Hapani, S.; Chu, D.; Wu, S. Risk of gastrointestinal perforation in patients with cancer treated with bevacizumab: A meta-analysis. *Lancet Oncol.* **2009**, *10*, 559–568. [CrossRef]
79. Coriat, R.; Mir, O.; Leblanc, S.; Ropert, S.; Brezault, C.; Chaussade, S.; Goldwasser, F. Feasibility of anti-VEGF agent bevacizumab in patients with Crohn's disease. *Inflamm. Bowel Dis.* **2010**, *17*, 1632. [CrossRef]

80. Tanaka, M.; Ishii, H.; Azuma, K.; Saisho, C.; Matsuo, N.; Imamura, Y.; Tokito, T.; Kinoshita, T.; Yamada, K.; Takedatsu, H.; et al. Ulcerative colitis in a patient with non-small-cell lung cancer receiving bevacizumab. *Investig. New Drugs* **2015**, *33*, 1133–1135. [CrossRef]
81. Herrera-Gómez, R.G.; Grecea, M.; Gallois, C.; Boige, V.; Pautier, P.; Pistilli, B.; Planchard, D.; Malka, D.; Ducreux, M.; Mir, O. Safety and Efficacy of Bevacizumab in Cancer Patients with Inflammatory Bowel Disease. *Cancers* **2022**, *14*, 2914. [CrossRef]
82. Loriot, Y.; Boudou-Rouquette, P.; Billemont, B.; Ropert, S.; Goldwasser, F. Acute exacerbation of hemorrhagic rectocolitis during antiangiogenic therapy with sunitinib and sorafenib. *Ann. Oncol.* **2008**, *19*, 1975. [CrossRef] [PubMed]
83. Fukunaga, S.; Mori, A.; Ohuchi, A.; Yoshioka, S.; Akiba, J.; Mistuyama, K.; Tsuruta, O.; Torimura, T. Gastrointestinal: Abdominal pain, diarrhea, and bloody stools in a patient treated for renal cell carcinoma with sunitinib. *J. Gastroenterol. Hepatol.* **2020**, *35*, 10. [CrossRef] [PubMed]
84. Gündoğdu, Y.; Deniz, O.C.; Saka, D.; Şişman, G.; Erdamar, S.; Köksal, İ. Sunitinib induced colitis manifesting as invasive diarrhea in a patient with renal cell carcinoma. *J. Oncol. Pharm. Pract.* **2022**, *28*, 516–518. [CrossRef] [PubMed]
85. Guenzi, E.; Töpolt, K.; Cornali, E.; Lubeseder-Martellato, C.; Jörg, A.; Matzen, K.; Zietz, C.; Kremmer, E.; Nappi, F.; Schwemmle, M.; et al. The helical domain of GBP-1 mediates the inhibition of endothelial cell proliferation by inflammatory cytokines. *EMBO J.* **2001**, *20*, 5568–5577. [CrossRef] [PubMed]
86. Guenzi, E.; Töpolt, K.; Lubeseder-Martellato, C.; Jörg, A.; Naschberger, E.; Benelli, R.; Albini, A.; Stürzl, M. The guanylate binding protein-1 GTPase controls the invasive and angiogenic capability of endothelial cells through inhibition of MMP-1 expression. *EMBO J.* **2003**, *22*, 3772–3782. [CrossRef]
87. Lubeseder-Martellato, C.; Guenzi, E.; Jörg, A.; Töpolt, K.; Naschberger, E.; Kremmer, E.; Zietz, C.; Tschachler, E.; Hutzler, P.; Schwemmle, M.; et al. Guanylate-binding protein-1 expression is selectively induced by inflammatory cytokines and is an activation marker of endothelial cells during inflammatory diseases. *Am. J. Pathol.* **2002**, *161*, 1749–1759. [CrossRef]
88. Cornelius, L.A.; Nehring, L.C.; Harding, E.; Bolanowski, M.; Welgus, H.G.; Kobayashi, D.K.; Pierce, R.A.; Shapiro, S.D. Matrix metalloproteinases generate angiostatin: Effects on neovascularization. *J. Immunol.* **1998**, *161*, 6845–6852. [CrossRef]
89. Danese, S. Negative regulators of angiogenesis in inflammatory bowel disease: Thrombospondin in the spotlight. *Pathobiology* **2008**, *75*, 22–24. [CrossRef]
90. Punekar, S.; Zak, S.; Kalter, V.G.; Dobransky, L.; Punekar, I.; Lawler, J.W.; Gutierrez, L.S. Thrombospondin 1 and its mimetic peptide ABT-510 decrease angiogenesis and inflammation in a murine model of inflammatory bowel disease. *Pathobiology* **2008**, *75*, 9–21. [CrossRef]
91. Sandor, Z.; Deng, X.M.; Khomenko, T.; Tarnawski, A.S.; Szabo, S. Altered angiogenic balance in ulcerative colitis: A key to impaired healing? *Biochem. Biophys. Res. Commun.* **2006**, *350*, 147–150. [CrossRef]
92. Singh, U.P.; Singh, N.P.; Murphy, E.A.; Price, R.L.; Fayad, R.; Nagarkatti, M.; Nagarkatti, P.S. Chemokine and cytokine levels in inflammatory bowel disease patients. *Cytokine* **2016**, *77*, 44–49. [CrossRef] [PubMed]
93. Ozawa, C.R.; Banfi, A.; Glazer, N.L.; Thurston, G.; Springer, M.L.; Kraft, P.E.; McDonald, D.M.; Blau, H.M. Microenvironmental VEGF concentration, not total dose, determines a threshold between normal and aberrant angiogenesis. *J. Clin. Investig.* **2004**, *113*, 516–527. [CrossRef] [PubMed]
94. Xing, S.; Luo, Y.; Liu, Z.; Bu, P.; Duan, H.; Liu, D.; Wang, P.; Yang, J.; Song, L.; Feng, J.; et al. Targeting endothelial CD146 attenuates colitis and prevents colitis-associated carcinogenesis. *Am. J. Pathol.* **2014**, *184*, 1604–1616. [CrossRef] [PubMed]
95. Yan, H.; Zhang, C.; Wang, Z.; Tu, T.; Duan, H.; Luo, Y.; Feng, J.; Liu, F.; Yan, X. CD146 is required for VEGF-C-induced lymphatic sprouting during lymphangiogenesis. *Sci. Rep.* **2017**, *7*, 7442. [CrossRef] [PubMed]
96. Tsiolakidou, G.; Koutroubakis, I.E.; Tzardi, M.; Kouroumalis, E.A. Increased expression of VEGF and CD146 in patients with inflammatory bowel disease. *Dig. Liver Dis.* **2008**, *40*, 673–679. [CrossRef]
97. Danese, S.; de la Motte, C.; Sturm, A.; Vogel, J.D.; West, G.A.; Strong, S.A.; Katz, J.A.; Fiocchi, C. Platelets trigger a CD40-dependent inflammatory response in the microvasculature of inflammatory bowel disease patients. *Gastroenterology* **2003**, *124*, 1249–1264. [CrossRef]
98. Vogel, J.D.; West, G.A.; Danese, S.; De La Motte, C.; Phillips, M.H.; Strong, S.A.; Willis, J.; Fiocchi, C. CD40-mediated immune-nonimmune cell interactions induce mucosal fibroblast chemokines leading to T-cell transmigration. *Gastroenterology* **2004**, *126*, 63–80. [CrossRef]
99. Danese, S.; Scaldaferri, F.; Vetrano, S.; Stefanelli, T.; Graziani, C.; Repici, A.; Ricci, R.; Straface, G.; Sgambato, A.; Malesci, A.; et al. Critical role of the CD40 CD40-ligand pathway in regulating mucosal inflammation-driven angiogenesis in inflammatory bowel disease. *Gut* **2007**, *56*, 1248–1256. [CrossRef]
100. Konerding, M.A.; Turhan, A.; Ravnic, D.J.; Lin, M.; Fuchs, C.; Secomb, T.W.; Tsuda, A.; Mentzer, S.J. Inflammation-induced intussusceptive angiogenesis in murine colitis. *Anat. Rec.* **2010**, *293*, 849–857. [CrossRef]
101. Djonov, V.; Baum, O.; Burri, P.H. Vascular remodeling by intussusceptive angiogenesis. *Cell Tissue Res.* **2003**, *314*, 107–117. [CrossRef]
102. Burri, P.H.; Hlushchuk, R.; Djonov, V. Intussusceptive angiogenesis: Its emergence, its characteristics, and its significance. *Dev. Dyn.* **2004**, *231*, 474–488. [CrossRef]
103. Styp-Rekowska, B.; Hlushchuk, R.; Pries, A.R.; Djonov, V. Intussusceptive angiogenesis: Pillars against the blood flow. *Acta Physiol.* **2011**, *202*, 213–223. [CrossRef] [PubMed]

104. Hlushchuk, R.; Styp-Rekowska, B.; Dzambazi, J.; Wnuk, M.; Huynh-Do, U.; Makanya, A.; Djonov, V. Endoglin inhibition leads to intussusceptive angiogenesis via activation of factors related to COUP-TFII signaling pathway. *PLoS ONE* **2017**, *12*, e0182813. [CrossRef] [PubMed]
105. Groppa, E.; Brkic, S.; Uccelli, A.; Wirth, G.; Korpisalo-Pirinen, P.; Filippova, M.; Dasen, B.; Sacchi, V.; Muraro, M.G.; Trani, M.; et al. EphrinB2/EphB4 signaling regulates non-sprouting angiogenesis by VEGF. *EMBO Rep.* **2018**, *19*, e45054. [CrossRef] [PubMed]
106. Ackermann, M.; Tsuda, A.; Secomb, T.W.; Mentzer, S.J.; Konerding, M.A. Intussusceptive remodeling of vascular branch angles in chemically-induced murine colitis. *Microvasc. Res.* **2013**, *87*, 75–82. [CrossRef]
107. Esteban, S.; Clemente, C.; Koziol, A.; Gonzalo, P.; Rius, C.; Martínez, F.; Linares, P.M.; Chaparro, M.; Urzainqui, A.; Andrés, V.; et al. Endothelial MT1-MMP targeting limits intussusceptive angiogenesis and colitis via TSP1/nitric oxide axis. *EMBO Mol. Med.* **2020**, *12*, e10862. [CrossRef]
108. Betto, T.; Amano, H.; Ito, Y.; Eshima, K.; Yoshida, T.; Matsui, Y.; Yamane, S.; Inoue, T.; Otaka, F.; Kobayashi, K.; et al. Vascular endothelial growth factor receptor 1 tyrosine kinase signaling facilitates healing of DSS-induced colitis by accumulation of Tregs in ulcer area. *Biomed. Pharm.* **2019**, *111*, 131–141. [CrossRef]
109. Yoshimi, K.; Tanaka, T.; Serikawa, T.; Kuramoto, T. Tumor suppressor APC protein is essential in mucosal repair from colonic inflammation through angiogenesis. *Am. J. Pathol.* **2013**, *182*, 1263–1274. [CrossRef]
110. Jerkic, M.; Peter, M.; Ardelean, D.; Fine, M.; Konerding, M.A.; Letarte, M. Dextran sulfate sodium leads to chronic colitis and pathological angiogenesis in endoglin heterozygous mice. *Inflamm. Bowel Dis.* **2010**, *16*, 1859–1870. [CrossRef]
111. Ardelean, D.S.; Yin, M.; Jerkic, M.; Peter, M.; Ngan, B.; Kerbel, R.S.; Foster, F.S.; Letarte, M. Anti-VEGF therapy reduces intestinal inflammation in Endoglin heterozygous mice subjected to experimental colitis. *Angiogenesis* **2014**, *17*, 641–659. [CrossRef]
112. Kobayashi, M.; Fukuda, M.; Nakayama, J. Role of sulfated O-glycans expressed by high endothelial venule-like vessels in pathogenesis of chronic inflammatory gastrointestinal diseases. *Biol. Pharm. Bull.* **2009**, *32*, 774–779. [CrossRef] [PubMed]
113. Horjus Talabur Horje, C.S.; Smids, C.; Meijer, J.W.; Groenen, M.J.; Rijnders, M.K.; van Lochem, E.G.; Wahab, P.J. High endothelial venules associated with T cell subsets in the inflamed gut of newly diagnosed inflammatory bowel disease patients. *Clin. Exp. Immunol.* **2017**, *188*, 163–173. [CrossRef] [PubMed]
114. Roosenboom, B.; Lochem, E.G.V.; Meijer, J.; Smids, C.; Nierkens, S.; Brand, E.C.; Erp, L.W.V.; Kemperman, L.; Groenen, M.J.M.; Horje, C.; et al. Development of Mucosal PNAd+ and MAdCAM-1+ Venules during Disease Course in Ulcerative Colitis. *Cells* **2020**, *9*, 891. [CrossRef] [PubMed]
115. Kobayashi, M.; Hoshino, H.; Masumoto, J.; Fukushima, M.; Suzawa, K.; Kageyama, S.; Suzuki, M.; Ohtani, H.; Fukuda, M.; Nakayama, J. GlcNAc6ST-1-mediated decoration of MAdCAM-1 protein with L-selectin ligand carbohydrates directs disease activity of ulcerative colitis. *Inflamm. Bowel Dis.* **2009**, *15*, 697–706. [CrossRef]
116. Nakai, D.; Miyake, M. The change of the electrophysiological parameters using human intestinal tissues from ulcerative colitis and Crohn's disease. *J. Pharmacol. Sci.* **2022**, *150*, 90–93. [CrossRef]
117. Jergens, A.E.; Parvinroo, S.; Kopper, J.; Wannemuehler, M.J. Rules of Engagement: Epithelial—Microbe Interactions and Inflammatory Bowel Disease. *Front. Med.* **2021**, *8*, 669913. [CrossRef]
118. Neurath, M.F. Cytokines in inflammatory bowel disease. *Nat. Rev. Immunol.* **2014**, *14*, 329–342. [CrossRef]
119. Buda, A.; Hatem, G.; Neumann, H.; D'Incà, R.; Mescoli, C.; Piselli, P.; Jackson, J.; Bruno, M.; Sturniolo, G.C. Confocal laser endomicroscopy for prediction of disease relapse in ulcerative colitis: A pilot study. *J. Crohn's Colitis* **2014**, *8*, 304–311. [CrossRef]
120. Taniguchi, T.; Inoue, A.; Okahisa, T.; Kimura, T.; Gohji, T.; Niki, M.; Kitamura, S.; Takeuchi, H.; Okamoto, K.; Kaji, M.; et al. Increased Angiogenesis and Vascular Permeability in Patient with Ulcerative Colitis. *Gastrointest. Endosc.* **2009**, *69*, AB365. [CrossRef]
121. Oshima, T.; Laroux, F.S.; Coe, L.L.; Morise, Z.; Kawachi, S.; Bauer, P.; Grisham, M.B.; Specian, R.D.; Carter, P.; Jennings, S.; et al. Interferon-gamma and interleukin-10 reciprocally regulate endothelial junction integrity and barrier function. *Microvasc. Res.* **2001**, *61*, 130–143. [CrossRef]
122. Bardin, N.; Reumaux, D.; Geboes, K.; Colombel, J.F.; Blot-Chabaud, M.; Sampol, J.; Duthilleul, P.; Dignat-George, F. Increased expression of CD146, a new marker of the endothelial junction in active inflammatory bowel disease. *Inflamm. Bowel Dis.* **2006**, *12*, 16–21. [CrossRef] [PubMed]
123. Tolstanova, G.; Deng, X.; French, S.W.; Lungo, W.; Paunovic, B.; Khomenko, T.; Ahluwalia, A.; Kaplan, T.; Dacosta-Iyer, M.; Tarnawski, A.; et al. Early endothelial damage and increased colonic vascular permeability in the development of experimental ulcerative colitis in rats and mice. *Lab. Investig.* **2012**, *92*, 9–21. [CrossRef] [PubMed]
124. Laroux, F.S.; Grisham, M.B. Immunological basis of inflammatory bowel disease: Role of the microcirculation. *Microcirculation* **2001**, *8*, 283–301. [CrossRef] [PubMed]
125. Vestweber, D.; Wessel, F.; Nottebaum, A.F. Similarities and differences in the regulation of leukocyte extravasation and vascular permeability. *Semin. Immunopathol.* **2014**, *36*, 177–192. [CrossRef] [PubMed]
126. Wautier, J.L.; Wautier, M.P. Vascular Permeability in Diseases. *Int. J. Mol. Sci.* **2022**, *23*, 3645. [CrossRef] [PubMed]
127. Tolstanova, G.; Khomenko, T.; Deng, X.; Szabo, S.; Sandor, Z. New molecular mechanisms of the unexpectedly complex role of VEGF in ulcerative colitis. *Biochem. Biophys. Res. Commun.* **2010**, *399*, 613–616. [CrossRef] [PubMed]
128. Weis, S.M.; Cheresh, D.A. Pathophysiological consequences of VEGF-induced vascular permeability. *Nature* **2005**, *437*, 497–504. [CrossRef]

129. Gavard, J.; Gutkind, J.S. VEGF controls endothelial-cell permeability by promoting the beta-arrestin-dependent endocytosis of VE-cadherin. *Nat. Cell Biol.* **2006**, *8*, 1223–1234. [CrossRef]
130. Zhang, C.; Chen, H.; He, Q.; Luo, Y.; He, A.; Tao, A.; Yan, J. Fibrinogen/AKT/Microfilament Axis Promotes Colitis by Enhancing Vascular Permeability. *Cell. Mol. Gastroenterol. Hepatol.* **2021**, *11*, 683–696. [CrossRef]
131. Matsumoto, K.; Yamaba, R.; Inoue, K.; Utsumi, D.; Tsukahara, T.; Amagase, K.; Tominaga, M.; Kato, S. Transient receptor potential vanilloid 4 channel regulates vascular endothelial permeability during colonic inflammation in dextran sulphate sodium-induced murine colitis. *Br. J. Pharmacol.* **2018**, *175*, 84–99. [CrossRef]
132. Dejana, E.; Orsenigo, F.; Lampugnani, M.G. The role of adherens junctions and VE-cadherin in the control of vascular permeability. *J. Cell Sci.* **2008**, *121*, 2115–2122. [CrossRef]
133. Vestweber, D. VE-cadherin: The major endothelial adhesion molecule controlling cellular junctions and blood vessel formation. *Arter. Thromb. Vasc. Biol.* **2008**, *28*, 223–232. [CrossRef] [PubMed]
134. Giannotta, M.; Trani, M.; Dejana, E. VE-cadherin and endothelial adherens junctions: Active guardians of vascular integrity. *Dev. Cell* **2013**, *26*, 441–454. [CrossRef] [PubMed]
135. Xiao, K.; Allison, D.F.; Kottke, M.D.; Summers, S.; Sorescu, G.P.; Faundez, V.; Kowalczyk, A.P. Mechanisms of VE-cadherin processing and degradation in microvascular endothelial cells. *J. Biol. Chem.* **2003**, *278*, 19199–19208. [CrossRef]
136. Schulz, B.; Pruessmeyer, J.; Maretzky, T.; Ludwig, A.; Blobel, C.P.; Saftig, P.; Reiss, K. ADAM10 regulates endothelial permeability and T-Cell transmigration by proteolysis of vascular endothelial cadherin. *Circ. Res.* **2008**, *102*, 1192–1201. [CrossRef]
137. Arihiro, S.; Ohtani, H.; Hiwatashi, N.; Torii, A.; Sorsa, T.; Nagura, H. Vascular smooth muscle cells and pericytes express MMP-1, MMP-9, TIMP-1 and type I procollagen in inflammatory bowel disease. *Histopathology* **2001**, *39*, 50–59. [CrossRef] [PubMed]
138. Angelini, D.J.; Hyun, S.W.; Grigoryev, D.N.; Garg, P.; Gong, P.; Singh, I.S.; Passaniti, A.; Hasday, J.D.; Goldblum, S.E. TNF-alpha increases tyrosine phosphorylation of vascular endothelial cadherin and opens the paracellular pathway through fyn activation in human lung endothelia. *Am. J. Physiol. Lung Cell. Mol. Physiol.* **2006**, *291*, L1232–L1245. [CrossRef]
139. Baugh, M.D.; Perry, M.J.; Hollander, A.P.; Davies, D.R.; Cross, S.S.; Lobo, A.J.; Taylor, C.J.; Evans, G.S. Matrix metalloproteinase levels are elevated in inflammatory bowel disease. *Gastroenterology* **1999**, *117*, 814–822. [CrossRef]
140. Matusiewicz, M.; Neubauer, K.; Mierzchala-Pasierb, M.; Gamian, A.; Krzystek-Korpacka, M. Matrix metalloproteinase-9: Its interplay with angiogenic factors in inflammatory bowel diseases. *Dis. Mark.* **2014**, *2014*, 643645. [CrossRef]
141. Meijer, M.J.; Mieremet-Ooms, M.A.; van der Zon, A.M.; van Duijn, W.; van Hogezand, R.A.; Sier, C.F.; Hommes, D.W.; Lamers, C.B.; Verspaget, H.W. Increased mucosal matrix metalloproteinase-1, -2, -3 and -9 activity in patients with inflammatory bowel disease and the relation with Crohn's disease phenotype. *Dig. Liver Dis.* **2007**, *39*, 733–739. [CrossRef] [PubMed]
142. Santana, A.; Medina, C.; Paz-Cabrera, M.C.; Díaz-Gonzalez, F.; Farré, E.; Salas, A.; Radomski, M.W.; Quintero, E. Attenuation of dextran sodium sulphate induced colitis in matrix metalloproteinase-9 deficient mice. *World J. Gastroenterol.* **2006**, *12*, 6464–6472. [CrossRef] [PubMed]
143. Medina, C.; Santana, A.; Paz, M.C.; Díaz-Gonzalez, F.; Farre, E.; Salas, A.; Radomski, M.W.; Quintero, E. Matrix metalloproteinase-9 modulates intestinal injury in rats with transmural colitis. *J. Leukoc. Biol.* **2006**, *79*, 954–962. [CrossRef] [PubMed]
144. Nighot, P.; Al-Sadi, R.; Rawat, M.; Guo, S.; Watterson, D.M.; Ma, T. Matrix metalloproteinase 9-induced increase in intestinal epithelial tight junction permeability contributes to the severity of experimental DSS colitis. *Am. J. Physiol. Gastrointest. Liver Physiol.* **2015**, *309*, G988–G997. [CrossRef]
145. Sidibé, A.; Mannic, T.; Arboleas, M.; Subileau, M.; Gulino-Debrac, D.; Bouillet, L.; Jan, M.; Vandhuick, T.; Le Loet, X.; Vittecoq, O.; et al. Soluble VE-cadherin in rheumatoid arthritis patients correlates with disease activity: Evidence for tumor necrosis factor alpha-induced VE-cadherin cleavage. *Arthritis Rheum.* **2012**, *64*, 77–87. [CrossRef] [PubMed]
146. Flemming, S.; Burkard, N.; Renschler, M.; Vielmuth, F.; Meir, M.; Schick, M.A.; Wunder, C.; Germer, C.T.; Spindler, V.; Waschke, J.; et al. Soluble VE-cadherin is involved in endothelial barrier breakdown in systemic inflammation and sepsis. *Cardiovasc. Res.* **2015**, *107*, 32–44. [CrossRef] [PubMed]
147. Polena, H.; Creuzet, J.; Dufies, M.; Sidibé, A.; Khalil-Mgharbel, A.; Salomon, A.; Deroux, A.; Quesada, J.L.; Roelants, C.; Filhol, O.; et al. The tyrosine-kinase inhibitor sunitinib targets vascular endothelial (VE)-cadherin: A marker of response to antitumoural treatment in metastatic renal cell carcinoma. *Br. J. Cancer* **2018**, *118*, 1179–1188. [CrossRef] [PubMed]
148. Wallez, Y.; Cand, F.; Cruzalegui, F.; Wernstedt, C.; Souchelnytskyi, S.; Vilgrain, I.; Huber, P. Src kinase phosphorylates vascular endothelial-cadherin in response to vascular endothelial growth factor: Identification of tyrosine 685 as the unique target site. *Oncogene* **2007**, *26*, 1067–1077. [CrossRef]
149. Nottebaum, A.F.; Cagna, G.; Winderlich, M.; Gamp, A.C.; Linnepe, R.; Polaschegg, C.; Filippova, K.; Lyck, R.; Engelhardt, B.; Kamenyeva, O.; et al. VE-PTP maintains the endothelial barrier via plakoglobin and becomes dissociated from VE-cadherin by leukocytes and by VEGF. *J. Exp. Med.* **2008**, *205*, 2929–2945. [CrossRef]
150. Gioelli, N.; Neilson, L.J.; Wei, N.; Villari, G.; Chen, W.; Kuhle, B.; Ehling, M.; Maione, F.; Willox, S.; Brundu, S.; et al. Neuropilin 1 and its inhibitory ligand mini-tryptophanyl-tRNA synthetase inversely regulate VE-cadherin turnover and vascular permeability. *Nat. Commun.* **2022**, *13*, 4188. [CrossRef]
151. Wong, R.K.; Baldwin, A.L.; Heimark, R.L. Cadherin-5 redistribution at sites of TNF-alpha and IFN-gamma-induced permeability in mesenteric venules. *Am. J. Physiol.* **1999**, *276*, H736–H748.
152. Gavard, J. Endothelial permeability and VE-cadherin: A wacky comradeship. *Cell Adhes. Migr.* **2013**, *7*, 455–461. [CrossRef] [PubMed]

153. Abu Taha, A.; Schnittler, H.J. Dynamics between actin and the VE-cadherin/catenin complex: Novel aspects of the ARP2/3 complex in regulation of endothelial junctions. *Cell Adhes. Migr.* **2014**, *8*, 125–135. [CrossRef] [PubMed]
154. Brandt, M.; Gerke, V.; Betz, T. Human endothelial cells display a rapid tensional stress increase in response to tumor necrosis factor-α. *PLoS ONE* **2022**, *17*, e0270197. [CrossRef] [PubMed]
155. Morales-Ruiz, M.; Fulton, D.; Sowa, G.; Languino, L.R.; Fujio, Y.; Walsh, K.; Sessa, W.C. Vascular endothelial growth factor-stimulated actin reorganization and migration of endothelial cells is regulated via the serine/threonine kinase Akt. *Circ. Res.* **2000**, *86*, 892–896. [CrossRef] [PubMed]
156. Ostler, N.; Britzen-Laurent, N.; Liebl, A.; Naschberger, E.; Lochnit, G.; Ostler, M.; Forster, F.; Kunzelmann, P.; Ince, S.; Supper, V.; et al. Gamma interferon-induced guanylate binding protein 1 is a novel actin cytoskeleton remodeling factor. *Mol. Cell. Biol.* **2014**, *34*, 196–209. [CrossRef]
157. Liu, P.; Bian, Y.; Fan, Y.; Zhong, J.; Liu, Z. Protective Effect of Naringin on In Vitro Gut-Vascular Barrier Disruption of Intestinal Microvascular Endothelial Cells Induced by TNF-α. *J. Agric. Food Chem.* **2020**, *68*, 168–175. [CrossRef]
158. Carloni, S.; Bertocchi, A.; Mancinelli, S.; Bellini, M.; Erreni, M.; Borreca, A.; Braga, D.; Giugliano, S.; Mozzarelli, A.M.; Manganaro, D.; et al. Identification of a choroid plexus vascular barrier closing during intestinal inflammation. *Science* **2021**, *374*, 439–448. [CrossRef]
159. Armulik, A.; Abramsson, A.; Betsholtz, C. Endothelial/pericyte interactions. *Circ. Res.* **2005**, *97*, 512–523. [CrossRef]
160. Ganta, V.C.; Cromer, W.; Mills, G.L.; Traylor, J.; Jennings, M.; Daley, S.; Clark, B.; Mathis, J.M.; Bernas, M.; Boktor, M.; et al. Angiopoietin-2 in experimental colitis. *Inflamm. Bowel Dis.* **2010**, *16*, 1029–1039. [CrossRef]
161. Sweeney, M.; Foldes, G. It Takes Two: Endothelial-Perivascular Cell Cross-Talk in Vascular Development and Disease. *Front. Cardiovasc. Med.* **2018**, *5*, 154. [CrossRef]
162. Armulik, A.; Genove, G.; Mae, M.; Nisancioglu, M.H.; Wallgard, E.; Niaudet, C.; He, L.; Norlin, J.; Lindblom, P.; Strittmatter, K.; et al. Pericytes regulate the blood-brain barrier. *Nature* **2010**, *468*, 557–561. [CrossRef]
163. Alexander, J.S.; Chaitanya, G.V.; Grisham, M.B.; Boktor, M. Emerging roles of lymphatics in inflammatory bowel disease. *Ann. N. Y. Acad. Sci.* **2010**, *1207* (Suppl. 1), E75–E85. [CrossRef] [PubMed]
164. Regensburger, D.; Tenkerian, C.; Pürzer, V.; Schmid, B.; Wohlfahrt, T.; Stolzer, I.; López-Posadas, R.; Günther, C.; Waldner, M.J.; Becker, C.; et al. Matricellular Protein SPARCL1 Regulates Blood Vessel Integrity and Antagonizes Inflammatory Bowel Disease. *Inflamm. Bowel Dis.* **2021**, *27*, 1491–1502. [CrossRef] [PubMed]
165. Suzuki, H.; Shibano, K.; Okane, M.; Kono, I.; Matsui, Y.; Yamane, K.; Kashiwagi, H. Interferon-gamma modulates messenger RNA levels of c-sis (PDGF-B chain), PDGF-A chain, and IL-1 beta genes in human vascular endothelial cells. *Am. J. Pathol.* **1989**, *134*, 35–43. [PubMed]
166. Darden, J.; Payne, L.B.; Zhao, H.; Chappell, J.C. Excess vascular endothelial growth factor-A disrupts pericyte recruitment during blood vessel formation. *Angiogenesis* **2019**, *22*, 167–183. [CrossRef] [PubMed]
167. Sprague, A.H.; Khalil, R.A. Inflammatory cytokines in vascular dysfunction and vascular disease. *Biochem. Pharmacol.* **2009**, *78*, 539–552. [CrossRef]
168. Hatoum, O.A.; Binion, D.G.; Gutterman, D.D. Paradox of simultaneous intestinal ischaemia and hyperaemia in inflammatory bowel disease. *Eur. J. Clin. Investig.* **2005**, *35*, 599–609. [CrossRef]
169. Binion, D.G.; Rafiee, P.; Ramanujam, K.S.; Fu, S.; Fisher, P.J.; Rivera, M.T.; Johnson, C.P.; Otterson, M.F.; Telford, G.L.; Wilson, K.T. Deficient iNOS in inflammatory bowel disease intestinal microvascular endothelial cells results in increased leukocyte adhesion. *Free Radic. Biol. Med.* **2000**, *29*, 881–888. [CrossRef]
170. Horowitz, S.; Binion, D.G.; Nelson, V.M.; Kanaa, Y.; Javadi, P.; Lazarova, Z.; Andrekopoulos, C.; Kalyanaraman, B.; Otterson, M.F.; Rafiee, P. Increased arginase activity and endothelial dysfunction in human inflammatory bowel disease. *Am. J. Physiol. Gastrointest. Liver Physiol.* **2007**, *292*, G1323–G1336. [CrossRef]
171. Hatoum, O.A.; Binion, D.G.; Otterson, M.F.; Gutterman, D.D. Acquired microvascular dysfunction in inflammatory bowel disease: Loss of nitric oxide-mediated vasodilation. *Gastroenterology* **2003**, *125*, 58–69. [CrossRef]
172. Hatoum, O.A.; Gauthier, K.M.; Binion, D.G.; Miura, H.; Telford, G.; Otterson, M.F.; Campbell, W.B.; Gutterman, D.D. Novel mechanism of vasodilation in inflammatory bowel disease. *Arter. Thromb. Vasc. Biol.* **2005**, *25*, 2355–2361. [CrossRef] [PubMed]
173. Thibeault, S.; Rautureau, Y.; Oubaha, M.; Faubert, D.; Wilkes, B.C.; Delisle, C.; Gratton, J.P. S-nitrosylation of beta-catenin by eNOS-derived NO promotes VEGF-induced endothelial cell permeability. *Mol. Cell* **2010**, *39*, 468–476. [CrossRef] [PubMed]
174. Di Lorenzo, A.; Lin, M.I.; Murata, T.; Landskroner-Eiger, S.; Schleicher, M.; Kothiya, M.; Iwakiri, Y.; Yu, J.; Huang, P.L.; Sessa, W.C. eNOS-derived nitric oxide regulates endothelial barrier function through VE-cadherin and Rho GTPases. *J. Cell Sci.* **2013**, *126*, 5541–5552. [CrossRef] [PubMed]
175. Seerapu, H.; Subramaniam, G.P.; Majumder, S.; Sinha, S.; Bisana, S.; Mahajan, S.; Kolluru, G.K.; Muley, A.; Siamwala, J.H.; Illavazagan, G.; et al. Inhibition of dynamin-2 confers endothelial barrier dysfunctions by attenuating nitric oxide production. *Cell Biol. Int.* **2010**, *34*, 755–761. [CrossRef] [PubMed]
176. Beck, P.L.; Xavier, R.; Wong, J.; Ezedi, I.; Mashimo, H.; Mizoguchi, A.; Mizoguchi, E.; Bhan, A.K.; Podolsky, D.K. Paradoxical roles of different nitric oxide synthase isoforms in colonic injury. *Am. J. Physiol. Gastrointest. Liver Physiol.* **2004**, *286*, G137–G147. [CrossRef] [PubMed]

177. Hokari, R.; Kato, S.; Matsuzaki, K.; Kuroki, M.; Iwai, A.; Kawaguchi, A.; Nagao, S.; Miyahara, T.; Itoh, K.; Sekizuka, E.; et al. Reduced sensitivity of inducible nitric oxide synthase-deficient mice to chronic colitis. *Free Radic. Biol. Med.* **2001**, *31*, 153–163. [CrossRef]
178. Sasaki, M.; Bharwani, S.; Jordan, P.; Elrod, J.W.; Grisham, M.B.; Jackson, T.H.; Lefer, D.J.; Alexander, J.S. Increased disease activity in eNOS-deficient mice in experimental colitis. *Free Radic. Biol. Med.* **2003**, *35*, 1679–1687. [CrossRef]
179. Vallance, B.A.; Dijkstra, G.; Qiu, B.; van der Waaij, L.A.; van Goor, H.; Jansen, P.L.; Mashimo, H.; Collins, S.M. Relative contributions of NOS isoforms during experimental colitis: Endothelial-derived NOS maintains mucosal integrity. *Am. J. Physiol. Gastrointest. Liver Physiol.* **2004**, *287*, G865–G874. [CrossRef]
180. Collins, C.E.; Rampton, D.S.; Rogers, J.; Williams, N.S. Platelet aggregation and neutrophil sequestration in the mesenteric circulation in inflammatory bowel disease. *Eur. J. Gastroenterol. Hepatol.* **1997**, *9*, 1213–1217.
181. Tekelioglu, Y.; Uzun, H.; Sisman, G. Activated platelets in patients suffering from inflammatory bowel disease. *Bratisl. Lek. Listy* **2014**, *115*, 83–85. [CrossRef]
182. Koutroubakis, I.E.; Theodoropoulou, A.; Xidakis, C.; Sfiridaki, A.; Notas, G.; Kolios, G.; Kouroumalis, E.A. Association between enhanced soluble CD40 ligand and prothrombotic state in inflammatory bowel disease. *Eur. J. Gastroenterol. Hepatol.* **2004**, *16*, 1147–1152. [CrossRef] [PubMed]
183. Danese, S.; Katz, J.A.; Saibeni, S.; Papa, A.; Gasbarrini, A.; Vecchi, M.; Fiocchi, C. Activated platelets are the source of elevated levels of soluble CD40 ligand in the circulation of inflammatory bowel disease patients. *Gut* **2003**, *52*, 1435–1441. [CrossRef] [PubMed]
184. Yoshida, H.; Russell, J.; Stokes, K.Y.; Yilmaz, C.E.; Esmon, C.T.; Granger, D.N. Role of the protein C pathway in the extraintestinal thrombosis associated with murine colitis. *Gastroenterology* **2008**, *135*, 882–888. [CrossRef] [PubMed]
185. Scaldaferri, F.; Sans, M.; Vetrano, S.; Graziani, C.; De Cristofaro, R.; Gerlitz, B.; Repici, A.; Arena, V.; Malesci, A.; Panes, J.; et al. Crucial role of the protein C pathway in governing microvascular inflammation in inflammatory bowel disease. *J. Clin. Investig.* **2007**, *117*, 1951–1960. [CrossRef]
186. Faioni, E.M.; Ferrero, S.; Fontana, G.; Gianelli, U.; Ciulla, M.M.; Vecchi, M.; Saibeni, S.; Biguzzi, E.; Cordani, N.; Franchi, F.; et al. Expression of endothelial protein C receptor and thrombomodulin in the intestinal tissue of patients with inflammatory bowel disease. *Crit. Care Med.* **2004**, *32*, S266–S270. [CrossRef]
187. Vetrano, S.; Ploplis, V.A.; Sala, E.; Sandoval-Cooper, M.; Donahue, D.L.; Correale, C.; Arena, V.; Spinelli, A.; Repici, A.; Malesci, A.; et al. Unexpected role of anticoagulant protein C in controlling epithelial barrier integrity and intestinal inflammation. *Proc. Natl. Acad. Sci. USA* **2011**, *108*, 19830–19835. [CrossRef]
188. Ogawa, H.; Rafiee, P.; Heidemann, J.; Fisher, P.J.; Johnson, N.A.; Otterson, M.F.; Kalyanaraman, B.; Pritchard, K.A., Jr.; Binion, D.G. Mechanisms of endotoxin tolerance in human intestinal microvascular endothelial cells. *J. Immunol.* **2003**, *170*, 5956–5964. [CrossRef]
189. Heidemann, J.; Domschke, W.; Kucharzik, T.; Maaser, C. Intestinal microvascular endothelium and innate immunity in inflammatory bowel disease: A second line of defense? *Infect. Immun.* **2006**, *74*, 5425–5432. [CrossRef]
190. Maaser, C.; Heidemann, J.; von Eiff, C.; Lugering, A.; Spahn, T.W.; Binion, D.G.; Domschke, W.; Lugering, N.; Kucharzik, T. Human intestinal microvascular endothelial cells express Toll-like receptor 5: A binding partner for bacterial flagellin. *J. Immunol.* **2004**, *172*, 5056–5062. [CrossRef]
191. Vijay-Kumar, M.; Aitken, J.D.; Gewirtz, A.T. Toll like receptor-5: Protecting the gut from enteric microbes. *Semin. Immunopathol.* **2008**, *30*, 11–21. [CrossRef]
192. Heidemann, J.; Rüther, C.; Kebschull, M.; Domschke, W.; Brüwer, M.; Koch, S.; Kucharzik, T.; Maaser, C. Expression of IL-12-related molecules in human intestinal microvascular endothelial cells is regulated by TLR3. *Am. J. Physiol. Gastrointest. Liver Physiol.* **2007**, *293*, G1315–G1324. [CrossRef] [PubMed]
193. Lodes, M.J.; Cong, Y.; Elson, C.O.; Mohamath, R.; Landers, C.J.; Targan, S.R.; Fort, M.; Hershberg, R.M. Bacterial flagellin is a dominant antigen in Crohn disease. *J. Clin. Investig.* **2004**, *113*, 1296–1306. [CrossRef] [PubMed]
194. Sitaraman, S.V.; Klapproth, J.M.; Moore, D.A., 3rd; Landers, C.; Targan, S.; Williams, I.R.; Gewirtz, A.T. Elevated flagellin-specific immunoglobulins in Crohn's disease. *Am. J. Physiol. Gastrointest. Liver Physiol.* **2005**, *288*, G403–G406. [CrossRef] [PubMed]
195. Targan, S.R.; Landers, C.J.; Yang, H.; Lodes, M.J.; Cong, Y.; Papadakis, K.A.; Vasiliauskas, E.; Elson, C.O.; Hershberg, R.M. Antibodies to CBir1 flagellin define a unique response that is associated independently with complicated Crohn's disease. *Gastroenterology* **2005**, *128*, 2020–2028. [CrossRef]
196. Vijay-Kumar, M.; Sanders, C.J.; Taylor, R.T.; Kumar, A.; Aitken, J.D.; Sitaraman, S.V.; Neish, A.S.; Uematsu, S.; Akira, S.; Williams, I.R.; et al. Deletion of TLR5 results in spontaneous colitis in mice. *J. Clin. Investig.* **2007**, *117*, 3909–3921. [CrossRef] [PubMed]
197. Vijay-Kumar, M.; Wu, H.; Aitken, J.; Kolachala, V.L.; Neish, A.S.; Sitaraman, S.V.; Gewirtz, A.T. Activation of toll-like receptor 3 protects against DSS-induced acute colitis. *Inflamm. Bowel Dis.* **2007**, *13*, 856–864. [CrossRef]
198. Hu, G.; Xue, J.; Duan, H.; Yang, Z.; Gao, L.; Luo, H.; Mu, X.; Cui, S. IFN-γ induces IFN-α and IFN-β expressions in cultured rat intestinal mucosa microvascular endothelial cells. *Immunopharmacol. Immunotoxicol.* **2010**, *32*, 656–662. [CrossRef]
199. Stürzl, M.; Kunz, M.; Krug, S.M.; Naschberger, E. Angiocrine Regulation of Epithelial Barrier Integrity in Inflammatory Bowel Disease. *Front. Med.* **2021**, *8*, 643607. [CrossRef]
200. Imaizumi, T.; Yoshida, H.; Satoh, K. Regulation of CX3CL1/fractalkine expression in endothelial cells. *J. Atheroscler. Thromb.* **2004**, *11*, 15–21. [CrossRef]

201. Nishimura, M.; Kuboi, Y.; Muramoto, K.; Kawano, T.; Imai, T. Chemokines as novel therapeutic targets for inflammatory bowel disease. *Ann. N. Y. Acad. Sci.* **2009**, *1173*, 350–356. [CrossRef]
202. Sans, M.; Danese, S.; de la Motte, C.; de Souza, H.S.; Rivera-Reyes, B.M.; West, G.A.; Phillips, M.; Katz, J.A.; Fiocchi, C. Enhanced recruitment of CX3CR1+ T cells by mucosal endothelial cell-derived fractalkine in inflammatory bowel disease. *Gastroenterology* **2007**, *132*, 139–153. [CrossRef] [PubMed]
203. Wu, X.; Sun, M.; Yang, Z.; Lu, C.; Wang, Q.; Wang, H.; Deng, C.; Liu, Y.; Yang, Y. The Roles of CCR9/CCL25 in Inflammation and Inflammation-Associated Diseases. *Front. Cell Dev. Biol.* **2021**, *9*, 686548. [CrossRef] [PubMed]
204. Bernier-Latmani, J.; Petrova, T.V. Intestinal lymphatic vasculature: Structure, mechanisms and functions. *Nat. Rev. Gastroenterol. Hepatol.* **2017**, *14*, 510–526. [CrossRef]
205. Kim, H.; Kataru, R.P.; Koh, G.Y. Inflammation-associated lymphangiogenesis: A double-edged sword? *J. Clin. Investig.* **2014**, *124*, 936–942. [CrossRef]
206. Geleff, S.; Schoppmann, S.F.; Oberhuber, G. Increase in podoplanin-expressing intestinal lymphatic vessels in inflammatory bowel disease. *Virchows Arch.* **2003**, *442*, 231–237. [CrossRef] [PubMed]
207. Fogt, F.; Pascha, T.L.; Zhang, P.J.; Gausas, R.E.; Rahemtulla, A.; Zimmerman, R.L. Proliferation of D2-40-expressing intestinal lymphatic vessels in the lamina propria in inflammatory bowel disease. *Int. J. Mol. Med.* **2004**, *13*, 211–214. [CrossRef]
208. Rahier, J.F.; De Beauce, S.; Dubuquoy, L.; Erdual, E.; Colombel, J.F.; Jouret-Mourin, A.; Geboes, K.; Desreumaux, P. Increased lymphatic vessel density and lymphangiogenesis in inflammatory bowel disease. *Aliment. Pharmacol. Ther.* **2011**, *34*, 533–543. [CrossRef] [PubMed]
209. Wu, T.F.; MacNaughton, W.K.; von der Weid, P.Y. Lymphatic vessel contractile activity and intestinal inflammation. *Mem. Inst. Oswaldo Cruz* **2005**, *100* (Suppl. 1), 107–110. [CrossRef]
210. Von Der Weid, P.Y.; Rehal, S. Lymphatic pump function in the inflamed gut. *Ann. N. Y. Acad. Sci.* **2010**, *1207* (Suppl. 1), E69–E74. [CrossRef]
211. Nikolakis, D.; de Voogd, F.A.E.; Pruijt, M.J.; Grootjans, J.; van de Sande, M.G.; D'Haens, G.R. The Role of the Lymphatic System in the Pathogenesis and Treatment of Inflammatory Bowel Disease. *Int. J. Mol. Sci.* **2022**, *23*, 1854. [CrossRef]
212. Zhang, L.; Ocansey, D.K.W.; Liu, L.; Olovo, C.V.; Zhang, X.; Qian, H.; Xu, W.; Mao, F. Implications of lymphatic alterations in the pathogenesis and treatment of inflammatory bowel disease. *Biomed Pharm.* **2021**, *140*, 111752. [CrossRef]
213. von der Weid, P.Y.; Rainey, K.J. Review article: Lymphatic system and associated adipose tissue in the development of inflammatory bowel disease. *Aliment. Pharmacol. Ther.* **2010**, *32*, 697–711. [CrossRef] [PubMed]
214. Agollah, G.D.; Wu, G.; Peng, H.L.; Kwon, S. Dextran sulfate sodium-induced acute colitis impairs dermal lymphatic function in mice. *World J. Gastroenterol.* **2015**, *21*, 12767–12777. [CrossRef] [PubMed]
215. Ott, C.; Schölmerich, J. Extraintestinal manifestations and complications in IBD. *Nat. Rev. Gastroenterol. Hepatol.* **2013**, *10*, 585–595. [CrossRef] [PubMed]
216. Navabi, S.; Gorrepati, V.S.; Yadav, S.; Chintanaboina, J.; Maher, S.; Demuth, P.; Stern, B.; Stuart, A.; Tinsley, A.; Clarke, K.; et al. Influences and Impact of Anxiety and Depression in the Setting of Inflammatory Bowel Disease. *Inflamm. Bowel Dis.* **2018**, *24*, 2303–2308. [CrossRef] [PubMed]
217. Gupta, G.; Gelfand, J.M.; Lewis, J.D. Increased Risk for Demyelinating Diseases in Patients With Inflammatory Bowel Disease. *Gastroenterology* **2005**, *129*, 819–826. [CrossRef]
218. Ferro, J.M.; Oliveira, S.N.; Correia, L. Neurologic manifestations of inflammatory bowel diseases. *Handb. Clin. Neurol.* **2014**, *120*, 595–605. [CrossRef]
219. Mouries, J.; Brescia, P.; Silvestri, A.; Spadoni, I.; Sorribas, M.; Wiest, R.; Mileti, E.; Galbiati, M.; Invernizzi, P.; Adorini, L.; et al. Microbiota-driven gut vascular barrier disruption is a prerequisite for non-alcoholic steatohepatitis development. *J. Hepatol.* **2019**, *71*, 1216–1228. [CrossRef]
220. Bertocchi, A.; Carloni, S.; Ravenda, P.S.; Bertalot, G.; Spadoni, I.; Lo Cascio, A.; Gandini, S.; Lizier, M.; Braga, D.; Asnicar, F.; et al. Gut vascular barrier impairment leads to intestinal bacteria dissemination and colorectal cancer metastasis to liver. *Cancer Cell* **2021**, *39*, 708–724.e11. [CrossRef]
221. Golan, D.; Gross, B.; Miller, A.; Klil-Drori, S.; Lavi, I.; Shiller, M.; Honigman, S.; Almog, R.; Segol, O. Cognitive Function of Patients with Crohn's Disease is Associated with Intestinal Disease Activity. *Inflamm. Bowel Dis.* **2016**, *22*, 364–371. [CrossRef]
222. Byrne, G.; Rosenfeld, G.; Leung, Y.; Qian, H.; Raudzus, J.; Nunez, C.; Bressler, B. Prevalence of Anxiety and Depression in Patients with Inflammatory Bowel Disease. *Can. J. Gastroenterol. Hepatol.* **2017**, *2017*, 6496727. [CrossRef]
223. Tadin Hadjina, I.; Zivkovic, P.M.; Matetic, A.; Rusic, D.; Vilovic, M.; Bajo, D.; Puljiz, Z.; Tonkic, A.; Bozic, J. Impaired neurocognitive and psychomotor performance in patients with inflammatory bowel disease. *Sci. Rep.* **2019**, *9*, 13740. [CrossRef] [PubMed]
224. Cluny, N.L.; Nyuyki, K.D.; Almishri, W.; Griffin, L.; Lee, B.H.; Hirota, S.A.; Pittman, Q.J.; Swain, M.G.; Sharkey, K.A. Recruitment of α4β7 monocytes and neutrophils to the brain in experimental colitis is associated with elevated cytokines and anxiety-like behavior. *J. Neuroinflammation* **2022**, *19*, 73. [CrossRef] [PubMed]
225. Do, J.; Woo, J. From Gut to Brain: Alteration in Inflammation Markers in the Brain of Dextran Sodium Sulfate-induced Colitis Model Mice. *Clin. Psychopharmacol. Neurosci.* **2018**, *16*, 422–433. [CrossRef] [PubMed]
226. Nyuyki, K.D.; Cluny, N.L.; Swain, M.G.; Sharkey, K.A.; Pittman, Q.J. Altered Brain Excitability and Increased Anxiety in Mice With Experimental Colitis: Consideration of Hyperalgesia and Sex Differences. *Front. Behav. Neurosci.* **2018**, *12*, 58. [CrossRef] [PubMed]

227. Dempsey, E.; Abautret-Daly, Á.; Docherty, N.G.; Medina, C.; Harkin, A. Persistent central inflammation and region specific cellular activation accompany depression- and anxiety-like behaviours during the resolution phase of experimental colitis. *Brain Behav. Immun.* **2019**, *80*, 616–632. [CrossRef]
228. Natah, S.S.; Mouihate, A.; Pittman, Q.J.; Sharkey, K.A. Disruption of the blood-brain barrier during TNBS colitis. *Neurogastroenterol. Motil.* **2005**, *17*, 433–446. [CrossRef]
229. Bernstein, C.N.; Nugent, Z.; Targownik, L.E.; Singh, H.; Lix, L.M. Predictors and risks for death in a population-based study of persons with IBD in Manitoba. *Gut* **2015**, *64*, 1403–1411. [CrossRef]
230. Ludvigsson, J.F.; Holmgren, J.; Grip, O.; Halfvarson, J.; Askling, J.; Sachs, M.C.; Olén, O. Adult-onset inflammatory bowel disease and rate of serious infections compared to the general population: A nationwide register-based cohort study 2002-2017. *Scand. J. Gastroenterol.* **2021**, *56*, 1152–1162. [CrossRef]
231. Ocón, B.; Aranda, C.J.; Gámez-Belmonte, R.; Suárez, M.D.; Zarzuelo, A.; Martínez-Augustin, O.; Sánchez de Medina, F. The glucocorticoid budesonide has protective and deleterious effects in experimental colitis in mice. *Biochem. Pharm.* **2016**, *116*, 73–88. [CrossRef]
232. Gutiérrez, A.; Francés, R.; Amorós, A.; Zapater, P.; Garmendia, M.; Ndongo, M.; Cano, R.; Jover, R.; Such, J.; Perez-Mateo, M. Cytokine association with bacterial DNA in serum of patients with inflammatory bowel disease. *Inflamm. Bowel Dis.* **2009**, *15*, 508–514. [CrossRef] [PubMed]
233. Gutiérrez, A.; Zapater, P.; Juanola, O.; Sempere, L.; Garcia, M.; Laveda, R.; Martinez, A.; Scharl, M.; Gonzalez-Navajas, J.M.; Such, J.; et al. Gut Bacterial DNA Translocation is an Independent Risk Factor of Flare at Short Term in Patients With Crohn's Disease. *Am. J. Gastroenterol.* **2016**, *111*, 529–540. [CrossRef] [PubMed]
234. Pasternak, B.A.; D'Mello, S.; Jurickova, I.I.; Han, X.; Willson, T.; Flick, L.; Petiniot, L.; Uozumi, N.; Divanovic, S.; Traurnicht, A.; et al. Lipopolysaccharide exposure is linked to activation of the acute phase response and growth failure in pediatric Crohn's disease and murine colitis. *Inflamm. Bowel Dis.* **2010**, *16*, 856–869. [CrossRef] [PubMed]
235. Rojo, Ó.P.; Román, A.L.S.; Arbizu, E.A.; de la Hera Martínez, A.; Sevillano, E.R.; Martínez, A.A. Serum lipopolysaccharide-binding protein in endotoxemic patients with inflammatory bowel disease. *Inflamm. Bowel Dis.* **2006**, *13*, 269–277. [CrossRef] [PubMed]
236. Luchetti, M.M.; Ciccia, F.; Avellini, C.; Benfaremo, D.; Rizzo, A.; Spadoni, T.; Svegliati, S.; Marzioni, D.; Santinelli, A.; Costantini, A.; et al. Gut epithelial impairment, microbial translocation and immune system activation in inflammatory bowel disease-associated spondyloarthritis. *Rheumatology* **2021**, *60*, 92–102. [CrossRef]
237. Pastorelli, L.; Dozio, E.; Pisani, L.F.; Boscolo-Anzoletti, M.; Vianello, E.; Munizio, N.; Spina, L.; Tontini, G.E.; Peyvandi, F.; Corsi Romanelli, M.M.; et al. Procoagulatory state in inflammatory bowel diseases is promoted by impaired intestinal barrier function. *Gastroenterol. Res. Pract.* **2015**, *2015*, 189341. [CrossRef]
238. Tulkens, J.; Vergauwen, G.; Van Deun, J.; Geeurickx, E.; Dhondt, B.; Lippens, L.; De Scheerder, M.A.; Miinalainen, I.; Rappu, P.; De Geest, B.G.; et al. Increased levels of systemic LPS-positive bacterial extracellular vesicles in patients with intestinal barrier dysfunction. *Gut* **2020**, *69*, 191–193. [CrossRef]
239. Marques, F.; Sousa, J.C.; Coppola, G.; Falcao, A.M.; Rodrigues, A.J.; Geschwind, D.H.; Sousa, N.; Correia-Neves, M.; Palha, J.A. Kinetic profile of the transcriptome changes induced in the choroid plexus by peripheral inflammation. *J. Cereb. Blood Flow Metab.* **2009**, *29*, 921–932. [CrossRef]
240. Marques, F.; Sousa, J.C.; Coppola, G.; Geschwind, D.H.; Sousa, N.; Palha, J.A.; Correia-Neves, M. The choroid plexus response to a repeated peripheral inflammatory stimulus. *BMC Neurosci.* **2009**, *10*, 135. [CrossRef]
241. Neuendorf, R.; Harding, A.; Stello, N.; Hanes, D.; Wahbeh, H. Depression and anxiety in patients with Inflammatory Bowel Disease: A systematic review. *J. Psychosom. Res.* **2016**, *87*, 70–80. [CrossRef]
242. Aloi, M.; Tromba, L.; Di Nardo, G.; Dilillo, A.; Del Giudice, E.; Marocchi, E.; Viola, F.; Civitelli, F.; Berni, A.; Cucchiara, S. Premature subclinical atherosclerosis in pediatric inflammatory bowel disease. *J. Pediatr.* **2012**, *161*, 589–594.e1. [CrossRef] [PubMed]
243. Aloi, M.; Tromba, L.; Rizzo, V.; D'Arcangelo, G.; Dilillo, A.; Blasi, S.; Civitelli, F.; Kiltzanidi, D.; Redler, A.; Viola, F. Aortic Intima-Media Thickness as an Early Marker of Atherosclerosis in Children With Inflammatory Bowel Disease. *J. Pediatr. Gastroenterol. Nutr.* **2015**, *61*, 41–46. [CrossRef] [PubMed]
244. Caliskan, Z.; Gokturk, H.S.; Caliskan, M.; Gullu, H.; Ciftci, O.; Ozgur, G.T.; Guven, A.; Selcuk, H. Impaired coronary microvascular and left ventricular diastolic function in patients with inflammatory bowel disease. *Microvasc. Res.* **2015**, *97*, 25–30. [CrossRef]
245. Cappello, M.; Licata, A.; Calvaruso, V.; Bravatà, I.; Aiello, A.; Torres, D.; Della Corte, V.; Tuttolomondo, A.; Perticone, M.; Licata, G.; et al. Increased expression of markers of early atherosclerosis in patients with inflammatory bowel disease. *Eur. J. Intern. Med.* **2017**, *37*, 83–89. [CrossRef] [PubMed]
246. Erolu, E.; Polat, E. Cardiac functions and aortic elasticity in children with inflammatory bowel disease: Effect of age at disease onset. *Cardiol. Young* **2020**, *30*, 313–317. [CrossRef]
247. Triantafyllou, C.; Nikolaou, M.; Ikonomidis, I.; Bamias, G.; Papaconstantinou, I. Endothelial and Cardiac Dysfunction in Inflammatory Bowel Diseases: Does Treatment Modify the Inflammatory Load on Arterial and Cardiac Structure and Function? *Curr. Vasc. Pharmacol.* **2020**, *18*, 27–37. [CrossRef]
248. Kakuta, K.; Dohi, K.; Yamamoto, T.; Fujimoto, N.; Shimoyama, T.; Umegae, S.; Ito, M. Coronary Microvascular Dysfunction Restored After Surgery in Inflammatory Bowel Disease: A Prospective Observational Study. *J. Am. Heart Assoc.* **2021**, *10*, e019125. [CrossRef]

249. Sy, A.; Khalidi, N.; Dehghan, N.; Barra, L.; Carette, S.; Cuthbertson, D.; Hoffman, G.S.; Koening, C.L.; Langford, C.A.; McAlear, C.; et al. Vasculitis in patients with inflammatory bowel diseases: A study of 32 patients and systematic review of the literature. *Semin. Arthritis Rheum.* **2016**, *45*, 475–482. [CrossRef]
250. Ho, T.; Orenstein, L.A.V.; Boos, M.D.; White, K.P.; Fett, N. Cutaneous Small-Vessel Vasculitis in Two Children with Inflammatory Bowel Disease: Case Series and Review of the Literature. *Pediatr. Dermatol.* **2017**, *34*, e235–e240. [CrossRef]
251. Romas, E.; Paspaliaris, B.; d'Apice, A.J.; Elliott, P.R. Autoantibodies to neutrophil cytoplasmic (ANCA) and endothelial cell surface antigens (AECA) in chronic inflammatory bowel disease. *Aust. N. Z. J. Med.* **1992**, *22*, 652–659. [CrossRef]
252. Stevens, T.R.; Harley, S.L.; Groom, J.S.; Cambridge, G.; Leaker, B.; Blake, D.R.; Rampton, D.S. Anti-endothelial cell antibodies in inflammatory bowel disease. *Dig. Dis. Sci.* **1993**, *38*, 426–432. [CrossRef] [PubMed]
253. Aldebert, D.; Notteghem, B.; Reumaux, D.; Lassalle, P.; Lion, G.; Desreumaux, P.; Duthilleul, P.; Colombel, J.F. Anti-endothelial cell antibodies in sera from patients with inflammatory bowel disease. *Gastroenterol. Clin. Biol.* **1995**, *19*, 867–870. [PubMed]
254. Agnoletti, D.; Piani, F.; Cicero, A.F.G.; Borghi, C. The Gut Microbiota and Vascular Aging: A State-of-the-Art and Systematic Review of the Literature. *J. Clin. Med.* **2022**, *11*, 3557. [CrossRef] [PubMed]
255. Yoshida, H.; Russell, J.; Granger, D.N. Thrombin mediates the extraintestinal thrombosis associated with experimental colitis. *Am. J. Physiol. Gastrointest. Liver Physiol.* **2008**, *295*, G904–G908. [CrossRef]
256. Papay, P.; Miehsler, W.; Tilg, H.; Petritsch, W.; Reinisch, W.; Mayer, A.; Haas, T.; Kaser, A.; Feichtenschlager, T.; Fuchssteiner, H.; et al. Clinical presentation of venous thromboembolism in inflammatory bowel disease. *J. Crohn's Colitis* **2013**, *7*, 723–729. [CrossRef]
257. Di Fabio, F.; Obrand, D.; Satin, R.; Gordon, P.H. Intra-abdominal venous and arterial thromboembolism in inflammatory bowel disease. *Dis. Colon Rectum* **2009**, *52*, 336–342. [CrossRef]
258. Cognat, E.; Crassard, I.; Denier, C.; Vahedi, K.; Bousser, M.G. Cerebral venous thrombosis in inflammatory bowel diseases: Eight cases and literature review. *Int. J. Stroke* **2011**, *6*, 487–492. [CrossRef]
259. Awab, A.; Elahmadi, B.; Elmoussaoui, R.; Elhijri, A.; Alilou, M.; Azzouzi, A. Cerebral venous thrombosis and inflammatory bowel disease: Reflections on pathogenesis. *Colorectal. Dis.* **2012**, *14*, 1153–1154. [CrossRef]
260. Tan, V.P.; Chung, A.; Yan, B.P.; Gibson, P.R. Venous and arterial disease in inflammatory bowel disease. *J. Gastroenterol. Hepatol.* **2013**, *28*, 1095–1113. [CrossRef]
261. Principi, M.; Mastrolonardo, M.; Scicchitano, P.; Gesualdo, M.; Sassara, M.; Guida, P.; Bucci, A.; Zito, A.; Caputo, P.; Albano, F.; et al. Endothelial function and cardiovascular risk in active inflammatory bowel diseases. *J. Crohn's Colitis* **2013**, *7*, e427–e433. [CrossRef]
262. Orfei, M.; Gasparetto, M.; Torrente, F. Headache and inflammatory bowel disease: Think cerebral vein! *BMJ Case Rep.* **2019**, *12*, e227228. [CrossRef] [PubMed]
263. Rohani, P.; Taraghikhah, N.; Naseh, M.M.; Alimadadi, H.; Assadzadeh Aghdaei, H. Cerebrovascular Events in Pediatric Inflammatory Bowel Disease: A Review of Published Cases. *Pediatr. Gastroenterol. Hepatol. Nutr.* **2022**, *25*, 180–193. [CrossRef] [PubMed]
264. Carty, E.; MacEy, M.; Rampton, D.S. Inhibition of platelet activation by 5-aminosalicylic acid in inflammatory bowel disease. *Aliment. Pharmacol. Ther.* **2000**, *14*, 1169–1179. [CrossRef] [PubMed]
265. Hommes, D.W.; van Dullemen, H.M.; Levi, M.; van der Ende, A.; Woody, J.; Tytgat, G.N.; van Deventer, S.J. Beneficial effect of treatment with a monoclonal anti-tumor necrosis factor-alpha antibody on markers of coagulation and fibrinolysis in patients with active Crohn's disease. *Haemostasis* **1997**, *27*, 269–277. [CrossRef]
266. Schinzari, F.; Armuzzi, A.; De Pascalis, B.; Mores, N.; Tesauro, M.; Melina, D.; Cardillo, C. Tumor necrosis factor-alpha antagonism improves endothelial dysfunction in patients with Crohn's disease. *Clin. Pharmacol. Ther.* **2008**, *83*, 70–76. [CrossRef]
267. Danese, S.; Sans, M.; Scaldaferri, F.; Sgambato, A.; Rutella, S.; Cittadini, A.; Piqué, J.M.; Panes, J.; Katz, J.A.; Gasbarrini, A.; et al. TNF-alpha blockade down-regulates the CD40/CD40L pathway in the mucosal microcirculation: A novel anti-inflammatory mechanism of infliximab in Crohn's disease. *J. Immunol.* **2006**, *176*, 2617–2624. [CrossRef]
268. Löwenberg, M.; D'Haens, G. Next-Generation Therapeutics for IBD. *Curr. Gastroenterol. Rep.* **2015**, *17*, 21. [CrossRef]
269. Neurath, M.F. Current and emerging therapeutic targets for IBD. *Nat. Rev. Gastroenterol. Hepatol.* **2017**, *14*, 269–278. [CrossRef]
270. Park, S.C.; Jeen, Y.T. Anti-integrin therapy for inflammatory bowel disease. *World J. Gastroenterol.* **2018**, *24*, 1868–1880. [CrossRef]
271. Feagan, B.G.; Rutgeerts, P.; Sands, B.E.; Hanauer, S.; Colombel, J.F.; Sandborn, W.J.; Van Assche, G.; Axler, J.; Kim, H.J.; Danese, S.; et al. Vedolizumab as induction and maintenance therapy for ulcerative colitis. *N. Engl. J. Med.* **2013**, *369*, 699–710. [CrossRef]
272. Sandborn, W.J.; Feagan, B.G.; Rutgeerts, P.; Hanauer, S.; Colombel, J.F.; Sands, B.E.; Lukas, M.; Fedorak, R.N.; Lee, S.; Bressler, B.; et al. Vedolizumab as induction and maintenance therapy for Crohn's disease. *N. Engl. J. Med.* **2013**, *369*, 711–721. [CrossRef] [PubMed]
273. Zundler, S.; Schillinger, D.; Fischer, A.; Atreya, R.; Lopez-Posadas, R.; Watson, A.; Neufert, C.; Atreya, I.; Neurath, M.F. Blockade of alphaEbeta7 integrin suppresses accumulation of CD8+ and Th9 lymphocytes from patients with IBD in the inflamed gut in vivo. *Gut* **2017**, *66*, 1936–1948. [CrossRef] [PubMed]
274. Picardo, S.; Panaccione, R. Anti-MADCAM therapy for ulcerative colitis. *Expert Opin. Biol. Ther.* **2020**, *20*, 437–442. [CrossRef] [PubMed]

275. Reinisch, W.; Sandborn, W.J.; Danese, S.; Hébuterne, X.; Kłopocka, M.; Tarabar, D.; Vaňásek, T.; Greguš, M.; Hellstern, P.A.; Kim, J.S.; et al. Long-term Safety and Efficacy of the Anti-MAdCAM-1 Monoclonal Antibody Ontamalimab [SHP647] for the Treatment of Ulcerative Colitis: The Open-label Study TURANDOT II. *J. Crohn's Colitis* **2021**, *15*, 938–949. [CrossRef]
276. Lightner, A.L.; Sklow, B.; Click, B.; Regueiro, M.; McMichael, J.J.; Jia, X.; Vaidya, P.; Delaney, C.P.; Cohen, B.; Wexner, S.D.; et al. Venous Thromboembolism in Admitted Patients with Inflammatory Bowel Disease: An Enterprise—Wide Experience of 86,000 Hospital Encounters. *Dis. Colon Rectum* **2022**, *66*, 410–418. [CrossRef]
277. Chande, N.; Wang, Y.; McDonald, J.W.; MacDonald, J.K. Unfractionated or low-molecular weight heparin for induction of remission in ulcerative colitis. *Cochrane Database Syst. Rev.* **2015**, *8*, Cd006774. [CrossRef]
278. Hong, L.; Chen, G.; Cai, Z.; Liu, H.; Zhang, C.; Wang, F.; Xiao, Z.; Zhong, J.; Wang, L.; Wang, Z.; et al. Balancing Microthrombosis and Inflammation via Injectable Protein Hydrogel for Inflammatory Bowel Disease. *Adv. Sci.* **2022**, *9*, e2200281. [CrossRef]
279. Prajapati, D.N.; Newcomer, J.R.; Emmons, J.; Abu-Hajir, M.; Binion, D.G. Successful treatment of an acute flare of steroid-resistant Crohn's colitis during pregnancy with unfractionated heparin. *Inflamm. Bowel Dis.* **2002**, *8*, 192–195. [CrossRef]
280. Chande, N.; MacDonald, J.K.; Wang, J.J.; McDonald, J.W. Unfractionated or low molecular weight heparin for induction of remission in ulcerative colitis: A Cochrane inflammatory bowel disease and functional bowel disorders systematic review of randomized trials. *Inflamm. Bowel Dis.* **2011**, *17*, 1979–1986. [CrossRef]
281. Day, R.; Forbes, A. Heparin, cell adhesion, and pathogenesis of inflammatory bowel disease. *Lancet* **1999**, *354*, 62–65. [CrossRef]
282. Papa, A.; Danese, S.; Gasbarrini, A.; Gasbarrini, G. Review article: Potential therapeutic applications and mechanisms of action of heparin in inflammatory bowel disease. *Aliment. Pharmacol. Ther.* **2000**, *14*, 1403–1409. [CrossRef] [PubMed]
283. Yazeji, T.; Moulari, B.; Beduneau, A.; Stein, V.; Dietrich, D.; Pellequer, Y.; Lamprecht, A. Nanoparticle-based delivery enhances anti-inflammatory effect of low molecular weight heparin in experimental ulcerative colitis. *Drug Deliv.* **2017**, *24*, 811–817. [CrossRef] [PubMed]
284. Zhang, S.; Cho, W.J.; Jin, A.T.; Kok, L.Y.; Shi, Y.; Heller, D.E.; Lee, Y.L.; Zhou, Y.; Xie, X.; Korzenik, J.R.; et al. Heparin-Coated Albumin Nanoparticles for Drug Combination in Targeting Inflamed Intestine. *Adv. Healthc. Mater.* **2020**, *9*, e2000536. [CrossRef]
285. Wang, S.Y.; Tao, P.; Hu, H.Y.; Yuan, J.Y.; Zhao, L.; Sun, B.Y.; Zhang, W.J.; Lin, J. Effects of initiating time and dosage of Panax notoginseng on mucosal microvascular injury in experimental colitis. *World J. Gastroenterol.* **2017**, *23*, 8308–8320. [CrossRef]
286. Zhang, X.; Song, L.; Li, L.; Zhu, B.; Huo, H.; Hu, Z.; Wang, X.; Wang, J.; Gao, M.; Zhang, J.; et al. Phosphatidylserine externalized on the colonic capillaries as a novel pharmacological target for IBD therapy. *Signal Transduct. Target. Ther.* **2021**, *6*, 235. [CrossRef] [PubMed]
287. Adzemovic, M.V.; Zeitelhofer, M.; Eriksson, U.; Olsson, T.; Nilsson, I. Imatinib ameliorates neuroinflammation in a rat model of multiple sclerosis by enhancing blood-brain barrier integrity and by modulating the peripheral immune response. *PLoS ONE* **2013**, *8*, e56586. [CrossRef]
288. Aman, J.; van Bezu, J.; Damanafshan, A.; Huveneers, S.; Eringa, E.C.; Vogel, S.M.; Groeneveld, A.B.; Vonk Noordegraaf, A.; van Hinsbergh, V.W.; van Nieuw Amerongen, G.P. Effective treatment of edema and endothelial barrier dysfunction with imatinib. *Circulation* **2012**, *126*, 2728–2738. [CrossRef] [PubMed]
289. Hosaka, K.; Yang, Y.; Seki, T.; Nakamura, M.; Andersson, P.; Rouhi, P.; Yang, X.; Jensen, L.; Lim, S.; Feng, N.; et al. Tumour PDGF-BB expression levels determine dual effects of anti-PDGF drugs on vascular remodelling and metastasis. *Nat. Commun.* **2013**, *4*, 2129. [CrossRef] [PubMed]
290. Magro, F.; Costa, C. Long-standing remission of Crohn's disease under imatinib therapy in a patient with Crohn's disease. *Inflamm. Bowel Dis.* **2006**, *12*, 1087–1089. [CrossRef]
291. Gonzalez-Cabrera, P.J.; Brown, S.; Studer, S.M.; Rosen, H. S1P signaling: New therapies and opportunities. *F1000Prime Rep.* **2014**, *6*, 109. [CrossRef]
292. Verstockt, B.; Vetrano, S.; Salas, A.; Nayeri, S.; Duijvestein, M.; Vande Casteele, N. Sphingosine 1-phosphate modulation and immune cell trafficking in inflammatory bowel disease. *Nat. Rev. Gastroenterol. Hepatol.* **2022**, *19*, 351–366. [CrossRef] [PubMed]
293. Obinata, H.; Hla, T. Sphingosine 1-phosphate and inflammation. *Int. Immunol.* **2019**, *31*, 617–625. [CrossRef] [PubMed]
294. Oo, M.L.; Chang, S.H.; Thangada, S.; Wu, M.T.; Rezaul, K.; Blaho, V.; Hwang, S.I.; Han, D.K.; Hla, T. Engagement of S1P$_1$-degradative mechanisms leads to vascular leak in mice. *J. Clin. Investig.* **2011**, *121*, 2290–2300. [CrossRef] [PubMed]
295. Jeya Paul, J.; Weigel, C.; Müller, T.; Heller, R.; Spiegel, S.; Gräler, M.H. Inflammatory Conditions Disrupt Constitutive Endothelial Cell Barrier Stabilization by Alleviating Autonomous Secretion of Sphingosine 1-Phosphate. *Cells* **2020**, *9*, 928. [CrossRef]
296. Ziegler, A.C.; Gräler, M.H. Barrier maintenance by S1P during inflammation and sepsis. *Tissue Barriers* **2021**, *9*, 1940069. [CrossRef]

Disclaimer/Publisher's Note: The statements, opinions and data contained in all publications are solely those of the individual author(s) and contributor(s) and not of MDPI and/or the editor(s). MDPI and/or the editor(s) disclaim responsibility for any injury to people or property resulting from any ideas, methods, instructions or products referred to in the content.

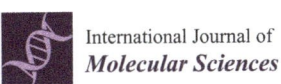

Article

Identification of Novel Core Genes Involved in Malignant Transformation of Inflamed Colon Tissue Using a Computational Biology Approach and Verification in Murine Models

Andrey V. Markov *, Innokenty A. Savin, Marina A. Zenkova and Aleksandra V. Sen'kova

Institute of Chemical Biology and Fundamental Medicine, Siberian Branch of the Russian Academy of Sciences, Lavrent'ev Ave., 8, 630090 Novosibirsk, Russia
* Correspondence: andmrkv@gmail.com; Tel.: +7-383-363-51-61

Abstract: Inflammatory bowel disease (IBD) is a complex and multifactorial systemic disorder of the gastrointestinal tract and is strongly associated with the development of colorectal cancer. Despite extensive studies of IBD pathogenesis, the molecular mechanism of colitis-driven tumorigenesis is not yet fully understood. In the current animal-based study, we report a comprehensive bioinformatics analysis of multiple transcriptomics datasets from the colon tissue of mice with acute colitis and colitis-associated cancer (CAC). We performed intersection of differentially expressed genes (DEGs), their functional annotation, reconstruction, and topology analysis of gene association networks, which, when combined with the text mining approach, revealed that a set of key overexpressed genes involved in the regulation of colitis (*C3*, *Tyrobp*, *Mmp3*, *Mmp9*, *Timp1*) and CAC (*Timp1*, *Adam8*, *Mmp7*, *Mmp13*) occupied hub positions within explored colitis- and CAC-related regulomes. Further validation of obtained data in murine models of dextran sulfate sodium (DSS)-induced colitis and azoxymethane/DSS-stimulated CAC fully confirmed the association of revealed hub genes with inflammatory and malignant lesions of colon tissue and demonstrated that genes encoding matrix metalloproteinases (acute colitis: *Mmp3*, *Mmp9*; CAC: *Mmp7*, *Mmp13*) can be used as a novel prognostic signature for colorectal neoplasia in IBD. Finally, using publicly available transcriptomics data, translational bridge interconnecting of listed colitis/CAC-associated core genes with the pathogenesis of ulcerative colitis, Crohn's disease, and colorectal cancer in humans was identified. Taken together, a set of key genes playing a core function in colon inflammation and CAC was revealed, which can serve both as promising molecular markers and therapeutic targets to control IBD and IBD-associated colorectal neoplasia.

Keywords: colitis; colitis-associated cancer; inflammatory bowel disease; colorectal cancer; colon adenocarcinoma; ulcerative colitis; Crohn's disease; cDNA microarray; transcriptomics analysis; microarray

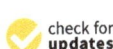

Citation: Markov, A.V.; Savin, I.A.; Zenkova, M.A.; Sen'kova, A.V. Identification of Novel Core Genes Involved in Malignant Transformation of Inflamed Colon Tissue Using a Computational Biology Approach and Verification in Murine Models. *Int. J. Mol. Sci.* **2023**, *24*, 4311. https://doi.org/10.3390/ijms24054311

Academic Editor: Susanne M. Krug

Received: 3 February 2023
Revised: 18 February 2023
Accepted: 20 February 2023
Published: 21 February 2023

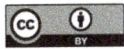

Copyright: © 2023 by the authors. Licensee MDPI, Basel, Switzerland. This article is an open access article distributed under the terms and conditions of the Creative Commons Attribution (CC BY) license (https://creativecommons.org/licenses/by/4.0/).

1. Introduction

Colorectal cancer (CRC) is the third most common malignancy and the second leading cause of cancer-related deaths worldwide [1,2]. Colon inflammation, along with the particular host and environmental factors, plays a crucial role in the initiation and progression of CRC [3]. Colitis-associated cancer (CAC) is a type of CRC, which is preceded by clinically detectable inflammatory bowel disease (IBD), including Crohn's disease (CD) and ulcerative colitis (UC), two highly heterogeneous, incurable, persistent, relapsing/worsening, and immune-arbitrated inflammatory pathologies of the digestive system [4,5]. Epidemiologic studies have showed that patients with IBD have a predisposition to CRC, and cancer risk is highly correlated with the duration and severity of colon inflammation [6,7].

In IBD, chronic long-term colon inflammation accompanied by oxidative stress can alter the expression patterns of key carcinogenesis-associated genes [8]. Moreover, persistent stimulation of epithelial proliferation in the colon by the pro-inflammatory stimuli and excessive cell damage with increased epithelial cell turnover result in detrimental genetic and immunological alterations, making patients with IBD prone to developing CRC [9]. Despite the proven involvement of "inflammation-dysplasia-carcinoma" axis in the malignant transformation of cells in IBD-related CRC [10], the molecular mechanism underlying this process is not yet fully understood. In particular, it remains rather unclear which core genes are involved in the regulation of acute colitis and how markedly their profiles change during colitis-associated malignant transformation of the colon tissue. In addition, the proven complexity of the colitis/CAC-related regulome underlies the low efficacy of conventional IBD/CRC therapy, making it inevitable that surgery is recommended for treating these pathologies [5,11]. Given the known adverse impact of the surgical management of colonic diseases on the quality of life, mental health, and work productivity of patients [5,11], the search for novel key genes involved in the inflammation-related tumor transformation, which can be used as potential molecular targets for IBD therapy, is urgently needed. Moreover, such regulatory genes can be considered as biomarkers of inflammation-driven tumorigenesis and serve as predictors for surveillance strategies and chemoprevention of colitis-related dysplasia and CRC in IBD patients.

To date, extensive exploration of colitis- and CAC-associated regulomes has been performed using transcriptomics-based approaches [12–21]. Reported bioinformatics studies have revealed some candidate biomarker genes and key signaling pathways susceptible to the development of the mentioned disorders [14–23], colitis-induced changes in the landscape of immune infiltration of colon tissue [14,16], and a range of hub genes probably involved in the development of CAC [15,20,23]. Despite a plethora of published studies, obtained results are still uncertain and are not well correlated with each other, probably due to insufficient usage of a multiple microarray analysis algorithm (the exploration of three or more independent microarray datasets in the same study, which gives more valid results [18,20,21]), ineffective manual searching of the published literature on the topic of study [14–21], and, in some cases, the absence of proper experimental validation [18]. Since the obtained data still remain insufficient for a thorough understanding of colitis/CAC-associated gene signature, further comprehensive bioinformatics analysis of colitis/CAC-related core genes is required.

In this study, deep re-analysis of multiple microarray datasets related to murine acute colitis (GSE42768, GSE35609, GSE64658, GSE71920, GSE35609) and CAC (GSE31106, GSE5605, GSE64658, GSE42768) was performed. Firstly, the differentially expressed genes (DEGs) were computed between injured and healthy colon tissues, followed by their functional annotation and Venn diagram analysis to identify acute colitis- and CAC-associated core genes. Next, the changes in the sets of core genes associated with the transition from colon inflammation to CRC were identified. Further reconstruction and analysis of gene association networks revealed a range of hub regulators among core genes, subsequent exploration of which by the text mining approach identified a list of candidate genes, which can be used as novel promising biomarkers and therapeutic targets for colitis and CAC. The obtained results were finally validated using an in vivo model of dextran sulfate sodium (DSS)-induced acute colitis and azoxymethane (AOM)/DSS-induced CAC. Furthermore, the role of identified core genes in the colonic carcinogenesis in the backstage of chronic long-term inflammation was analyzed with respect to IBD and CRC in humans.

2. Results

2.1. Identification of Core Genes Related to Colitis and Colitis-Associated Cancer

To reveal key genes involved in the regulation of acute colitis and its transformation to CAC in mice, a range of independent expression profiles of murine colon tissue were retrieved from the GEO database, including samples of mice of both sexes and different strains with acute colitis stimulated by DSS (GSE42768, GSE35609, GSE64658, GSE71920) or dinitrobenzene sulfonic acid (DNBS) (GSE35609), or chronic colitis driven by azoxymethane (AOM)/DSS accompanied by the development of colorectal cancer (GSE31106, GSE5605, GSE64658, GSE42768). The analysis of selected transcriptomic datasets using the GEO2R tool revealed the sets of differentially expressed genes (DEGs) (colitis vs. control and CAC vs. control) susceptible to the mentioned pathologies, further overlapping of which identified 54 and 109 common DEGs specific to colitis and CAC, respectively (hereafter referred to as core genes) (Figure 1A).

2.1.1. Hierarchical Clustering and Functional Analysis of DEGs

Hierarchical clustering of the expression profiles of identified colitis-associated core genes revealed two main clades separating up- and down-regulated DEGs from each other (Figure 1B). The sub-clade of the most overexpressed DEGs included genes related to immune response (*Ccl3, S100a9, S100a8, Cxcl2*) and heme metabolism (*Hp*), whereas the most suppressed core genes in the colitis group were *Hao2* and *Slc26a3*, associated with fatty acid metabolism and chloride ion transport, respectively (Figure 1B). Further functional analysis of colitis-specific core genes revealed high enrichment of inflammatory-related terms, including the production of pro-inflammatory cytokines IL-1 and TNF-α, IL-17, IGF1-Akt and Tyrobp signaling pathways, antiviral response, matrix metalloproteinases (MMPs), lung fibrosis, and rheumatoid arthritis (Figure 1C, upper panel).

Hierarchical clustering of CAC-specific core genes (Figure 1D) revealed two main clades, grouping activated and suppressed DEGs separately, and one outgroup consisted of the most overexpressed CAC-associated DEGs, notably, regulators of host-microbiota interplay (*Reg3b, Reg3g*), immune response (*S100a9*), and extracellular matrix (ECM) remodeling (*Mmp7*). In turn, the most suppressed core genes in the CAC group were involved in the regulation of cell adhesion (*Zan*), pH homeostasis (*Car4*), and ion transport (*Slc26a3, Slc37a2, Aqp8*) (Figure 1D). Performed gene set enrichment analysis revealed that CAC-specific core genes are tightly associated with cell invasiveness (wound healing involved in inflammatory response and MMPs), immune response (acute inflammatory response, antimicrobial peptides, etc.), redox imbalance, ion transport, bile secretion, and numerous metabolic processes (Figure 1C, lower panel). Interestingly, the retrieved functional annotation map specific for CAC was significantly less interconnected compared with the acute colitis-associated GO term/pathways network (Figure 1C, upper panel), which can be explained by the more discrete disposition of identified core genes in the CAC-related regulome.

2.1.2. Analysis of Interconnection between Acute Colitis- and CAC-Specific Core Genes

To explore how strongly identified core genes are interconnected in acute and chronic (CAC) phases of colitis, their Venn diagram analysis and the reconstruction of the gene association network were performed. Overlapping of acute colitis- and CAC-related genes demonstrated that 22 of the core genes, playing a regulatory role in acute inflammation, were involved in CAC pathogenesis (Figure 1E), including immune genes (*Ifitm1, Ifitm3, Il1a, Lcn2, S100a9, Saa3, Tnf*), genes encoding protease inhibitors (*Serpina3n, Slpi, Wfdc18*), ion transporters (*Slc26a2, Slc26a3, Trpm6*), ECM remodeling proteins (*Mmp10, Timp1, Mep1a*), signal transduction components (*Igfbp4, Lrg1*) and regulators of cell motility (*Capg*), fatty acid homeostasis (*Hao2*), host-microbiota interplay (*Sult1a1*), and heme metabolism (*Hp*).

Analysis of the gene association network generated from acute colitis- and CAC-associated core genes using the STRING database [24] demonstrated their relatively high interconnection: 72 of 141 uploaded core genes (51%) formed interactions with each other within the network (Figure 1F). Interestingly, only 34 of 87 CAC-specific genes (39%) were involved in the network, whereas the shares of acute colitis-specific and common genes in the reconstructed interactome were 66% (21 of 32 genes) and 73% (16 of 22 genes), respectively. Considering that highly interconnected genes can be involved in the same or similar biological processes [25], revealed low enrichment of the analyzed network by

CAC-specific genes (Figure 1F) was in line with the discrete structure of the CAC-related functional annotation map shown above (Figure 1C).

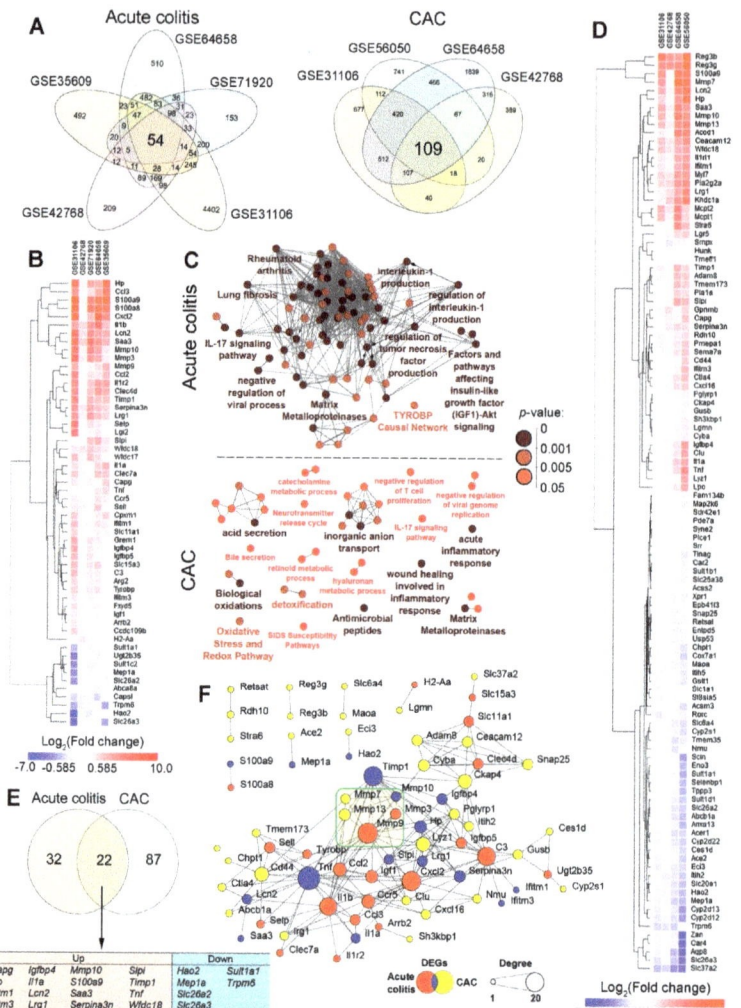

Figure 1. Core genes involved in the development of acute colitis and CAC in mice revealed by bioinformatics analysis. (**A**) Venn diagrams overlapping differentially expressed genes (DEGs) identified by re-analysis of cDNA microarray datasets of colon tissue of mice with colitis and CAC. (**B**) Heatmap demonstrating expression levels of DEGs in acute colitis-related GSE datasets (acute colitis vs. healthy control). (**C**) Functional analysis of overlapped DEGs associated with acute colitis and CAC. Enrichment for Gene Ontology (Biological Processes), KEGG, REACTOME, and WikiPathways terms performed using ClueGO plugin in Cytoscape. Only pathways with $p < 0.05$ after Bonferroni correction for multiple testing were included in the functional annotation map. (**D**) Heatmap demonstrating expression levels of DEGs in CAC-related GSE datasets (CAC vs. healthy control). (**E**) Venn diagrams overlapping revealed acute colitis- and CAC-associated core genes. (**F**) Gene association network retrieved from identified core genes associated with acute colitis and CAC reconstructed using STRING database (confidence score ≥ 0.7). Degree—the number of first neighbors (gene partners) within the gene network.

Further computing of degree centrality scores of explored core genes revealed a range of genes occupying hub positions in the analyzed network (Figure 1F). It was found that the most interconnected nodes were acute colitis-specific or common genes involved in immune response (*C3*, *Cxcl2*, *Il1b*, *Tnf*) and ECM remodeling (*Mmp9*, *Timp1*). Among CAC-specific genes, the highest degree was identified for stabilizer of endoplasmic reticulum structure *Ckap4*, regulator of cell–cell interaction *Cd44*, and gene *Lyz1* encoding lysozyme (Figure 1F). Given the hub position of *Mmp9* and *Timp1* and the formation of a highly connected cluster of MMPs in the core gene-retrieved network (Figure 1F), the changes in the MMPs profile can be involved in the regulation of malignant transformation of colon tissue during chronic colitis. This pattern needs further clarification.

2.2. Identification of Novel Acute Colitis- and CAC-Specific Hub Genes

2.2.1. Acute Colitis-Associated Hub Genes

To identify novel candidate genes for acute colitis and CAC, which can be used as both diagnostic markers and promising therapeutic targets, next we questioned how strongly evaluated core genes can be involved in the regulation of the mentioned pathologies and how well these genes have been studied in the field of inflammatory and neoplastic disorders of the colon.

To address the first issue, the degree centrality scores of the core genes in gene association networks created for each analyzed transcriptomic dataset were computed. Given that hub genes can exert key regulatory functions in reconstructed gene networks [26], the top 20 acute colitis-specific hub genes were identified and are shown in Figure 2A. The obtained results demonstrated that the most interconnected genes associated with acute colitis included genes encoding cytokines (*Tnf*, *Il1a*, *Il1b*), chemokines and its receptors (*Ccl2*, *Cxcl2*, *Ccl3*, *Ccr5*), growth factors and signal transduction components (*Igf1*, *Tyrobp*, *Arrb2*), ECM remodeling regulators (*Mmp3*, *Mmp9*, *Timp1*), and immune (*C3*, *Clec7a*, *H2-Aa*, *Sell*, *Selp*) and protective (*Hp*, *Ugt2b35*) proteins.

Next, to select genes poorly characterized for their role in colitis and colitis-associated disorders, a text mining approach was performed. Analysis of the mention of acute colitis-related core genes (Figure 1B) alongside the keywords "Colitis", "Crohn's", "Dysplasia", and "Colon cancer" in scientific texts deposited in the MEDLINE database revealed the most studied genes in the field of colitis (*Tnf*, *Il1b*, *Mmp9*, *Igf1*, *Ccl2*, *Slc26a2*, *Timp1*, *Lcn2*, *Il1a*, and *Sell*); the majority of them occupied hub positions in retrieved colitis-associated gene networks (key nodes) (Figure 2A). The rest of the genes were found to be less explored as colitis-related ones (Figure 2B), and, therefore, could be used as a source of novel promising markers/regulators of colitis. To experimentally verify the obtained data, *Mmp3*, *C3*, and *Tyrobp*, displaying, on the one hand, little connection with colitis in the published reports (Figure 2B), and, on the other hand, high degree centrality scores in colitis-associated gene networks (Figure 2A), were selected for further qRT-PCR analysis. Since the profile of MMPs was identified as hypothetically susceptible to transforming acute colitis into CAC (Figure 1F), expressions of *Mmp9* and *Timp1* (known inhibitor of MMPs) were also further validated.

2.2.2. CAC-Associated Hub Genes

The ranking of CAC-specific core genes according to their degree centrality scores in CAC-related gene networks identified the top 20 genes occupying hub positions, including genes encoding cyto- and chemokines (*Tnf*, *Il1a*, *Cxcl16*), regulators of ECM remodeling (*Timp1*, *Mmp7*, *Mmp13*, *Gusb*), immune (*Ctla4*, *Cyba*) and protective (*Gstt1*, *Hp*, *Clu*, *Cyp2s1*) response, lipid homeostasis (*Acss2*, *Chpt1*), ROS production (*Maoa*), cell–cell interaction (*Cd44*), membrane fusion (*Snap25*), and signal transduction (*Plce1*, *Lgr5*) (Figure 2C). Further text mining study, combined with the computing of the association of CAC-related core genes with the overall survival of patients with colon (COAD) and rectal (READ) adenocarcinomas, clearly confirmed the credibility of our bioinformatics analysis: the most reported CAC-related genes (*Tnf*, *Cd44*, *Timp1*, *Mmp7*, *Ctla4*, *Clu*, *Il1a*, *Hp*) were not only associated with poor prognosis in COAD and READ patients but also occupied the hub positions in the networks retrieved from CAC-associated DEGs (Figure 2D). These results indicate a probable important regulatory function of the listed core genes in colitis-associated neoplastic transformation of colon tissue.

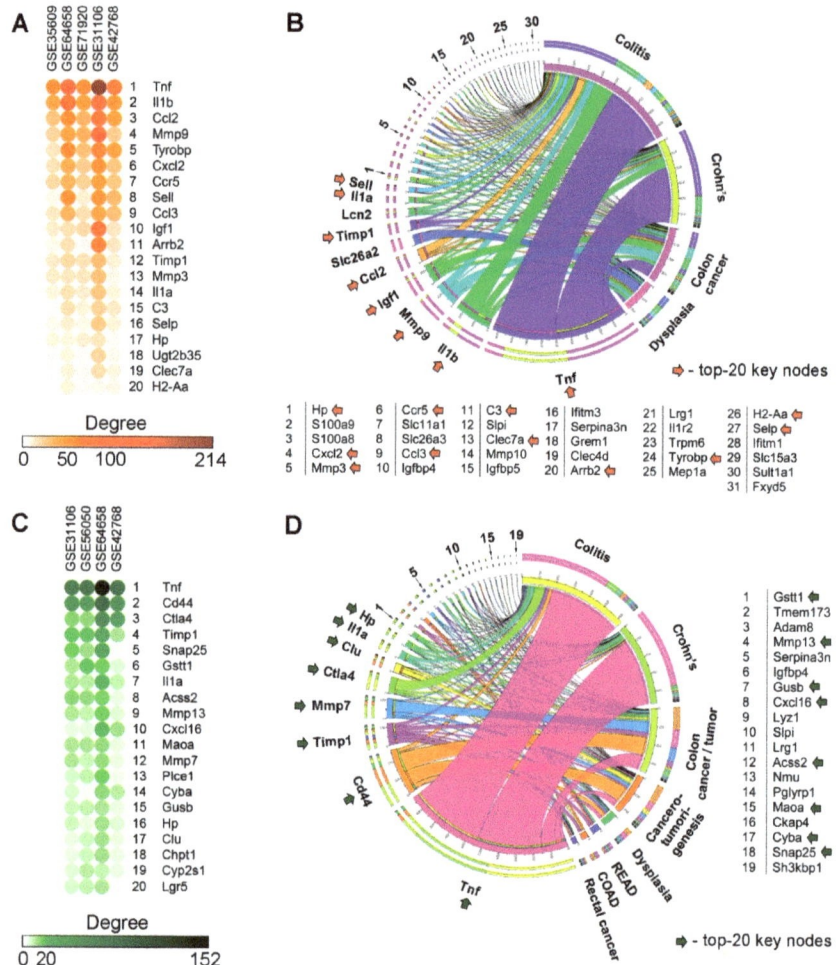

Figure 2. Core genes characterized by hub position within acute colitis- and CAC-related regulomes. (A,C) Heatmaps demonstrating interconnection of core genes in gene association networks reconstructed for each acute colitis- (A) and CAC-related (C) dataset using the STRING database (confidence score ≥ 0.7). Only the top 20 of the most interconnected hub genes are represented. (B,D) Co-occurrence of revealed hub genes with keywords associated with colitis (B) and CAC (D) in the scientific literature deposited in the MEDLINE database. Analysis was performed using the GenClip3 tool. Data were visualized using Circos. COAD and READ-association of the aberrant expression of hub genes with poor prognosis in patients with colon and rectal adenocarcinomas, respectively, according to the TCGA database.

To identify novel candidate genes for CAC, our attention was centered on the core genes that are, on the one hand, poorly characterized in the field of CAC, and, on the other hand, associated with ECM remodeling susceptible to "inflammation-dysplasia-carcinoma" axis (Figure 1C,F), notably, *Mmp13* (key node) and *Adam8* (extracellular metalloprotease-disintegrin involved in ECM digestion and markedly associated with pathogenesis of gastrointestinal malignancies [27]) (Figure 2D). In addition, the key nodes *Timp1* and *Mmp7* previously reported as probable regulators of CRC were also selected for qRT-PCR analysis.

2.3. Validation of Novel Candidate Genes for Colitis and CAC

2.3.1. Murine Model of DSS-Induced Colitis and CAC

Acute colitis was induced in mice by administration of 2.5% DSS solution in drinking water for 7 days, followed by a 3 day recovery (Figure 3A). CAC was induced in mice by single intraperitoneal (i.p.) injection of AOM 1 week before DSS administration. Furthermore, mice were exposed to 3 consecutive cycles of 1.5% DSS instillations for 7 days, followed by 2 weeks of recovery (Figure 3A). After the experiment termination, the colons were separated from the proximal rectum, mechanically cleaned with saline buffer, and collected for subsequent histological analysis and qRT-PCR.

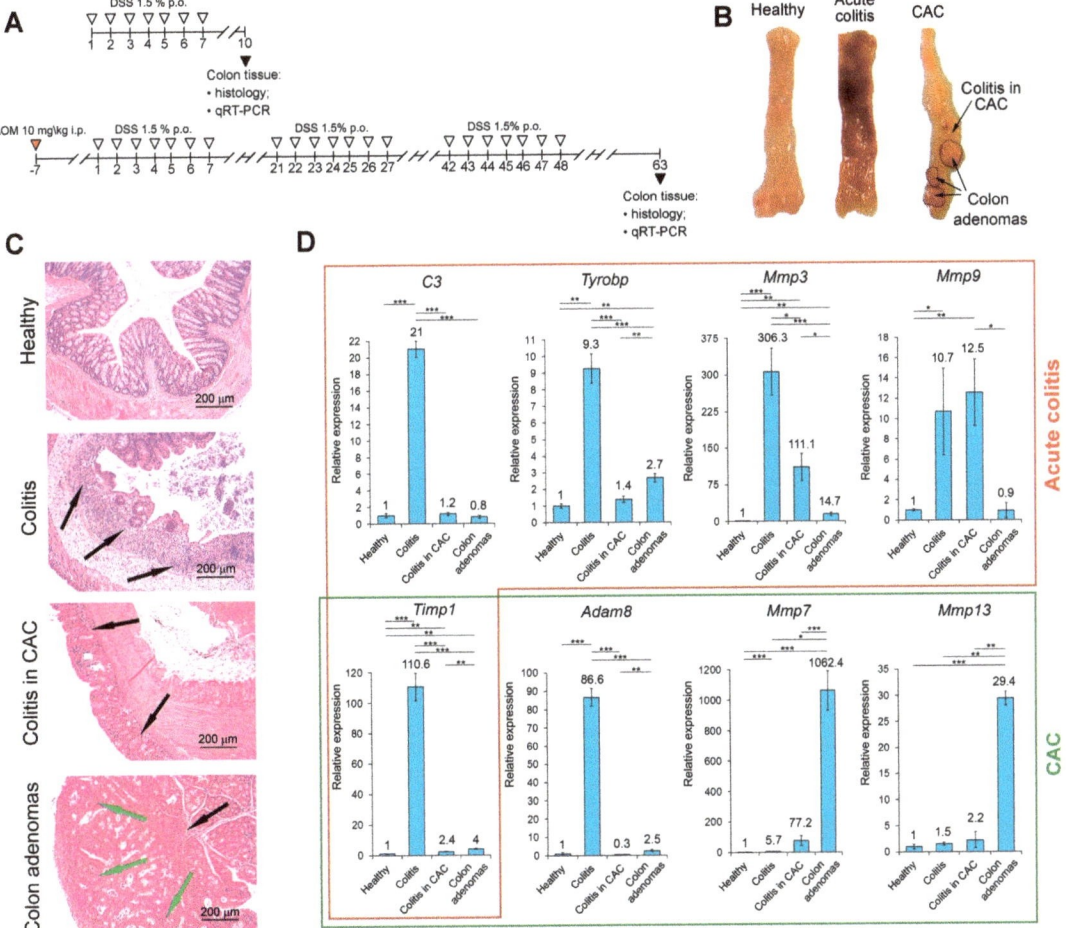

Figure 3. Morphological changes and expression levels of key genes identified by the bioinformatics

analysis in the colon tissues of healthy mice and mice with acute colitis and colitis-associated cancer (CAC). (**A**) Experimental setup. Acute colitis was induced by the administration of 2.5% dextran sulfate sodium (DSS) solution in drinking water for 7 days followed by a 3 day recovery (upper panel) ($n = 10$). CAC was induced in mice by single intraperitoneal (i.p.) injection of azoxymethane (AOM) 1 week before DSS administration. Mice were then exposed to 3 consecutive cycles of 1.5% DSS instillations for 7 days followed by 2 weeks recovery (lower panel) ($n = 10$). At the end of the experiment, the colons were collected for subsequent histological analysis and qRT-PCR. (**B**,**C**) Gross morphology (**B**) and histology (**C**) of the colon tissue of healthy mice and mice with acute colitis and CAC. Hematoxylin and eosin staining. Original magnification ×100. Black arrows indicate inflammatory infiltration. Green arrows indicate adenomatous transformation of colon epithelium. (**D**) Expression levels of identified genes in the colon tissues measured by qRT-PCR. HPRT was used as a reference gene. Healthy—healthy colon tissue, colitis—colon tissue with acute colitis, colitis in CAC—colon tissue with chronic colitis adjacent to adenomas. The data are expressed as the mean ± SD ($n = 6$). * $p < 0.05$, ** $p < 0.01$, *** $p < 0.001$.

Gross morphological analysis of healthy colons revealed the normal thickness of the colonic wall and mucosa structure (Figure 3B). Administration of 2.5% DSS for one week led to acute inflammatory changes in the colonic tissues, clearly demonstrating the development of acute colitis and represented by thickening of the colonic wall, hyperemia, hemorrhages, and scattered ulcers (Figure 3B). Long-term cyclic administration of 1.5% DSS with prior injections of carcinogen AOM caused the development of multiple adenomas in the distal part of mice colons with a significant decrease in the intensity of acute inflammatory changes in the colonic tissues (Figure 3B).

Histologically, the colon tissue of healthy mice demonstrated intact colon architecture, non-disrupted crypts, and goblet cells with active mucus vacuoles (Figure 3C). Acute administration of DSS caused severe colon tissue damage, represented by massive epithelium disruption with erosions and ulcerations, diffuse destruction of crypts, and loss of mucosal architecture (Figure 3C). Pronounced inflammatory infiltration through the whole colonic wall, due to neutrophils and lymphocytes as well as mucosa edema, was revealed (Figure 3C). In the case of CAC, chronic administration of DSS after AOM injection caused adenomatous transformation of the colon mucosa, represented by multiple adenomas in the colonic tissue with epithelial hyperproliferation and hyperplastic crypts (Figure 3C). Residual inflammatory infiltration located in the mucosa and submucosa of colon tissue with adenomas and represented by lymphocytes and macrophages was detected (Figure 3C). In the colon tissue adjacent to adenomas (colitis in CAC), signs of chronic colonic inflammation with moderate destruction of the mucosal architecture and crypt damage were found (Figure 3C).

Thus, we reproduced the process of colon carcinogenesis, starting with acute inflammation in the colon tissue, transitioning to chronic inflammation, and eventually ending up with the colonic tumor formation.

2.3.2. Core Genes Expression in the Colonic Tissue of Mice with Acute Colitis and CAC

Finally, the expression of the revealed hub genes related to acute colitis (*C3*, *Tyrobp*, *Mmp3*, *Mmp9*, *Timp1*) and CAC (*Timp1*, *Adam8*, *Mmp7*, *Mmp13*) was validated by qRT-PCR in the colon tissue of mice with acute colitis and colitis-driven adenomas (Figure 3D). As expected, the expression of colitis-related genes *C3*, *Tyrobp*, *Mmp3*, *Mmp9*, and *Timp1* was significantly up-regulated in inflamed colon tissue compared with healthy controls; among them, *Mmp3* and *Timp1* were found to be the most susceptible to acute colitis induction, demonstrating 306.3- and 110.6-fold increases in the expression, respectively, in DSS-treated mice compared with healthy controls (Figure 3D). The chronification of colonic inflammation led to significant reduction in the expression of *C3*, *Tyrobp*, *Mmp3*, and *Timp1* in the adjacent to adenomas colonic tissue by 17.5, 6.6, 2.8 and 46.1 times compared with the samples from acute colitis group, and, moreover, the expression of *C3* and *Tyrobp* in this compartment decreased to the healthy level (Figure 3D). Interestingly, chronification of colitis had no obvious effect on the expression of *Mmp9*: comparable induction of this gene in both DSS- and AOM/DSS-inflamed colon tissues was observed (Figure 3D), which could indicate the important role of *Mmp9* in both acute and chronic colon inflammation, agreeing with [28]. The analysis of colonic adenomatous nodes revealed low expression of all the explored acute colitis-associated key genes: the expression levels of *C3*, *Tyrobp*, *Mmp3*, *Mmp9*, and *Timp1* in adenoma tissue were 26.3, 3.4, 20.8, 11.9, and 27.7 times lower than those in the samples with acute colitis (Figure 3D). Note that adenomatous and adjacent tissues in mice with CAC mainly differed in the expression of the following genes: *Tyrobp* and *Timp1* were found to be 1.9 and 1.7 times overexpressed in adenomas compared with the adjacent counterparts, respectively, whereas *Mmp3* and *Mmp9* were 7.6 and 13.9 times suppressed in tumor tissue, respectively (Figure 3D). Taken together, the obtained results clearly demonstrated that selected key genes associated with acute colitis indeed reached the maximum expression in the acute phase of colon inflammation, whereas chronification of the latter led to a marked decline in this parameter.

As expected, all CAC-associated hub genes (*Adam8*, *Mmp7*, *Mmp13*, and *Timp1* (mentioned above)) were characterized by significant overexpression in tumor nodes compared with healthy tissue, which confirms the expediency of their further exploration as CAC-related marker genes (Figure 3D). Interestingly, only *Mmp7* and *Mmp13* displayed a significantly higher level of activation in colon adenomas compared with both the adjacent tissue (13.8- and 13.4-fold increase, respectively) and colon tissue with acute colitis (186.4- and 19.6-fold increase, respectively). *Adam8* and *Timp1* mentioned above were also up-regulated in adenomas by 8.3 and 1.7 times compared with the adjacent tissue; however, the maximum of their expression was revealed in the acute colitis samples (86.6- and 110.6-fold increase compared with the healthy group, respectively) (Figure 3D).

Thus, the performed qRT-PCR analysis successfully confirmed the expression of the acute colitis- and CAC-related hub genes identified by the in silico analysis in corresponding murine tissues and clearly demonstrated that colitis-driven colonic adenomatous transformation is accompanied by significant changes in the expression profiles of matrix metalloproteinases, which can be used as a novel prognostic signature for colorectal neoplasia in IBD.

3. Discussion

Despite the large collection of transcriptomics data from IBD and CAC studies, molecular regulators of the transition of colonic inflammatory lesions to cancer have not yet been clearly defined. The current study aimed to reveal core genes involved in the regulation of acute colitis and CAC development in mice and to explore how far their expression profiles changed during the chronification of colon inflammation.

Performed bioinformatics analysis of multiple cDNA microarray datasets of acute colitis and CAC identified a range of core genes associated with the explored pathologies, further functional annotation of which clearly confirmed the reliability of the obtained data. Indeed, high enrichment of acute colitis-related functional terms with pro-inflammatory cytokines and IGF1-Akt signaling pathway (Figure 1C, upper network) agrees well with the proven regulatory role of the latter in colon inflammation and inflammation-induced mucosal injury [29,30]. Along with this, CAC-related core genes were associated with the processes which markedly changed during colitis-driven tumorigenesis (Figure 1C, lower network): it is known that dysplastic and malignant lesions of colon tissue markedly dysregulate sodium transport [31], bile acid secretion [32], and metabolic [33] and oxidative [34] homeostasis.

Interestingly, the analysis of core genes common for both acute colitis and CAC (Figure 1E) also demonstrated the credibility of the performed in silico study. According to the published reports, the acute-phase genes *Hp*, *Lcn2*, *Lrg1*, and *Serpina3n* included in this list are not only activated in response to inflammatory stimuli, but their aberrant expression is also strongly implicated in tumorigenesis: high levels of *Hp* and *Lcn2* resulted in glucose metabolic dysfunction, angiogenesis, and metastasis in different tumor types [35,36], and

Lrg1 and *Serpina3n* were associated with epithelial–mesenchymal transition in colorectal cancer [37,38]. In addition, the interferon-responsive gene *Ifitm3* is critical to early colon cancer development [12,39], along with *S100a9* and *Slpi*, which, when highly expressed in inflamed colon tissues in mice and patients with colitis and IBD, respectively, can be considered as potent amplifiers of tumor invasion [40,41].

Analysis of gene association networks with subsequent processing of obtained results using the text mining approach revealed a range of core genes occupied hub positions in the acute colitis- and CAC-associated regulomes, which had not yet been extensively studied in relation to the explored diseases (acute colitis: *C3*, *Tyrobp*, *Mmp3*; CAC: *Adam8*, *Mmp13*) (Figure 2). Further qRT-PCR analysis clearly confirmed the overexpression of the mentioned hub genes in the colon tissue of mice with acute colitis and CAC (Figure 3D) that indicated the expediency of further exploration of these genes as promising novel biomarkers of colon inflammation and colon tumorigenesis.

To independently examine how tightly revealed hub genes were associated with inflammation and colorectal cancer, their sub-networks with first gene neighbors from rodent inflammatome [42] and the gene network related to malignant tumors of the colon (DisGeNET ID: C00071202) were reconstructed and analyzed. As depicted in Figure 4, all explored hub genes, except for *Adam8*, indeed form tight modules with gene partners within the evaluated regulomes, and are related to diverse processes and signaling pathways important for the pathogenesis of colitis and CAC. For instance, the detection of the functional group "Interleukin-4 and 13 signaling" is in accordance with [43]: a marked IL-13 response from CD4+ natural killer T cells was previously detected in mice with oxazolone-induced colitis and its blockage was found to ameliorate intestinal inflammation and injury. The members of the integrin family (Figure 4A, Timp1-, C3- and Mmp3-centered sub-networks) play a crucial role in the intestinal homing of immune cells and in supporting the inflammatory mechanisms in the gut [44]. uPA-mediated signaling (Figure 4, Timp1-, Mmp3-, Mmp9-centered sub-networks) controls macrophage phagocytosis in intestinal inflammation, and uPA receptor deficiency leads to marked aggravation of experimental colitis in mice [45]. Moreover, uPA-/- mice demonstrated more severe colorectal neoplasia compared with their wild-type littermates [46]. In addition, remodeling of the extracellular matrix is a hallmark of both colitis/IBD [47] and CAC [48], and prostaglandin signaling is involved in the malignant transformation of inflamed intestinal tissue [49].

The detailed comparison of obtained results revealed a group of MMPs as key participants of acute colon inflammation and its transition to malignancy: functional term "Matrix Metalloproteinases" was identified as statistically significant in both acute colitis- and CAC-associated functional annotation maps (Figure 1C), the highly interconnected cluster of MMPs related to different phases of colitis was revealed in the gene network retrieved from computed core genes (Figure 1F), and MMPs occupied hub positions in all analyzed regulomes related to both acute colitis (Figure 2A: *Mmp3*, *Mmp9*) and CAC (Figure 2B: *Mmp7*, *Mmp13*). Interestingly, the tissue inhibitor of matrix metalloproteinase-1 (*Timp1*) was also detected as a hub gene specific to both acute colitis and CAC (Figures 1E and 2A,B) and tightly interconnected with MMPs module (Figure 1F), which clearly indicated the importance of Timp1/MMPs balance in colitis-induced tumorigenesis. Indeed, Timp1 is a known regulator of colitis, knockout of which markedly attenuated fibrosis in DSS-inflamed colon tissue [50], and, according to the recent report of Niu et al. [51], a hub gene in colorectal cancer regulome. High expression of MMP3 and MMP9 in mucosa-resident macrophages/neutrophils and IgG plasma cells was detected in patients with IBD [52,53]. According to Pedersen et al. [54], MMP3 and MMP9 are two key enzymes involved in the degradation of intestinal tissue during IBD. Interestingly, the silencing of Mmp3 by siRNA markedly ameliorated DSS-induced colitis in mice [55], whereas knockout of Mmp9 or its pharmacological inhibition surprisingly had no obvious effect on the progression of DSS- and TNBS-stimulated colitis in the murine model [56]. Thus, the master regulatory functions of MMPs in colitis pathogenesis require further clarification: in some cases, their overexpression can be considered as a consequence rather than a cause of intestinal inflammation [56]. In the case of CAC-associated MMPs (*Mmp7*, *Mmp13*) revealed in this study, focal high expression of *Mmp7* was previously observed in CAC-related dysplastic lesions [48] and its overexpression was associated with tumor growth, metastasis, and worse overall survival in patients with colon cancer [57]. According to Wernicke et al. [58], the up-regulation of MMP-13 was considered as an early predictive cancer biomarker in patients with colon adenoma, which agrees well with the results of our qRT-PCR analysis (Figure 3D). Despite the extensive studies of MMPs as candidate marker genes of colitis and CAC, to the best of our knowledge, the complex evaluation of the expression of *Mmp3*, *Mmp7*, *Mmp9*, and *Mmp13* in acutely inflamed, adenomatous, and adjacent colon tissues has not yet been reported. Revealed marked changes in their expression profiles during chronification of colitis (Figure 3D) can be considered as a novel gene signature for predicting CAC.

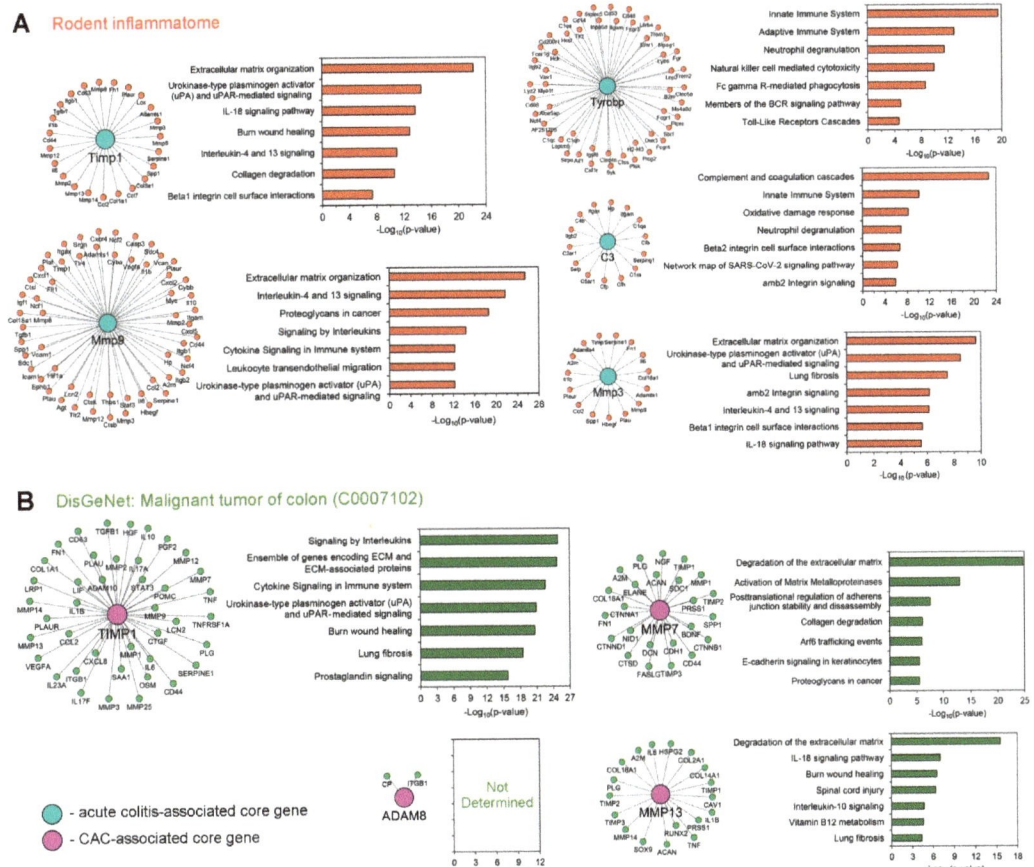

Figure 4. The involvement of the identified acute colitis- and CAC-related hub genes in murine inflammatome (**A**) and the gene network associated with malignant tumor of the colon, retrieved from DisGeNET (**B**). The modules containing the explored genes with their gene partners were extracted from gene networks created using the STRING database and visualized using Cytoscape, according to Section 4.3. Functional analysis of gene modules was performed using the ToppFun tool.

Besides MMPs, another ECM remodeling player, *Adam8*, a member of a disintegrin and metalloproteinase family (ADAMs), was identified as a core gene associated with

CAC development (Figures 1F, 2D and 3D). Surprisingly, high expression of *Adam8* was detected not only in CAC but also in DSS-inflamed colon tissue (Figure 3D). Along with the reorganization of ECM, ADAMs are engaged in the processing of various substrates, including cytokines, growth factors, cell adhesion molecules, and receptors, that determines their important role in a range of pathological processes [59]. The most studied ADAMs in IBD was Adam17, associated with EGFR and STAT3 signaling pathways crucial for the pathogenesis of colitis [60], high epithelial expression of which positively correlated with cell proliferation and goblet cell number in UC patients [61]. To the best of our knowledge, the involvement of *Adam8* in the regulation of acute colitis and colitis-induced adenomatous transformation of colon tissue had not yet been reported. Only Christophi et al. and Guo et al. have discussed the overexpression of *Adam8* in IBD patients [62] and AOM/DSS-induced colitis in mice [63]. Given the recently demonstrated ability of Adam8 to control neutrophil transmigration [64] and NLRP3 inflammasome activation [65], the processes tightly associated with colon inflammation [66,67], Adam8 can be considered as a novel promising master regulator of colitis and CAC; this requires further clarification. Interestingly, despite the revealed low interconnection of Adam8 with the colon cancer-associated gene network retrieved from DisGeNET (Figure 4), this gene seems to play an important role in the pathogenesis of CAC: Adam8 is involved in the activation of integrin, FAK, ERK1/2, and Akt/PKB signaling pathways related to cancer progression [68], its overexpression was identified in colorectal cancer compared with adjacent normal tissues [69], and the suppression of the expression of *Adam8* by knockout or siRNA approaches resulted in reduced proliferation and invasiveness of colon cancer cells [69,70].

Finally, *C3* and *Tyrobp* were also revealed as colitis-specific hub genes (Figures 2A and 3D), which is in line with published reports. Previously, a high level of C3 in the serum and jejunal secretion of IBD patients was identified [71,72]. Moreover, C3 was found to be up-regulated in intestinal epithelial cells in the DSS-induced colitis model [73], and its ablation promoted inflammatory responses in the mid colon [74] and significantly reinforced DSS-induced colitis in C3 knockout mice compared with wild-type littermates [72]. Tyrobp is a known regulator of the production of pro-inflammatory mediators in macrophages and neutrophils [75], and, thus, is implicated in pathogenesis of various inflammation-associated diseases [75–77]. According to recent studies, Tyrobp was identified as a probable upstream regulator of UC [78], and its knockout robustly attenuated the severity of DSS-induced colitis in mice, whereas its overexpression resulted in a striking exacerbation of colon damage caused by DSS [79].

The published works discussed above demonstrated the involvement of the revealed core genes in the regulation of inflammation and malignant lesion of the colon, not only in murine models but also in patients. To independently confirm the translational bridge between our findings and the pathogenesis of colitis/CAC in humans, expression of core genes (acute colitis: *C3*, *Tyrobp*, *Mmp3*, *Mmp9*, *Timp1*; CAC: *Timp1*, *Mmp7*, *Mmp13*, *Adam8*) was further evaluated in the transcriptomics profiles of colon tissue from patients with UC and CD collected from GEO (Figure 5A) and colorectal cancer retrieved from The Cancer Genome Atlas (TCGA) (Figure 5B). As depicted in Figure 5A, the majority of the explored key genes were overexpressed in IBD and demonstrated more pronounced susceptibility to the induction of UC compared with CD, except for *TYROBP*, expression of which was more up-regulated in CD patients. Interestingly, despite the proven association with CAC (Figure 2B,D), *TIMP1*, *MMP7*, and *ADAM8* were activated in IBD-affected colon tissues (Figure 5A), which is fully in line with our data: the high expression of these genes was demonstrated in DSS-inflamed and adjacent to adenomas colon tissues in mice (Figure 3D). In addition, similar to our results (Figure 3D), CAC-specific MMP13 was found to be slightly associated with IBD: its low activation in two of the four analyzed UC transcriptomics datasets and unchanged levels in CD samples were observed (Figure 5A). Presumably, Mmp13 plays a minor role in ECM remodeling in colitis, whereas CAC was associated with significant up-regulation of its expression, which makes *Mmp13* a promising gene candidate for the predicting of colitis-associated tumorigenesis; this requires further detailed study.

TCGA analysis of the identified CAC-related core genes revealed a significant association between high expression of *TIMP1* and *ADAM8* with low overall survival of patients with both colon (COAD) and rectal (READ) adenocarcinomas (Figure 5B). Despite the finding that Timp1 and Adam8 can play important regulatory functions in CAC, this supposition requires further detailed confirmation, since TCGA analysis was performed without consideration of the ratio of UC- and CD-associated CAC patients in COAD and READ cohorts. In addition, given recently reported sex disparities in the association of Timp1 expression with cancer progression [80], further exploration of its regulatory role in CAC in mice of both sexes is needed.

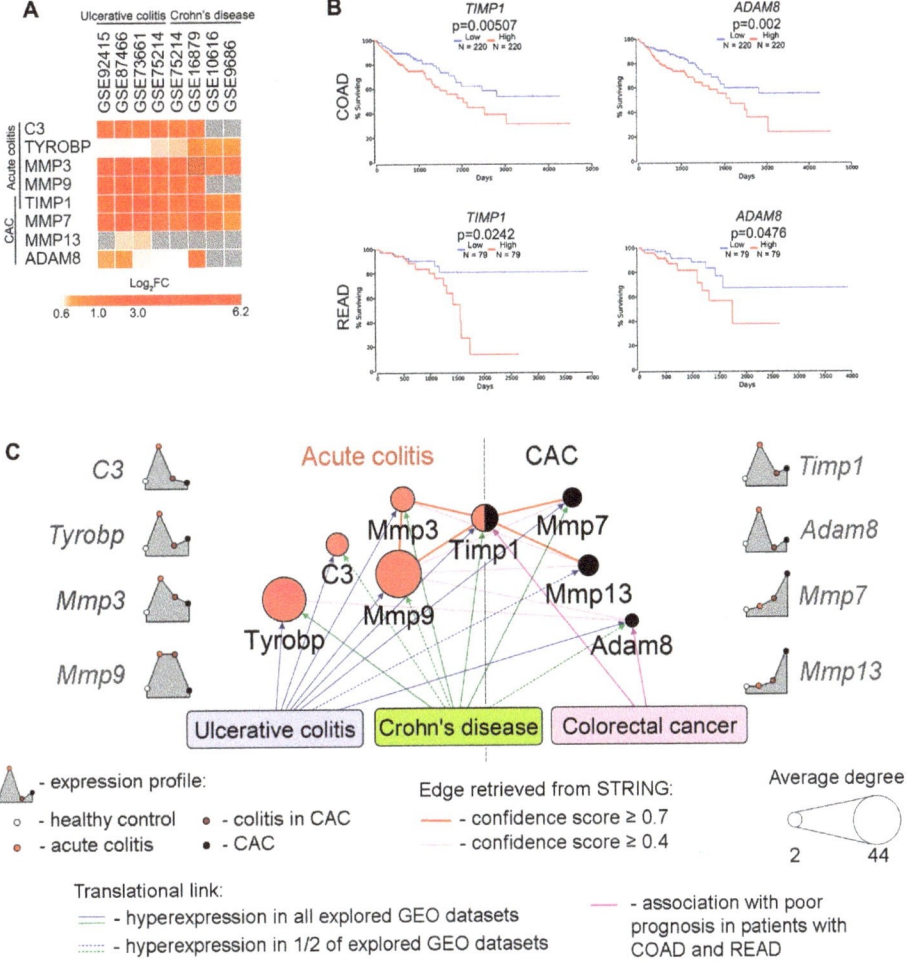

Figure 5. Expression levels of identified DEGs in human patients with inflammatory bowel diseases (ulcerative colitis and Crohn's disease) and their association with the survival of patients with colon adenocarcinoma (COAD) and rectal adenocarcinoma (READ). (**A**) Heatmap demonstrating the expression levels of identified acute colitis- and CAC-related hub genes in datasets of human patients

with ulcerative colitis and Crohn's disease. The differential analysis of cDNA microarray data was performed according to Section 4.1. The heat map was constructed using Morpheus. $Log_2 FC = Log_2$(fold change). In all datasets, biopsy samples were taken from the colon at the sites of active inflammation. (**B**) Survival of patients with COAD and READ depending on the expression levels of identified DEGs (*TIMP1* and *ADAM8*) in the colon tissue. Kaplan–Meier survival curves were constructed using TCGA data according to Section 4.8. (**C**) The final scheme of core genes associated with acute colitis and CAC revealed in the current study, their expression profiles in murine models, and association with IBD and colorectal cancer in humans.

The obtained results were finally summarized in the scheme depicted in Figure 5C. According to our findings, (a) revealed core genes not only occupy hub positions within explored acute colitis- and CAC-specific regulomes, but also are interconnected with each other, (b) *Timp1* is identified as a hub node in gene association networks retrieved for both acute colitis and CAC, which can indicate its crucial role in colitis-associated tumorigenesis, (c) chronification of colonic inflammation is accompanied by a switch in MMPs profile (acute colitis: *Mmp3*, *Mmp9*; CAC: *Mmp7*, *Mmp13*), which can serve as a gene signature panel for prognosis of malignant transformation of inflamed colon tissue; and (d) identified core genes are overexpressed in the colon tissue of patients with IBD (all explored genes) and highly aggressive colorectal cancer (*TIMP1*, *ADAM8*), confirming the interest in studying these genes within the framework of intestinal pathologies in humans (Figure 5C).

Limitations of the Study

The limitations of the study are as follows: First, given the relatively low number of mice used for experimental validation of the obtained data ($n = 6$), and their belonging to only one sex (female) and one strain (C57Bl6), further study is required to validate the results using a larger sample size obtained from mice of both sexes and different strains. Second, considering that our findings are predominantly animal-based, to more clearly elucidate how closely (if at all) the identified core genes are involved in the regulation of intestinal pathologies in humans, revealed translational bridge needs further large-scale verification study, using clinical samples of patients with UC, CD, and UC/CD-associated colorectal cancer. Third, despite the identification of high degree centrality scores of the explored key genes and their tight association with crucial colitis/CAC-related signaling pathways, the master regulatory functions of these genes in colitis and CAC should be further verified experimentally (for instance, using knockout models).

4. Materials and Methods

4.1. Microarray Data Collection and Differential Expression Analysis

The gene expression profiles associated with murine acute colitis and CAC, as well as ulcerative colitis and Crohn's disease, in patients were acquired from the Gene Expression Omnibus database [81] (Table 1). The fold changes between the mean expression values of the genes in the experimental (pathology) versus control groups were computed using the GEO2R tool [82]. The Benjamini–Hochberg false discovery rate method was selected for adjusting *p*-values. The genes with a *p*-value < 0.05 and |fold change| > 1.5 were identified as differentially expressed genes (DEGs) and were collected for further analysis. Overlapping of the DEGs from different datasets was performed using the InteractiVenn tool [83]. Hierarchical clustering of DEGs according to their expression profiles was carried out using the Euclidean distance metric, using the Morpheus tool (https://software.broadinstitute.org/morpheus, accessed on 12 December 2022).

Table 1. The GEO microarray datasets used in the study.

Object	Pathology	GEO ID	Murine Strain	Sex	Analyzed Groups	Number of DSS Cycles
Mice	Acute colitis	GSE31106	ICR	m	3 untreated mice, 3 AOM/DSS-treated mice	1
		GSE35609	ICR	f	4 untreated mice, 4 TNBS-treated mice	–
		GSE42768	C57Bl6	f	3 untreated mice, 3 DSS-treated mice	1
		GSE64658	C57Bl6	f	6 untreated mice, 3 AOM/DSS-treated mice	1
		GSE71920	C57Bl6	m	3 untreated mice, 3 DSS-treated mice	1
	CAC	GSE31106	ICR	m	3 untreated mice, 3 AOM/DSS-treated mice	3
		GSE42768	C57Bl6	f	3 untreated mice, 3 DSS-treated mice	3
		GSE56050	Lrg5-lacZ	m	2 untreated mice, 2 AOM/DSS-treated mice	3
		GSE64658	C57Bl6	f	6 untreated mice, 6 AOM/DSS-treated mice	3
Humans	Ulcerative colitis (UC)	GSE73661	–	f, m	12 healthy samples, 67 UC samples	–
		GSE75214	–	f, m	11 healthy samples, 74 UC samples	–
		GSE87466	–	f, m	21 healthy samples, 27 UC samples	–
		GSE92415	–	f, m	21 healthy samples, 87 UC samples	–
	Crohn's disease (CD)	GSE9686	–	f, m	8 healthy samples, 11 CD samples	–
		GSE10616	–	f, m	26 healthy samples, 18 CD samples	–
		GSE16879	–	f, m	6 healthy samples, 18 CD samples	–
		GSE75214	–	f, m	11 healthy samples, 59 CD samples	–

4.2. Functional Analysis of DEGs

Functional annotation of acute colitis- and CAC-associated DEGs was performed using the ClueGO 2.5.7 plugin in Cytoscape 3.7.2, using the latest updates of Gene Ontology (Biological Processes), Kyoto Encyclopedia of Genes and Genomes (KEGG), WikiPathways, and REACTOME databases. The GO Tree interval was ranged from 3 to 8 and the minimum number of genes per cluster was set to 3. Enrichment of functional terms was tested using the two-sided hypergeometric test corrected using the Bonferroni method, followed by selecting significantly enriched terms with a p-value < 0.05. To cluster similar functional groups retrieved from different databases in the common pathway-specific modules, the GO Term Fusion was used. Functional grouping of finally selected functional terms was performed using kappa statistics (kappa score $\geq$ 0.4). Functional annotation of gene modules, consisting of core genes and their first gene partners extracted from murine inflammatome and colon cancer-related regulome, was performed using the ToppFun tool (databases: KEGG, REACTOME, MSigDB C2 BIOCARTA, BioSystems: Pathway Interaction Database, Pathway Ontology; Bonferroni adjustment) [84].

4.3. Reconstruction of Gene Association Networks

Gene association networks were reconstructed from the genes of interest using the Search Tool for the Retrieval of Interaction Genes (STRING) database, using the stringApp 1.5.1 tool [85], and were visualized using Cytoscape 3.7.2. The cutoff criterion of the confidence score was set as >0.7 to eliminate inconsistent "gene–gene" pairs from the dataset. The number of neighbors of a gene of interest within reconstructed networks was calculated using the NetworkAnalyzer plugin [86] and visualized using the Morpheus platform [87].

4.4. Data Mining Analysis

The search for the co-occurrence of the names of core genes with various colitis- and CAC-related terms in the same sentences in abstracts of published reports deposited in the MEDLINE database was performed using the GenCLiP3 tool [88], with the following settings: impact factor of 0–50 and year of publication of 1992–2022. The results were visualized using Circos [89].

4.5. Murine Models of Acute Colitis and Colitis-Associated Cancer (CAC)

Eight-week-old female C57Bl6 mice with an average weight of 22–24 g were obtained from the Vivarium of the Institute of Chemical Biology and Fundamental Medicine SB RAS (Novosibirsk, Russia). Mice were housed in plastic cages (7 animals per cage) under normal daylight conditions. Water and food were provided ad libitum. Experiments were carried out in accordance with the European Communities Council Directive 86/609/CEE. The experimental protocols were approved by the Committee on the Ethics of Animal Experiments at the Institute of Cytology and Genetics SB RAS (Novosibirsk, Russia) (protocol No. 56 from 10 August 2019).

Acute colitis was induced in mice ($n = 10$) by administration of 2.5% DSS solution in drinking water for 7 days, followed by 3 days of recovery. Mice were sacrificed on day 10 after colitis initiation. CAC was induced in mice ($n = 10$) by a single intraperitoneal (i.p.) injection of carcinogen AOM (10 mg/kg) 1 week before DSS administration, as described in [90]. Furthermore, mice were exposed to 3 consecutive cycles of 1.5% DSS instillations with drinking water for 7 days, followed by 2 weeks of recovery. The mice were sacrificed 10 weeks after the start of the experiment. At the end of the study, the colons were separated from the proximal rectum, mechanically cleaned with saline buffer, and were then collected. Only 8 of 10 samples had well-formed adenomas in the colon, which were selected for the subsequent gross examination, histological analysis, and qRT–PCR.

4.6. Histology

For the histological study, colon specimens were fixed in 10% neutral-buffered formalin (BioVitrum, Moscow, Russia), dehydrated in ascending ethanol and xylols, and embedded in HISTOMIX paraffin (BioVitrum, Moscow, Russia). The paraffin sections (5 μm) were sliced on a Microm HM 355S microtome (Thermo Fisher Scientific, Waltham, MA, USA) and stained with haematoxylin and eosin. The images were examined and scanned using an Axiostar Plus microscope equipped with an Axiocam MRc5 digital camera (Zeiss, Oberkochen, Germany) at magnifications of $\times 100$.

4.7. Quantitative Real-Time PCR (qRT-PCR)

Total RNA was isolated from the colons of experimental animals using TRIzol reagent (Ambion, Austin, TX, USA) according to the manufacturer's instructions. Briefly, colon tissue was collected in 1.5 mL capped tubes, filled with 1 g of lysing matrix D (MP Biomedicals, Irvine, CA, USA) and 1 mL of TRIzol reagent, then homogenized using a FastPrep-24 TM 5G homogenizer (MP Biomedicals, Irvine, CA, USA) with QuickPrep 24 adapter. The homogenization was performed at 6.0 m/s for 40 s. After homogenization, the content of the tubes was transferred to the new 1.5 mL tubes without lysing matrix. Total RNA extraction was performed according to the TRIzol reagent protocol.

Due to the known ability of DSS to linger in the RNA extracted from the colon tissue, and, thus, interfere with both reverse transcription and PCR reactions, the extracted total RNA was diluted to a volume of 250 μL and purified using Microcon Centrifugal Filter Devices (MilliPore, Burlington, MA, USA) by centrifuging for 1 h at $14,000 \times g$.

The first strand of cDNA was synthesized from total RNA ($n = 6$ per group, the samples with the highest RNA purity and integrity) in 100 µL of reaction mixture containing 2.5 µg of total RNA, 20 µL of 5× RT buffer (Biolabmix, Novosibirsk, Russia), 250 U of M-MuLV-RH revertase (Biolabmix, Novosibirsk, Russia), and 100 µM of dT(15) diluted to a volume of 100 µL. Reverse transcription was performed at 25 °C for 10 min followed by the incubation at 42 °C for 60 min with subsequent termination at 70 °C for 10 min.

Amplification of cDNA was performed in a 25 µL PCR reaction mixture containing 5 µL of cDNA, 12.5 µL of HS-qPCR (2×) master mix (Biolabmix, Novosibirsk, Russia), 0.25 µM each of the forward and reverse primers to *Hprt* and *Hprt* specific ROX-labeled probe, 0.25 µM each of the forward and reverse gene-specific primers, and FAM-labeled probe (Table 2). Amplification was performed as follows: (1) 94 °C, 2 min; (2) 94 °C, 10 s; (3) 60 °C, 30 s (steps 2–3: 50 cycles). The relative level of gene expression was normalized to the level of *Hprt* expression according to the ∆∆Ct method.

Table 2. Primers used in the study.

Gene	Type	Sequence
Adam8	Forward	5′-TATGCAACCACAAGAGGGAG-3′
	Probe	5′-((5,6)-FAM)-TCATCTGATACATCTGCCAGCCGC-3′–BHQ1
	Reverse	5′-ACCAAGACCACAACCACAC-3′
C3	Forward	5′-GTTTATTCCTTCATTTCGCCTGG-3′
	Probe	5′-((5,6)-FAM)-ACACCCTGATTGGAGCTAGTGGC-3′–BHQ1
	Reverse	5′-GATGGTTATCTCTTGGGTCACC-3′
Timp1	Forward	5′-CTCAAAGACCTATAGTGCTGGC-3′
	Probe	5′-((5,6)-FAM)-ACTCACTGTTTGTGGACGGATCAGG-3′–BHQ1
	Reverse	5′-CAAAGTGACGGCTCTGGTAG-3′
Tyrobp	Forward	5′-GGTGACTTGGTGTTGACTCTG-3′
	Probe	5′-((5,6)-FAM)-CCTTCCGCTGTCCCTTGACCTC-3′–BHQ1
	Reverse	5′-GACCCTGAAGCTCCTGATAAG-3′
Mmp3	Forward	5′-TGCATATGAGGTTACTAACAGAGAC-3′
	Probe	((5,6)-FAM)-5′-AATCAGTTCTGGGCTATACGAGGGC-3′–BHQ1
	Reverse	5′-CAGGGTGTGAATGCTTTTAGG-3′
Mmp7	Forward	5′-CATAATTGGCTTCGCAAGGAG-3′
	Probe	((5,6)-FAM)-5′-TACTGGACTGATGGTGAGGACGCA-3′–BHQ1
	Reverse	5′-CAAATTCATGGGTGGCAGC-3′
Mmp9	Forward	5′-ACCTGAAAACCTCCAACCTC-3′
	Probe	((5,6)-FAM)-5′-TAGCGGTACAAGTATGCCTCTGCC-3′–BHQ1
	Reverse	5′-TCGAATGGCCTTTAGTGTCTG-3′
Mmp13	Forward	5′-GATTATCCCCGCCTCATAGAAG-3′
	Probe	((5,6)-FAM)-5′-CAGCATCTACTTTGTTGCCAATTCCAGG-3′–BHQ1
	Reverse	5′-CCCACCCCATACATCTGAAAG-3′

Amplification was performed using a C1000 Touch with CFX96 module Real-Time system (BioRad, Hercules, CA, USA), and the relative level of gene expression was calculated using BioRad CFX manager software (BioRad, Hercules, CA, USA). Three to five samples from each experimental group were analyzed in triplicate. The sequences of the primers used in the study are listed in Table 2.

4.8. The Association of DEGs Expression with Survival Rates of Patients with Colorectal Cancer

To explore the association of revealed core genes with the progression of colon (COAD) and rectal (READ) adenocarcinomas, analysis of the survival rates and their correlation with the expression of studied genes was performed using The Cancer Genome Atlas (TCGA) clinical data for patients with COAD and READ. Kaplan–Meier survival curves for

COAD and READ patients depending on the mRNA expression level of core genes were constructed using the OncoLnc tool [91].

4.9. Statistical Analysis

The statistical analysis was performed using Benjamini–Hochberg false discovery rate method (identification of DEGs; GEO2R tool), two-sided hypergeometric test with Bonferroni correction (functional analysis of DEGs; ClueGO plugin and ToppFunn tool), and two-tailed unpaired Student's *t*-test (qRT-PCR analysis; Microsoft Excel). *p*-values of less than 0.05 were considered statistically significant.

5. Conclusions

In summary, this animal-based research revealed a range of core genes associated with acute colitis (*C3*, *Tyrobp*, *Mmp3*, *Mmp9*, *Timp1*) and CAC (*Timp1*, *Mmp7*, *Mmp13*) in mice. The observed high rate of interconnection of these genes with gene networks retrieved for intestinal inflammation and malignancy, their significant association with key colitis/CAC-related signaling pathways, and probable involvement in the pathogenesis of IBD and colorectal cancer in patients demonstrated the expediency of further detailed studies of identified core genes as novel master regulators and promising therapeutic targets for colitis and CAC.

Author Contributions: Conceptualization, A.V.M.; methodology, A.V.M. and A.V.S.; software, A.V.M.; validation, I.A.S. and A.V.S.; formal analysis, A.V.M., I.A.S., and A.V.S.; investigation, A.V.M., I.A.S., and A.V.S.; resources, A.V.M. and M.A.Z.; data curation, A.V.M. and A.V.S.; writing—original draft preparation, A.V.M. and A.V.S.; writing—review and editing, M.A.Z.; visualization, A.V.M. and A.V.S.; supervision, M.A.Z.; project administration, A.V.M.; funding acquisition, M.A.Z. All authors have read and agreed to the published version of the manuscript.

Funding: This research was funded by the Russian Science Foundation (Grant No. 19–74–30011) and the Russian state-funded budget project of ICBFM SB RAS No. 121031300044–5.

Institutional Review Board Statement: Animal studies were carried out in accordance with the European Communities Council Directive 86/609/CEE. The experimental protocols were approved by the Committee on the Ethics of Animal Experiments at the Institute of Cytology and Genetics SB RAS (Novosibirsk, Russia) (protocol No. 56 from 10 August 2019).

Informed Consent Statement: Not applicable since only public cDNA microarray datasets deposited in the Gene Expression Omnibus database were used.

Data Availability Statement: The data presented in this study are openly available on the Gene Expression Omnibus database. Reference numbers: GSE31106, GSE35609, GSE42768, GSE64658, GSE71920, GSE31106, GSE42768, GSE56050, GSE64658, GSE73661, GSE75214, GSE87466, GSE92415, GSE9686, GSE10616, GSE16879, and GSE75214.

Acknowledgments: The authors gratefully thank Anton V. Filatov (Institute of Chemical Biology and Fundamental Medicine SB RAS, Novosibirsk, Russia) for help with the GEO datasets analysis.

Conflicts of Interest: The authors declare no conflict of interest.

References

1. Bardou, M.; Rouland, A.; Martel, M.; Loffroy, R.; Barkun, A.N.; Chapelle, N. Review: Obesity and colorectal cancer. *Aliment. Pharmacol. Ther.* **2022**, *56*, 407–418. [CrossRef]
2. Dai, Z.H.; Tang, M.; Chen, Y.L.; Zhang, T.L.; Li, J.; Lv, G.H.; Yan, Y.G.; Ouyang, Z.H.; Huang, W.; Zou, M.X. Incidence and Risk Factors for Cerebrovascular-Specific Mortality in Patients with Colorectal Cancer: A Registry-Based Cohort Study Involving 563,298 Patients. *Cancers* **2022**, *14*, 2053. [CrossRef]
3. Majumder, S.; Shivaji, U.N.; Kasturi, R.; Sigamani, A.; Ghosh, S.; Iacucci, M. Inflammatory bowel disease-related colorectal cancer: Past, present and future perspectives. *World J. Gastrointest. Oncol.* **2022**, *14*, 547. [CrossRef] [PubMed]
4. Grivennikov, S.I. Inflammation and colorectal cancer: Colitis-associated neoplasia. *Semin. Immunopathol.* **2013**, *35*, 229–244. [CrossRef] [PubMed]
5. M'koma, A.E. Inflammatory Bowel Disease: Clinical Diagnosis and Surgical Treatment-Overview. *Medicina* **2022**, *58*, 567. [CrossRef] [PubMed]

6. Hsiao, S.-W.; Yen, H.-H.; Chen, Y.-Y. Chemoprevention of Colitis-Associated Dysplasia or Cancer in Inflammatory Bowel Disease. *Gut Liver* **2022**, *16*, 840–848. [CrossRef] [PubMed]
7. Iwanaga, K.; Nakamura, T.; Maeda, S.; Aritake, K.; Hori, M.; Urade, Y.; Ozaki, H.; Murata, T. Mast cell-derived prostaglandin D2 inhibits colitis and colitis-associated colon cancer in mice. *Cancer Res.* **2014**, *74*, 3011–3019. [CrossRef]
8. Shah, S.C.; Itzkowitz, S.H. Colorectal Cancer in Inflammatory Bowel Disease: Mechanisms and Management. *Gastroenterology* **2022**, *162*, 715–730.e3. [CrossRef]
9. Frigerio, S.; Lartey, D.A.; D'haens, G.R.; Grootjans, J. The Role of the Immune System in IBD-Associated Colorectal Cancer: From Pro to Anti-Tumorigenic Mechanisms. *Int. J. Mol. Sci.* **2021**, *22*, 12739. [CrossRef]
10. Rogler, G. Chronic ulcerative colitis and colorectal cancer. *Cancer Lett.* **2014**, *345*, 235–241. [CrossRef]
11. Matson, J.; Ramamoorthy, S.; Lopez, N.E. The Role of Biomarkers in Surgery for Ulcerative Colitis: A Review. *J. Clin. Med.* **2021**, *10*, 3362. [CrossRef] [PubMed]
12. Suzuki, R.; Miyamoto, S.; Yasui, Y.; Sugie, S.; Tanaka, T. Global gene expression analysis of the mouse colonic mucosa treated with azoxymethane and dextran sodium sulfate. *BMC Cancer* **2007**, *7*, 84. [CrossRef] [PubMed]
13. Shi, L.; Han, X.; Li, J.-X.; Liao, Y.-T.; Kou, F.-S.; Wang, Z.-B.; Shi, R.; Zhao, X.-J.; Sun, Z.-M.; Hao, Y. Identification of differentially expressed genes in ulcerative colitis and verification in a colitis mouse model by bioinformatics analyses. *World J. Gastroenterol.* **2020**, *26*, 5983–5996. [CrossRef] [PubMed]
14. Xiu, M.; Liu, Y.; Chen, G.; Hu, C.; Kuang, B. Identifying Hub Genes, Key Pathways and Immune Cell Infiltration Characteristics in Pediatric and Adult Ulcerative Colitis by Integrated Bioinformatic Analysis. *Dig. Dis. Sci.* **2021**, *66*, 3002–3014. [CrossRef] [PubMed]
15. Lu, C.; Zhang, X.; Luo, Y.; Huang, J.; Yu, M. Identification of CXCL10 and CXCL11 as the candidate genes involving the development of colitis-associated colorectal cancer. *Front. Genet.* **2022**, *13*, 945414. [CrossRef] [PubMed]
16. Xu, M.; Kong, Y.; Chen, N.; Peng, W.; Zi, R.; Jiang, M.; Zhu, J.; Wang, Y.; Yue, J.; Lv, J.; et al. Identification of Immune-Related Gene Signature and Prediction of CeRNA Network in Active Ulcerative Colitis. *Front. Immunol.* **2022**, *13*, 855645. [CrossRef]
17. Cheng, C.; Hua, J.; Tan, J.; Qian, W.; Zhang, L.; Hou, X. Identification of differentially expressed genes, associated functional terms pathways, and candidate diagnostic biomarkers in inflammatory bowel diseases by bioinformatics analysis. *Exp. Ther. Med.* **2019**, *18*, 278–288. [CrossRef]
18. Hu, W.; Fang, T.; Chen, X. Identification of Differentially Expressed Genes and miRNAs for Ulcerative Colitis Using Bioinformatics Analysis. *Front. Genet.* **2022**, *13*, 914384. [CrossRef]
19. Zhang, J.; Wang, X.; Xu, L.; Zhang, Z.; Wang, F.; Tang, X. Investigation of Potential Genetic Biomarkers and Molecular Mechanism of Ulcerative Colitis Utilizing Bioinformatics Analysis. *Biomed. Res. Int.* **2020**, *2020*, 4921387. [CrossRef]
20. Shi, W.; Zou, R.; Yang, M.; Mai, L.; Ren, J.; Wen, J.; Liu, Z.; Lai, R. Analysis of Genes Involved in Ulcerative Colitis Activity and Tumorigenesis Through Systematic Mining of Gene Co-expression Networks. *Front. Physiol.* **2019**, *10*, 662. [CrossRef]
21. Chen, H.-M.; MacDonald, J.A. Molecular Network Analyses Implicate Death-Associated Protein Kinase 3 (DAPK3) as a Key Factor in Colitis-Associated Dysplasia Progression. *Inflamm. Bowel Dis.* **2022**, *28*, 1485–1496. [CrossRef]
22. Ding, H.; Liu, X.; Jian-ming, X.; Qiao, M. Identification of Crucial Genes and Related Transcription Factors in Ulcerative Colitis. *Ann. Clin. Lab. Sci.* **2021**, *51*, 245–254. [PubMed]
23. Huang, Y.; Zhang, X.; Wang, P.; Li, Y.; Yao, J. Identification of hub genes and pathways in colitis-associated colon cancer by integrated bioinformatic analysis. *BMC Genom. Data* **2022**, *23*, 48. [CrossRef] [PubMed]
24. Szklarczyk, D.; Gable, A.L.; Nastou, K.C.; Lyon, D.; Kirsch, R.; Pyysalo, S.; Doncheva, N.T.; Legeay, M.; Fang, T.; Bork, P.; et al. The STRING database in 2021: Customizable protein–protein networks, and functional characterization of user-uploaded gene/measurement sets. *Nucleic Acids Res.* **2021**, *49*, D605–D612. [CrossRef]
25. Markov, A.V.; Kel, A.E.; Salomatina, O.V.; Salakhutdinov, N.F.; Zenkova, M.A.; Logashenko, E.B. Deep insights into the response of human cervical carcinoma cells to a new cyano enone-bearing triterpenoid soloxolone methyl: A transcriptome analysis. *Oncotarget* **2019**, *10*, 5267–5297. [CrossRef] [PubMed]
26. Yu, D.; Lim, J.; Wang, X.; Liang, F.; Xiao, G. Enhanced construction of gene regulatory networks using hub gene information. *BMC Bioinform.* **2017**, *18*, 186. [CrossRef] [PubMed]
27. Łukaszewicz-Zając, M.; Pączek, S.; Mroczko, B. A Disintegrin and Metalloproteinase (ADAM) Family—Novel Biomarkers of Selected Gastrointestinal (GI) Malignancies? *Cancers* **2022**, *14*, 2307. [CrossRef]
28. Marônek, M.; Marafini, I.; Gardlík, R.; Link, R.; Troncone, E.; Monteleone, G. Metalloproteinases in Inflammatory Bowel Diseases. *J. Inflamm. Res.* **2021**, *14*, 1029–1041. [CrossRef] [PubMed]
29. Liu, D.; Saikam, V.; Skrada, K.A.; Merlin, D.; Iyer, S.S. Inflammatory bowel disease biomarkers. *Med. Res. Rev.* **2022**, *42*, 1856–1887. [CrossRef]
30. Guijarro, L.G.; Cano-Martínez, D.; Toledo-Lobo, M.V.; Salinas, P.S.; Chaparro, M.; Gómez-Lahoz, A.M.; Zoullas, S.; Rodríguez-Torres, R.; Román, I.D.; Monasor, L.S.; et al. Relationship between IGF-1 and body weight in inflammatory bowel diseases: Cellular and molecular mechanisms involved. *Biomed. Pharmacother.* **2021**, *144*, 112239. [CrossRef]
31. Prasad, H.; Visweswariah, S.S. Impaired Intestinal Sodium Transport in Inflammatory Bowel Disease: From the Passenger to the Driver's Seat. *Cell. Mol. Gastroenterol. Hepatol.* **2021**, *12*, 277–292. [CrossRef]
32. Camilleri, M. Bile acid detergency: Permeability, inflammation, and effects of sulfation. *Am. J. Physiol. Liver Physiol.* **2022**, *322*, G480–G488. [CrossRef] [PubMed]

33. Shen, Y.; Sun, M.; Zhu, J.; Wei, M.; Li, H.; Zhao, P.; Wang, J.; Li, R.; Tian, L.; Tao, Y.; et al. Tissue metabolic profiling reveals major metabolic alteration in colorectal cancer. *Mol. Omics* **2021**, *17*, 464–471. [CrossRef] [PubMed]
34. Cao, Y.; Deng, S.; Yan, L.; Gu, J.; Mao, F.; Xue, Y.; Zheng, C.; Yang, M.; Liu, H.; Liu, L.; et al. An Oxidative Stress Index-Based Score for Prognostic Prediction in Colorectal Cancer Patients Undergoing Surgery. *Oxid. Med. Cell. Longev.* **2021**, *2021*, 6693707. [CrossRef] [PubMed]
35. Chen, J.; Cheuk, I.W.-Y.; Siu, M.-T.; Yang, W.; Cheng, A.S.; Shin, V.Y.; Kwong, A. Human haptoglobin contributes to breast cancer oncogenesis through glycolytic activity modulation. *Am. J. Cancer Res.* **2020**, *10*, 2865–2877.
36. Santiago-Sánchez, G.S.; Pita-Grisanti, V.; Quiñones-Díaz, B.; Gumpper, K.; Cruz-Monserrate, Z.; Vivas-Mejía, P.E. Biological Functions and Therapeutic Potential of Lipocalin 2 in Cancer. *Int. J. Mol. Sci.* **2020**, *21*, 4365. [CrossRef]
37. Camilli, C.; Hoeh, A.E.; De Rossi, G.; Moss, S.E.; Greenwood, J. LRG1: An emerging player in disease pathogenesis. *J. Biomed. Sci.* **2022**, *29*, 6. [CrossRef]
38. Soman, A.; Asha Nair, S. Unfolding the cascade of SERPINA3: Inflammation to cancer. *Biochim. Biophys. Acta Rev. Cancer* **2022**, *1877*, 188760. [CrossRef]
39. Fan, J.; Peng, Z.; Zhou, C.; Qiu, G.; Tang, H.; Sun, Y.; Wang, X.; Li, Q.; Le, X.; Xie, K. Gene-expression profiling in Chinese patients with colon cancer by coupling experimental and bioinformatic genomewide gene-expression analyses. *Cancer* **2008**, *113*, 266–275. [CrossRef]
40. Shabani, F.; Farasat, A.; Mahdavi, M.; Gheibi, N. Calprotectin (S100A8/S100A9): A key protein between inflammation and cancer. *Inflamm. Res.* **2018**, *67*, 801–812. [CrossRef]
41. Nugteren, S.; Samsom, J.N. Secretory Leukocyte Protease Inhibitor (SLPI) in mucosal tissues: Protects against inflammation, but promotes cancer. *Cytokine Growth Factor Rev.* **2021**, *59*, 22–35. [CrossRef] [PubMed]
42. Wang, I.M.; Zhang, B.; Yang, X.; Zhu, J.; Stepaniants, S.; Zhang, C.; Meng, Q.; Peters, M.; He, Y.; Ni, C.; et al. Systems analysis of eleven rodent disease models reveals an inflammatome signature and key drivers. *Mol. Syst. Biol.* **2012**, *8*, 594. [CrossRef] [PubMed]
43. May, R.D.; Fung, M. Strategies targeting the IL-4/IL-13 axes in disease. *Cytokine* **2015**, *75*, 89–116. [CrossRef] [PubMed]
44. Garlatti, V.; Lovisa, S.; Danese, S.; Vetrano, S. The Multiple Faces of Integrin–ECM Interactions in Inflammatory Bowel Disease. *Int. J. Mol. Sci.* **2021**, *22*, 10439. [CrossRef]
45. Genua, M.; D'Alessio, S.; Cibella, J.; Gandelli, A.; Sala, E.; Correale, C.; Spinelli, A.; Arena, V.; Malesci, A.; Rutella, S.; et al. The urokinase plasminogen activator receptor (uPAR) controls macrophage phagocytosis in intestinal inflammation. *Gut* **2015**, *64*, 589–600. [CrossRef]
46. Karamanavi, E.; Angelopoulou, K.; Lavrentiadou, S.; Tsingotjidou, A.; Abas, Z.; Taitzoglou, I.; Vlemmas, I.; Erdman, S.E.; Poutahidis, T. Urokinase-Type Plasminogen Activator Deficiency Promotes Neoplasmatogenesis in the Colon of Mice. *Transl. Oncol.* **2014**, *7*, 174–187.e5. [CrossRef]
47. Derkacz, A.; Olczyk, P.; Olczyk, K.; Komosinska-Vassev, K. The Role of Extracellular Matrix Components in Inflammatory Bowel Diseases. *J. Clin. Med.* **2021**, *10*, 1122. [CrossRef]
48. Walter, L.; Harper, C.; Garg, P. Role of Matrix Metalloproteinases in Inflammation/Colitis-Associated Colon Cancer. *ImmunoGastroenterology* **2013**, *2*, 22. [CrossRef]
49. Wang, Q.; Morris, R.J.; Bode, A.M.; Zhang, T. Prostaglandin Pathways: Opportunities for Cancer Prevention and Therapy. *Cancer Res.* **2022**, *82*, 949–965. [CrossRef]
50. Breynaert, C.; de Bruyn, M.; Arijs, I.; Cremer, J.; Martens, E.; Van Lommel, L.; Geboes, K.; De Hertogh, G.; Schuit, F.; Ferrante, M.; et al. Genetic Deletion of Tissue Inhibitor of Metalloproteinase-1/TIMP-1 Alters Inflammation and Attenuates Fibrosis in Dextran Sodium Sulphate-induced Murine Models of Colitis. *J. Crohn's Colitis* **2016**, *10*, 1336–1350. [CrossRef]
51. Niu, L.; Gao, C.; Li, Y. Identification of potential core genes in colorectal carcinoma and key genes in colorectal cancer liver metastasis using bioinformatics analysis. *Sci. Rep.* **2021**, *11*, 23938. [CrossRef] [PubMed]
52. O'Sullivan, S.; Gilmer, J.F.; Medina, C. Matrix Metalloproteinases in Inflammatory Bowel Disease: An Update. *Mediat. Inflamm.* **2015**, *2015*, 964131. [CrossRef] [PubMed]
53. Nakov, R. New markers in ulcerative colitis. *Clin. Chim. Acta* **2019**, *497*, 141–146. [CrossRef] [PubMed]
54. Pedersen, G.; Saermark, T.; Kirkegaard, T.; Brynskov, J. Spontaneous and cytokine induced expression and activity of matrix metalloproteinases in human colonic epithelium. *Clin. Exp. Immunol.* **2009**, *155*, 257–265. [CrossRef]
55. Kobayashi, K.; Arimura, Y.; Goto, A.; Okahara, S.; Endo, T.; Shinomura, Y.; Imai, K. Therapeutic implications of the specific inhibition of causative matrix metalloproteinases in experimental colitis induced by dextran sulphate sodium. *J. Pathol.* **2006**, *209*, 376–383. [CrossRef]
56. de Bruyn, M.; Breynaert, C.; Arijs, I.; De Hertogh, G.; Geboes, K.; Thijs, G.; Matteoli, G.; Hu, J.; Van Damme, J.; Arnold, B.; et al. Inhibition of gelatinase B/MMP-9 does not attenuate colitis in murine models of inflammatory bowel disease. *Nat. Commun.* **2017**, *8*, 15384. [CrossRef]
57. Liao, H.-Y.; Da, C.-M.; Liao, B.; Zhang, H.-H. Roles of matrix metalloproteinase-7 (MMP-7) in cancer. *Clin. Biochem.* **2021**, *92*, 9–18. [CrossRef]
58. Wernicke, A.-K.; Churin, Y.; Sheridan, D.; Windhorst, A.; Tschuschner, A.; Gattenlöhner, S.; Roderfeld, M.; Roeb, E. Matrix metalloproteinase-13 refines pathological staging of precancerous colorectal lesions. *Oncotarget* **2016**, *7*, 73552–73557. [CrossRef]

59. Lambrecht, B.N.; Vanderkerken, M.; Hammad, H. The emerging role of ADAM metalloproteinases in immunity. *Nat. Rev. Immunol.* **2018**, *18*, 745–758. [CrossRef]
60. Calligaris, M.; Cuffaro, D.; Bonelli, S.; Spanò, D.P.; Rossello, A.; Nuti, E.; Scilabra, S.D. Strategies to Target ADAM17 in Disease: From Its Discovery to the iRhom Revolution. *Molecules* **2021**, *26*, 944. [CrossRef]
61. Blaydon, D.C.; Biancheri, P.; Di, W.-L.; Plagnol, V.; Cabral, R.M.; Brooke, M.A.; van Heel, D.A.; Ruschendorf, F.; Toynbee, M.; Walne, A.; et al. Inflammatory Skin and Bowel Disease Linked to ADAM17 Deletion. *N. Engl. J. Med.* **2011**, *365*, 1502–1508. [CrossRef] [PubMed]
62. Christophi, G.P.; Rong, R.; Holtzapple, P.G.; Massa, P.T.; Landas, S.K. Immune Markers and Differential Signaling Networks in Ulcerative Colitis and Crohn's Disease. *Inflamm. Bowel Dis.* **2012**, *18*, 2342–2356. [CrossRef] [PubMed]
63. Guo, Y.; Su, Z.-Y.; Zhang, C.; Gaspar, J.M.; Wang, R.; Hart, R.P.; Verzi, M.P.; Kong, A.-N.T. Mechanisms of colitis-accelerated colon carcinogenesis and its prevention with the combination of aspirin and curcumin: Transcriptomic analysis using RNA-seq. *Biochem. Pharmacol.* **2017**, *135*, 22–34. [CrossRef] [PubMed]
64. Conrad, C.; Yildiz, D.; Cleary, S.J.; Margraf, A.; Cook, L.; Schlomann, U.; Panaretou, B.; Bowser, J.L.; Karmouty-Quintana, H.; Li, J.; et al. ADAM8 signaling drives neutrophil migration and ARDS severity. *JCI Insight* **2022**, *7*, e87489. [CrossRef] [PubMed]
65. Lu, H.; Meng, Y.; Han, X.; Zhang, W. ADAM8 Activates NLRP3 Inflammasome to Promote Cerebral Ischemia-Reperfusion Injury. *J. Healthc. Eng.* **2021**, *2021*, 3097432. [CrossRef] [PubMed]
66. Wang, Y.; Wang, K.; Han, G.-C.; Wang, R.-X.; Xiao, H.; Hou, C.-M.; Guo, R.-F.; Dou, Y.; Shen, B.-F.; Li, Y.; et al. Neutrophil infiltration favors colitis-associated tumorigenesis by activating the interleukin-1 (IL-1)/IL-6 axis. *Mucosal Immunol.* **2014**, *7*, 1106–1115. [CrossRef]
67. Perera, A.P.; Sajnani, K.; Dickinson, J.; Eri, R.; Körner, H. NLRP3 inflammasome in colitis and colitis-associated colorectal cancer. *Mamm. Genome* **2018**, *29*, 817–830. [CrossRef]
68. Conrad, C.; Benzel, J.; Dorzweiler, K.; Cook, L.; Schlomann, U.; Zarbock, A.; Slater, E.P.; Nimsky, C.; Bartsch, J.W. ADAM8 in invasive cancers: Links to tumor progression, metastasis, and chemoresistance. *Clin. Sci.* **2019**, *133*, 83–99. [CrossRef]
69. Yang, Z.; Bai, Y.; Huo, L.; Chen, H.; Huang, J.; Li, J.; Fan, X.; Yang, Z.; Wang, L.; Wang, J. Expression of A disintegrin and metalloprotease 8 is associated with cell growth and poor survival in colorectal cancer. *BMC Cancer* **2014**, *14*, 568. [CrossRef]
70. Park Bin, B.; Choi, S.; Yoon Sang, Y.; Kim, D. TrkB/C-induced HOXC6 activation enhances the ADAM8-mediated metastasis of chemoresistant colon cancer cells. *Mol. Med. Rep.* **2021**, *23*, 423. [CrossRef]
71. Okada, K.; Itoh, H.; Ikemoto, M. Serum complement C3 and α2-macroglubulin are potentially useful biomarkers for inflammatory bowel disease patients. *Heliyon* **2021**, *7*, e06554. [CrossRef] [PubMed]
72. Sina, C.; Kemper, C.; Derer, S. The intestinal complement system in inflammatory bowel disease: Shaping intestinal barrier function. *Semin. Immunol.* **2018**, *37*, 66–73. [CrossRef] [PubMed]
73. Sünderhauf, A.; Skibbe, K.; Preisker, S.; Ebbert, K.; Verschoor, A.; Karsten, C.M.; Kemper, C.; Huber-Lang, M.; Basic, M.; Bleich, A.; et al. Regulation of epithelial cell expressed C3 in the intestine—Relevance for the pathophysiology of inflammatory bowel disease? *Mol. Immunol.* **2017**, *90*, 227–238. [CrossRef] [PubMed]
74. Choi, Y.J.; Kim, J.E.; Lee, S.J.; Gong, J.E.; Jin, Y.J.; Lee, H.; Hwang, D.Y. Promotion of the inflammatory response in mid colon of complement component 3 knockout mice. *Sci. Rep.* **2022**, *12*, 1700. [CrossRef]
75. Subramanian, S.; Pallati, P.K.; Sharma, P.; Agrawal, D.K.; Nandipati, K.C. Significant association of TREM-1 with HMGB1, TLRs and RAGE in the pathogenesis of insulin resistance in obese diabetic populations. *Am. J. Transl. Res.* **2017**, *9*, 3224–3244.
76. Fan, D.; He, X.; Bian, Y.; Guo, Q.; Zheng, K.; Zhao, Y.; Lu, C.; Liu, B.; Xu, X.; Zhang, G.; et al. Triptolide Modulates TREM-1 Signal Pathway to Inhibit the Inflammatory Response in Rheumatoid Arthritis. *Int. J. Mol. Sci.* **2016**, *17*, 498. [CrossRef]
77. Tammaro, A.; Stroo, I.; Rampanelli, E.; Blank, F.; Butter, L.M.; Claessen, N.; Takai, T.; Colonna, M.; Leemans, J.C.; Florquin, S.; et al. Role of TREM1-DAP12 in Renal Inflammation during Obstructive Nephropathy. *PLoS ONE* **2013**, *8*, e82498. [CrossRef] [PubMed]
78. Li, X.; Lee, E.J.; Gawel, D.R.; Lilja, S.; Schäfer, S.; Zhang, H.; Benson, M. Meta-Analysis of Expression Profiling Data Indicates Need for Combinatorial Biomarkers in Pediatric Ulcerative Colitis. *J. Immunol. Res.* **2020**, *2020*, 8279619. [CrossRef]
79. Biagioli, M.; Mencarelli, A.; Carino, A.; Cipriani, S.; Marchianò, S.; Fiorucci, C.; Donini, A.; Graziosi, L.; Baldelli, F.; Distrutti, E.; et al. Genetic and Pharmacological Dissection of the Role of Spleen Tyrosine Kinase (Syk) in Intestinal Inflammation and Immune Dysfunction in Inflammatory Bowel Diseases. *Inflamm. Bowel Dis.* **2018**, *24*, 123–135. [CrossRef]
80. Hermann, C.D.; Schoeps, B.; Eckfeld, C.; Munkhbaatar, E.; Kniep, L.; Prokopchuk, O.; Wirges, N.; Steiger, K.; Häußler, D.; Knolle, P.; et al. TIMP1 expression underlies sex disparity in liver metastasis and survival in pancreatic cancer. *J. Exp. Med.* **2021**, *218*, e20210911. [CrossRef]
81. Clough, E.; Barrett, T. *The Gene Expression Omnibus Database BT—Statistical Genomics: Methods and Protocols*; Mathé, E., Davis, S., Eds.; Springer: New York, NY, USA, 2016; pp. 93–110, ISBN 978-1-4939-3578-9.
82. Barrett, T.; Wilhite, S.E.; Ledoux, P.; Evangelista, C.; Kim, I.F.; Tomashevsky, M.; Marshall, K.A.; Phillippy, K.H.; Sherman, P.M.; Holko, M.; et al. NCBI GEO: Archive for functional genomics data sets—Update. *Nucleic Acids Res.* **2013**, *41*, D991–D995. [CrossRef] [PubMed]
83. Heberle, H.; Meirelles, V.G.; da Silva, F.R.; Telles, G.P.; Minghim, R. InteractiVenn: A web-based tool for the analysis of sets through Venn diagrams. *BMC Bioinform.* **2015**, *16*, 169. [CrossRef] [PubMed]
84. Chen, J.; Bardes, E.E.; Aronow, B.J.; Jegga, A.G. ToppGene Suite for gene list enrichment analysis and candidate gene prioritization. *Nucleic Acids Res.* **2009**, *37*, W.305–W.311. [CrossRef] [PubMed]

85. Doncheva, N.T.; Morris, J.H.; Gorodkin, J.; Jensen, L.J. Cytoscape StringApp: Network Analysis and Visualization of Proteomics Data. *J. Proteome Res.* **2019**, *18*, 623–632. [CrossRef]
86. Assenov, Y.; Ramírez, F.; Schelhorn, S.E.S.E.; Lengauer, T.; Albrecht, M. Computing topological parameters of biological networks. *Bioinformatics* **2008**, *24*, 282–284. [CrossRef]
87. MORPHEUS. Versatile Matrix Visualization and Analysis Software. Available online: https://software.broadinstitute.org/morpheus/ (accessed on 12 November 2022).
88. Wang, J.-H.; Zhao, L.-F.; Wang, H.-F.; Wen, Y.-T.; Jiang, K.-K.; Mao, X.-M.; Zhou, Z.-Y.; Yao, K.-T.; Geng, Q.-S.; Guo, D.; et al. GenCLiP 3: Mining human genes' functions and regulatory networks from PubMed based on co-occurrences and natural language processing. *Bioinformatics* **2019**, *36*, 1973–1975. [CrossRef]
89. Krzywinski, M.; Schein, J.; Birol, I.; Connors, J.; Gascoyne, R.; Horsman, D.; Jones, S.J.; Marra, M.A. Circos: An information aesthetic for comparative genomics. *Genome Res.* **2009**, *19*, 1639–1645. [CrossRef]
90. Tanaka, T.; Kohno, H.; Suzuki, R.; Yamada, Y.; Sugie, S.; Mori, H. A novel inflammation-related mouse colon carcinogenesis model induced by azoxymethane and dextran sodium sulfate. *Cancer Sci.* **2003**, *94*, 965–973. [CrossRef]
91. Anaya, J. OncoLnc: Linking TCGA survival data to mRNAs, miRNAs, and lncRNAs. *PeerJ Comput. Sci.* **2016**, *2016*, e67. [CrossRef]

Disclaimer/Publisher's Note: The statements, opinions and data contained in all publications are solely those of the individual author(s) and contributor(s) and not of MDPI and/or the editor(s). MDPI and/or the editor(s) disclaim responsibility for any injury to people or property resulting from any ideas, methods, instructions or products referred to in the content.

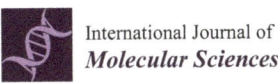

Article

Natural NADH and FAD Autofluorescence as Label-Free Biomarkers for Discriminating Subtypes and Functional States of Immune Cells

Sarah Lemire [1,2,*], Oana-Maria Thoma [1,2], Lucas Kreiss [1,3], Simon Völkl [4], Oliver Friedrich [3,5], Markus F. Neurath [1,2], Sebastian Schürmann [3,5] and Maximilian J. Waldner [1,2,5,*]

1. Department of Internal Medicine 1, University Hospital Erlangen, Friedrich-Alexander-Universität Erlangen-Nürnberg (FAU), 91052 Erlangen, Germany; oana-maria.thoma@uk-erlangen.de (O.-M.T.); lucas.kreiss@fau.de (L.K.); markus.neurath@uk-erlangen.de (M.F.N.)
2. Deutsches Zentrum Immuntherapie, University Hospital Erlangen, Friedrich-Alexander-Universität Erlangen-Nürnberg (FAU), 91054 Erlangen, Germany
3. Institute of Medical Biotechnology, Friedrich-Alexander-Universität Erlangen-Nürnberg (FAU), 91052 Erlangen, Germany; oliver.friedrich@fau.de (O.F.); sebastian.schuermann@fau.de (S.S.)
4. Department of Internal Medicine 5, Haematology and Oncology, University Hospital Erlangen, Friedrich-Alexander-Universität Erlangen-Nürnberg (FAU), 91054 Erlangen, Germany; simon.voelkl@uk-erlangen.de
5. Erlangen Graduate School in Advanced Optical Technologies, Friedrich-Alexander-Universität Erlangen-Nürnberg (FAU), 91052 Erlangen, Germany
* Correspondence: sarah.lemire@fau.de (S.L.); maximilian.waldner@uk-erlangen.de (M.J.W.); Tel.: +49-9131-8535894 (S.L.); +49-9131-8535000 (M.J.W.)

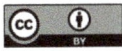

Citation: Lemire, S.; Thoma, O.-M.; Kreiss, L.; Völkl, S.; Friedrich, O.; Neurath, M.F.; Schürmann, S.; Waldner, M.J. Natural NADH and FAD Autofluorescence as Label-Free Biomarkers for Discriminating Subtypes and Functional States of Immune Cells. *Int. J. Mol. Sci.* **2022**, *23*, 2338. https://doi.org/10.3390/ijms23042338

Academic Editor: Susanne M. Krug

Received: 13 January 2022
Accepted: 17 February 2022
Published: 20 February 2022

Publisher's Note: MDPI stays neutral with regard to jurisdictional claims in published maps and institutional affiliations.

Copyright: © 2022 by the authors. Licensee MDPI, Basel, Switzerland. This article is an open access article distributed under the terms and conditions of the Creative Commons Attribution (CC BY) license (https://creativecommons.org/licenses/by/4.0/).

Abstract: Immune cell activity is a major factor for disease progression in inflammatory bowel diseases (IBD). Classifying the type and functional state of immune cells is therefore crucial in clinical diagnostics of IBD. Label-free optical technologies exploiting NADH and FAD autofluorescence, such as multiphoton microscopy, have been used to describe tissue morphology in healthy and inflamed colon samples. Nevertheless, a strategy for the identification of single immune cell subtypes within the tissue is yet to be developed. This work aims to initiate an understanding of autofluorescence changes depending on immune cell type and activation state. For this, NADH and FAD autofluorescence signals of different murine immune cell subtypes under native conditions, as well as upon in vitro stimulation and cell death, have been evaluated. Autofluorescence was assessed using flow cytometry and multiphoton microscopy. Our results reveal significantly increased NADH and FAD signals in innate immune cells compared to adaptive immune cells. This allowed identification of relative amounts of neutrophils and CD4+ T cells in mixed cell suspensions, by using NADH signals as a differentiation marker. Furthermore, in vitro stimulation significantly increased NADH and FAD autofluorescence in adaptive immune cells and macrophages. Cell death induced a significant drop in NADH autofluorescence, while FAD signals were hardly affected. Taken together, these results demonstrate the value of autofluorescence as a tool to characterize immune cells in different functional states, paving the way to the label-free clinical classification of IBD in the future.

Keywords: inflammatory bowel diseases; cell autofluorescence; immune cells; NADH; FAD; flow cytometry; multiphoton microscopy

1. Introduction

Immune cells are highly important for maintaining health and homeostasis and play a key role in the pathogenesis of inflammatory bowel diseases (IBD). Specific T-cell subtypes have been directly linked to disease progression in IBD. For example, helper T cells (Th1, Th2 and Th17 cells) trigger gut inflammation [1,2], while regulatory T cells (Treg) help to prevent the inflammation-related destruction of the mucosa [1]. Similarly, adaptive immune cells, such as macrophages and neutrophils, are involved in the pathogenesis of mucosal inflammation. For instance, pro-inflammatory M1 macrophages can support inflammation through the release of pro-inflammatory cytokines, whereas M2 macrophages have anti-inflammatory properties [3]. Neutrophil infiltration in the gut mucosa has been linked to high disease activity in ulcerative colitis (UC), while a lack of neutrophils leads to an uncontrolled invasion of bacteria that promote inflammation in Crohn's disease (CD) [4]. Understanding how immune cells modulate IBD is an important area of research. Therefore, a specific identification and evaluation of immune cell subtypes, activation states, proliferation and cell death could reveal important information on the current state and future course of disease in IBD.

Optical technologies, such as multiphoton microscopy (MPM), have lately received increasing interest as label-free options to investigate the native tissue morphology of healthy and inflamed colon based on autofluorescence [5,6]. Autofluorescence is a cell property that depends on the presence of endogenous fluorescent molecules, such as NADH and FAD [7]. Using this natural autofluorescence is highly advantageous, as label-free imaging strategies do not affect the state of individual cells. While MPM allows for the identification of intrastromal cells in colitis models [5], a clear classification of infiltrating immune cell subtypes and functional states is not yet available. Therefore, laying a foundation for understanding how autofluorescence signals differ in individual types of immune cells and their activation status is relevant for possible clinical applications in IBD patients.

This study analysed NADH and FAD signals of murine immune cells in different functional states using flow cytometry and MPM. Flow cytometry, on the one hand, is a broadly used method, able to analyse high numbers of cells in a short period of time [8]. Although usually used to characterize cells with the help of fluorescent markers, it has also shown its potential in detecting autofluorescent signals in different types of cells [9–11]. MPM is a promising optical imaging technique exploiting the non-linear excitation of fluorescent molecules including NADH and FAD [12]. This allows successful label-free evaluation of 3D tissue morphology, as we have described in previous studies [5]. The specific characteristics of NADH and FAD autofluorescence in single immune cell types and under different functional conditions, however, remain to be described. Therefore, the purpose of this study was to evaluate autofluorescence profiles in various types of innate and adaptive immune cells and how these are affected by different functional states. This might be a first step towards a label-free classification of infiltrating immune cells in the clinical diagnostics of IBD.

2. Results

2.1. Adaptive and Innate Immune Cells Show Different NADH and FAD Signals in Flow Cytometry

In Figure 1A, we schematically describe the workflow from immune cell isolation to autofluorescence measurements and NADH/FAD detection by flow cytometry. As explained in Section 4, the filters used for label-free flow cytometry of immune cells mainly collected NADH/FAD autofluorescence signals; however, autofluorescence signals from other endogenous fluorophores cannot be completely avoided. The respective intensities of NADH and FAD signals among different immune cell types (e.g., CD4+ T cells and dendritic cells) are illustrated in the exemplary NADH/FAD dot plots and histograms. Similar histograms for further immune cell subtypes are presented in Supplementary Figure S1. Quantification of NADH and FAD fluorescence revealed a considerable increase in both fluorescent molecules in innate immune cells compared to adaptive immune cells (Figure 1B).

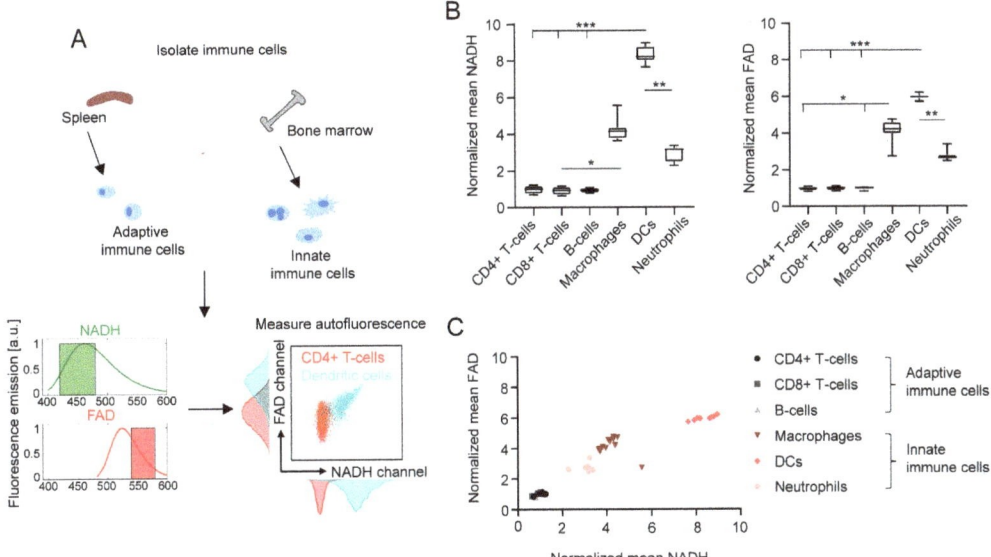

Figure 1. Immune cell subtypes can be differentiated by NADH and FAD autofluorescence signals in flow cytometry. (**A**) Schematic representation of immune cell isolation from murine spleen and bone marrow, and exemplary autofluorescence analysis in flow cytometry. (**B**) NADH and FAD signal mean values of different immune cell subtypes, normalized to the mean values of alive, unstimulated CD4+ T cells. For statistical analysis, a Kruskal–Wallis test with subsequent Dunn's multiple comparisons test was used (* $p < 0.05$, ** $p < 0.01$, *** $p < 0.001$). At least four samples per group were analysed. Each sample reflects either cells isolated from one mouse (CD4+ T cells, CD8+ T cells, B cells, neutrophils) or cells cultured in one culture dish (macrophages, dendritic cells). (**C**) Comparison of normalized mean NADH and FAD signals in different immune cell types.

Overall, dendritic cells showed the strongest NADH and FAD signals of all analysed cell types (eight-fold increase in NADH and six-fold increase in FAD compared to adaptive immune cells). Furthermore, NADH and FAD signals of dendritic cells were also significantly different to those of neutrophils (2.8-fold increase in NADH, 2.1-fold increase in FAD). The autofluorescence signals among CD4+ T cells, CD8+ T cells and B cells did not show any relevant differences. Interestingly, changes in NADH and FAD signals correlated with each other in the different cell types, as shown in Figure 1C.

2.2. In Vitro Stimulation Increases NADH and FAD Signals in Flow Cytometry

In addition to the type of cell, we identified in vitro stimulation as another important determinant of cell autofluorescence. As described in Figure 2A, we performed in vitro stimulation of all six immune cell types and analysed their NADH and FAD signals with flow cytometry. Histograms and dot plots of unstimulated and stimulated CD4+ T cells are shown exemplarily and illustrate a significant shift in NADH and FAD autofluorescence after stimulation. For instance, NADH increased six-fold in stimulated CD4+ T cells compared to unstimulated CD4+ T cells (Figure 2B).

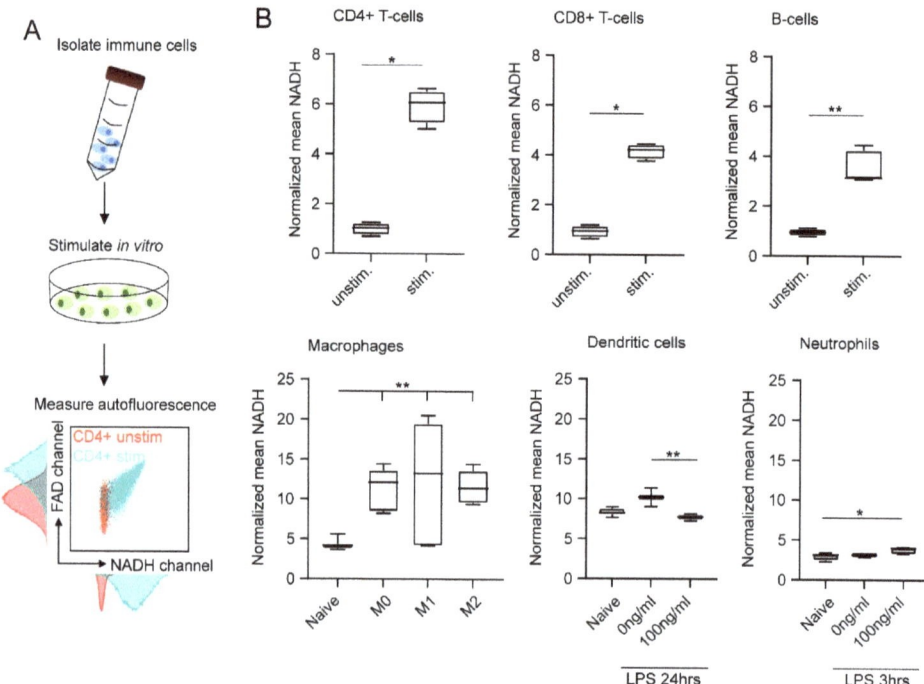

Figure 2. In vitro stimulation affects immune cell autofluorescence in flow cytometry. (**A**) After in vitro stimulation, immune cell autofluorescence was assessed by flow cytometry. (**B**) Boxplots showing NADH autofluorescence of adaptive and innate immune cells before and after in vitro stimulation. Statistical significance was analysed with a Mann–Whitney test for comparing two independent groups. For three independent groups, a Kruskal–Wallis test with subsequent Dunn's multiple comparisons test was used (* $p < 0.05$, ** $p < 0.01$). At least three samples per group were analysed. Each sample reflects either cells isolated from one mouse (unstimulated CD4+ T cells, CD8+ T cells, B cells, neutrophils) or cells cultured in one culture dish (stimulated CD4+ T cells, CD8+ T cells, B cells, neutrophils; unstimulated and stimulated macrophages, dendritic cells).

Significant differences were also observed when comparing unstimulated and stimulated CD8+ T cells (4.5-fold increase in NADH) and unstimulated and stimulated B cells (3.7-fold increase in NADH). Polarized macrophages showed similar results: all three polarization groups displayed significantly increased NADH signals compared to the unstimulated cells (2.9-fold increase in NADH). Interestingly, the type of polarization had no major effect on autofluorescence signals. Dendritic cells and neutrophils were only weakly affected by in vitro stimulation (Figure 2B). FAD values displayed similar results in all cases (data not shown). In conclusion, we observed clear effects of in vitro stimulation on autofluorescence signals of adaptive immune cells and macrophages.

2.3. NADH Autofluorescence Is Decreased in Dead Cells

To analyse the effect of cell death on immune cell autofluorescence, cells were stained with the cell death marker Sytox Red. Figure 3A exemplarily illustrates the effect of cell death on unstimulated CD4+ T cells: while NADH autofluorescence was shifted to decreased values in the Sytox+ dead cell population compared to the Sytox- alive cells, FAD signals remained constant. Heat maps in Figure 3B describe similar patterns for all the other immune cell types and show that cell death only had an impact on NADH autofluorescence signals, whereas FAD signals were not, or only slightly, affected. To illustrate this finding, we calculated the optical redox ratio as R = NADH/(NADH + FAD) and compared the results for dead and alive cells. As expected, this ratio was significantly decreased in Sytox+ dead cells due to the drop in NADH autofluorescence (Figure 3C). The strongest differences were observed within adaptive immune cell populations (three-fold decrease in ratio) and dendritic cells (1.7-fold decrease in ratio); macrophages showed the smallest decrease in the NADH autofluorescence of dead cells (1.3-fold decrease in ratio). Taken together, these findings show a considerable impact of cell death on NADH autofluorescence, while FAD signals were not significantly affected.

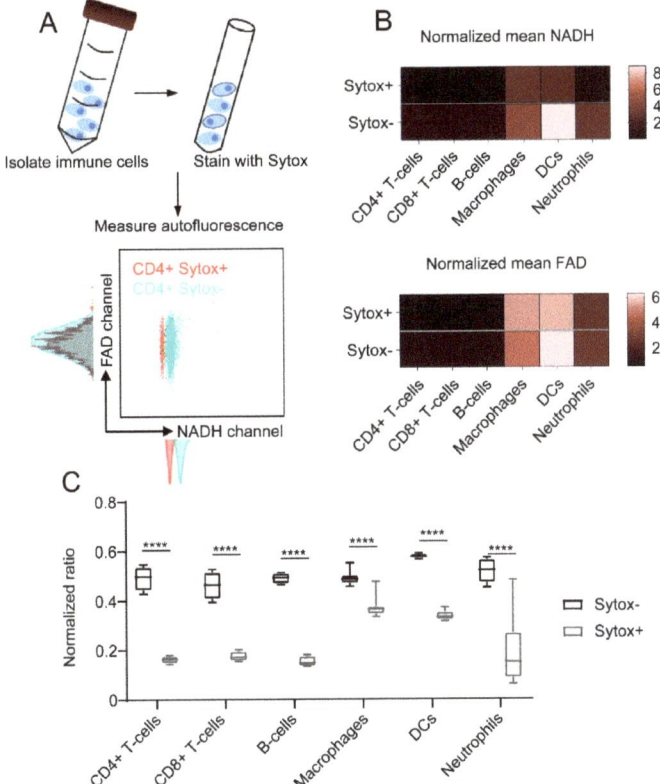

Figure 3. NADH autofluorescence decrease upon cell death as shown by flow cytometry. (**A**) To identify dead cells, the samples were stained with Sytox Red after isolation. Autofluorescence signals were measured using flow cytometry. (**B**) NADH and FAD signals of dead (Sytox+) and alive (Sytox−) cells, illustrated in a heat map. (**C**) Redox ratios calculated as R = NADH/(NADH + FAD). For statistical analysis, two-way ANOVA with Sidak's multiple comparisons test was used (**** $p < 0.0001$). At least four samples per group were analysed. Each sample reflects either cells isolated from one mouse (CD4+ T cells, CD8+ T cells, B cells, neutrophils) or cells cultured in one culture dish (macrophages, dendritic cells).

2.4. NADH and FAD Signals of Immune Cells Can Be Analysed with MPM

In the second part of our study, all immune cell subtypes were analysed with MPM (Figure 4A). According to the filter setup described in Section 4, NADH and FAD predominantly contributed to the autofluorescence signals measured in this study. Nevertheless, other autofluorescent molecules might also influence cell autofluorescence to a small extent. Figure 4B depicts the NADH and FAD signals of all six immune cell subtypes as shown by

MPM. NADH signals are illustrated in green, FAD signals are shown in red and signals from the DODT channel are displayed in grey. The immune cell subtypes morphologically differed in shape and size, but also revealed differences in the strength of NADH and FAD signals. Innate immune cells showed stronger autofluorescence, whereas the signal in adaptive immune cells was generally weak. Quantification of the data displayed similar trends to what we observed with flow cytometry: innate immune cells had higher NADH (1.6-fold increase) and FAD (1.7-fold increase) autofluorescence signals in comparison to adaptive immune cells (Figure 4C). Furthermore, signal intensities of NADH correlated with FAD signal intensities for all cell types (Figure 4D).

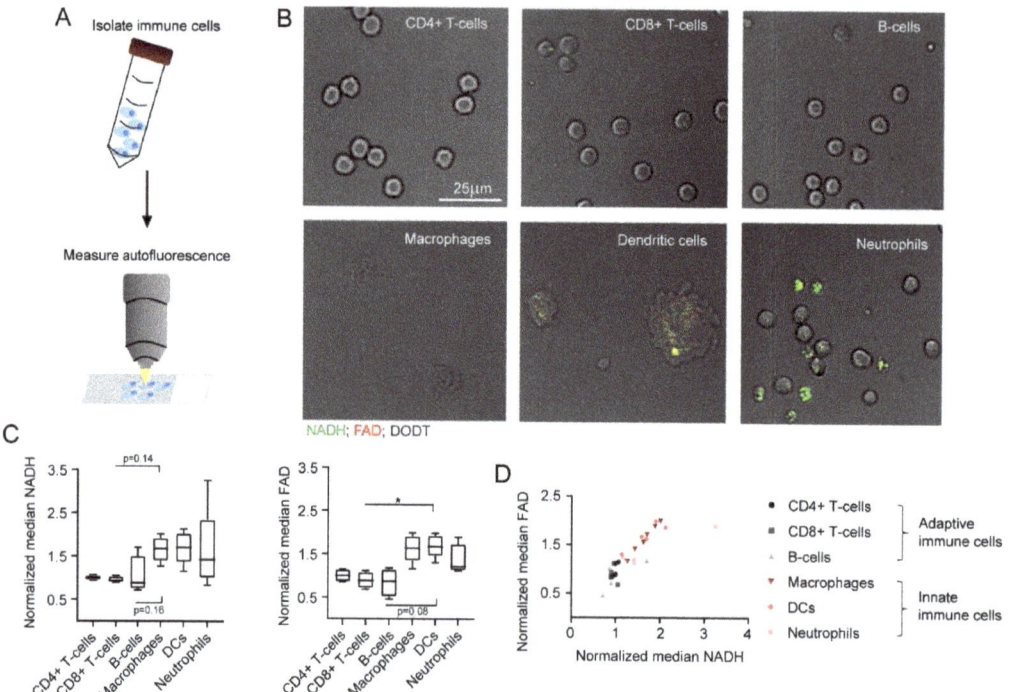

Figure 4. NADH and FAD autofluorescence changes as measured in multiphoton microscopy. (**A**) Schematic representation of MPM measurements after immune cell isolation from murine spleen and bone marrow. (**B**) Exemplary images of different immune cell types, as measured in MPM. NADH: green, FAD: red, DODT: grey (scalebar: 25 μm). (**C**) Median NADH and FAD signals of different immune cells, normalized to NADH and FAD signals of alive, unstimulated CD4+ T cells. For statistical analysis, a Kruskal–Wallis test with Dunn's multiple comparisons test was used (* $p < 0.05$). At least four samples per group were analysed. Each sample includes at least 30–500 cells and reflects either cells isolated from one mouse (CD4+ T cells, CD8+ T cells, B cells, neutrophils) or cells cultured in one culture dish (macrophages, dendritic cells). (**D**) Comparison of normalized median NADH and FAD signals.

2.5. NADH and FAD Signals Increase upon In Vitro Stimulation as Measured by MPM

Additionally, we analysed the effect of in vitro stimulation on immune cells in MPM. For this, autofluorescence signals of unstimulated and stimulated cells were compared, analogous to what we have described for flow cytometry measurements. The increase in NADH and FAD signals was especially visible in CD4+ T cells and macrophages (Figure 5A). This visual impression was confirmed by quantification in Figure 5B: we observed a significant increase in NADH signals in stimulated adaptive immune cells compared to unstimulated adaptive immune cells (1.9-fold increase in NADH). Furthermore, macrophage polarization induced a significant NADH increase (2.5-fold increase in NADH compared to unpolarized macrophages). No relevant effects of in vitro stimulation were observed among dendritic cells and neutrophils. FAD values showed similar results in all cases (data not shown). Overall, these findings correlate with our results from flow cytometry measurements and demonstrate the feasibility of assessing single cell autofluorescence with MPM.

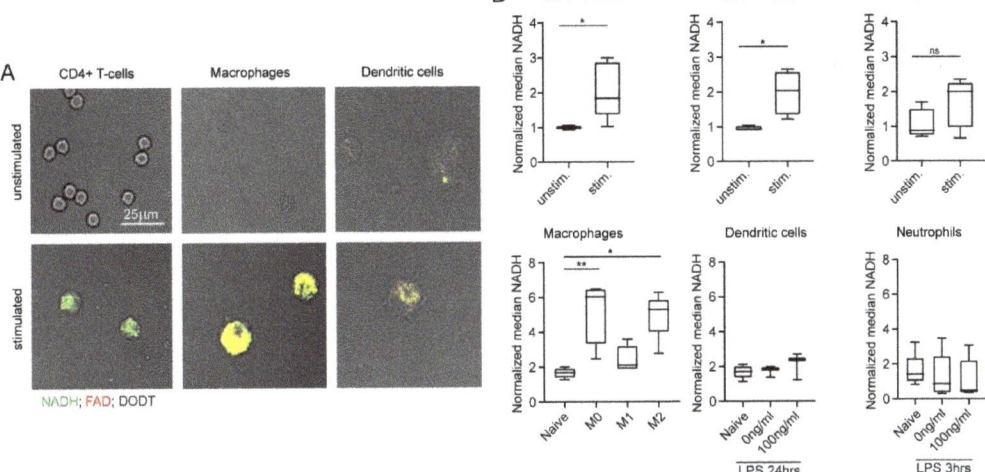

Figure 5. In vitro stimulation changes NADH and FAD autofluorescence signals, as measured by multiphoton microscopy. (**A**) Example images of unstimulated and stimulated CD4+ T cells, macrophages, and dendritic cells. NADH: green, FAD: red, DODT: grey (scalebar: 25 μm). (**B**) NADH autofluorescence signals of adaptive and innate immune cells after in vitro stimulation. Statistical significance was analysed with a Mann–Whitney test for comparing two independent groups. For three independent groups, a Kruskal–Wallis test with subsequent Dunn's multiple comparisons test was used (* $p < 0.05$, ** $p < 0.01$). At least three samples per group were analysed. Each sample includes at least 30–500 cells and reflects either cells isolated from one mouse (unstimulated CD4+ T cells, CD8+ T cells, B cells, neutrophils) or cells cultured in one culture dish (stimulated CD4+ T cells, CD8+ T cells, B cells, neutrophils; unstimulated and stimulated macrophages, dendritic cells).

2.6. Autofluorescence as a Tool to Distinguish Cell Types in a Mixed Cell Suspension

The final aim of this study was to detect relative amounts of two different immune cell types in a mixed suspension by quantifying autofluorescence signatures by flow cytometry and MPM. CD4+ T cells and neutrophils were chosen as the most suitable mixture, since they differ regarding their NADH signals, while showing similar morphology and size. As described in Section 4, NADH and APC values of single cells were measured for all four conditions of cell mixes. APC-labelled α-CD3 was used as a marker to identify CD4+ T cells. Results were visualized and quantified in dot plots for MPM and flow cytometry and dot plots were divided into four quadrants defined by high and low NADH and APC values. Exemplary dot plots are presented in Figure 6A,B. Furthermore, we calculated the percentage of cells found in each quadrant. In the samples that only contained CD4+ T cells, 94.88% of cells in flow cytometry and 73.98% of cells in MPM displayed low NADH and high APC. For neutrophils alone, most cells were defined by high NADH and low APC (78.7% flow cytometry, 68.37% MPM). In the mixed samples, both conditions occurred according to the mixing ratio in the sample. Interestingly, a cell population displaying low NADH and low APC was found in the samples containing isolated neutrophils. These cells were confirmed as B cells in flow cytometry (data not shown) and can hardly be avoided due to the isolation protocol used for neutrophils. Taken together, this experiment showed that NADH autofluorescence values may be used as a potential identification tool for different immune cell subtypes, without the need for additional staining or morphological characterization.

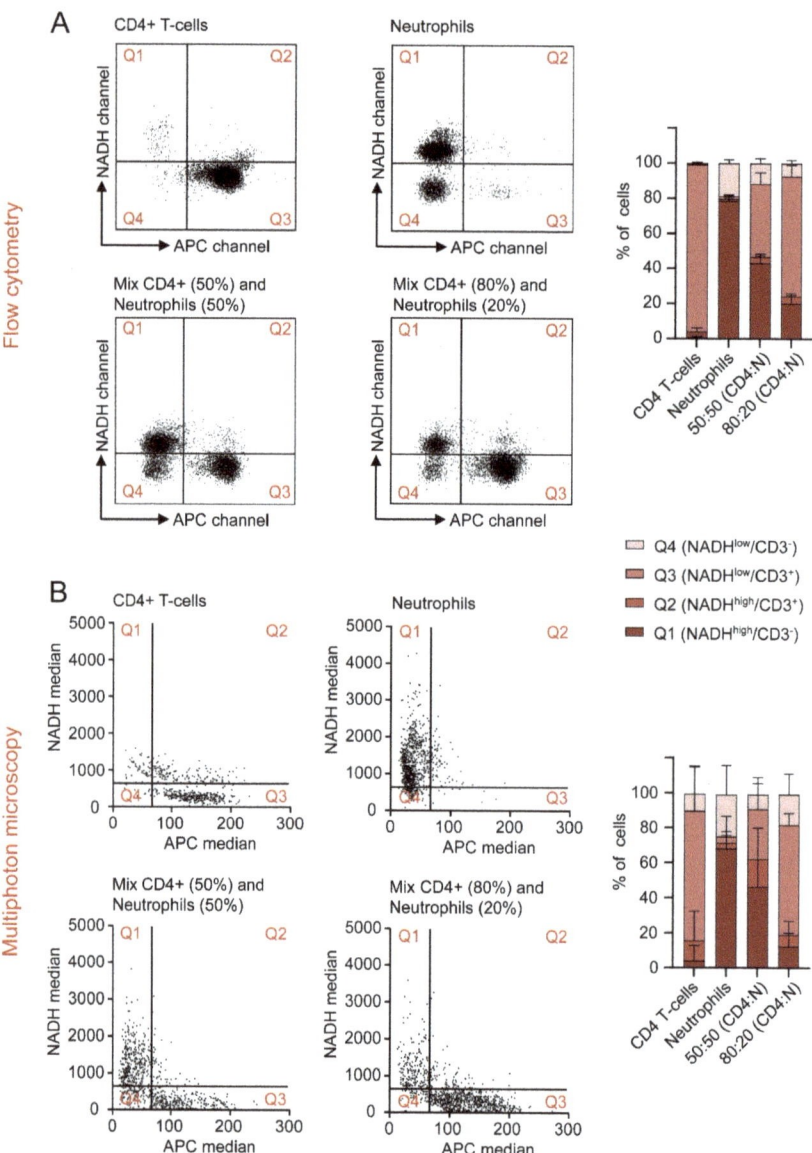

Figure 6. NADH autofluorescence signals may be used to differentiate between cell types in a mixed sample in flow cytometry and multiphoton microscopy. (**A**,**B**) Cells were divided into four quadrants, defined by high and low NADH and APC values. CD4+ T cells and neutrophils were analysed on their own and in mixed samples and the percentages of cells found in each quadrant were represented for both flow cytometry and MPM.

3. Discussion

This study was designed to evaluate label-free, optical differentiation of immune cell subtypes and functional states without relying on exogenous and artificial markers. This work is relevant to many inflammatory diseases, such as IBD, since it could allow semi-specific classification of immune cell groups based on native tissue samples. In the context of IBD, MPM has already been used to describe the 3D morphology of the gut mucosa in untreated tissue biopsies or during in vivo endomicroscopy. Thereby, it was suggested that increased numbers of stromal cells in different colitis models represent infiltrating immune cells [5]. Yet, a clear identification of single immune cell types and functional states within this tissue remained difficult, even though this knowledge can be valuable in the clinical diagnostics of IBD [3,13,14].

In unstimulated immune cells, we observed an increase in NADH and FAD signals in innate immune cells compared to adaptive immune cells in flow cytometry and MPM. Similar changes were previously described in macrophages and dendritic cells [15]. These findings might be explained by the increased cell granularity in innate immune cells due to high lysosome activity, which can contribute to cell autofluorescence [16–18]. Not surprisingly, the activation of immune cells also changes NADH and FAD autofluorescence. This might be the result of increased glycolysis and promotion of oxidative phosphorylation [19,20]. However, not all immune cells showed a change in autofluorescence upon in vitro stimulation. For example, in neutrophils, LPS is not able to directly activate the enzyme NAD(P)H oxidase and can therefore not induce extensive oxidation of NAD(P)H to NAD(P)+ [21–23].

Overall, changes in NADH and FAD signals in both steady state and activated immune cells might provide additional information about their behaviour in inflammatory diseases, such as IBD. For example, the recognition of stimulated T cells based on increased NADH and FAD signals may allow the differentiation of healthy and diseased colon tissue in the future. Furthermore, monitoring macrophage activation using the strong increase in NADH and FAD autofluorescence may help to identify early states of gut inflammation, as the activation of macrophages is a crucial step in the initiation of IBD [24]. Similarly, neutrophil infiltration in the gut could be tracked by high autofluorescence signals, as this is an important indicator of acute gut inflammation.

In this study, we report for the first time that cell death induces a decrease in NADH signals of different immune cell types, while hardly affecting FAD autofluorescence. One important cause of cell death is oxidative stress, which promotes the oxidation of NADH and $FADH_2$ to NAD+ and FAD [25]. Since NAD+ is not autofluorescent at the investigated wavelength [26], this explains the strong decrease in NADH signal during cell death. In the context of IBD, immune cell apoptosis plays an essential role in therapeutic strategies. For example, the mechanism of action in drugs, such as azathioprine and anti-TNF antibodies, relies on cell death induction in T cells [27]. Therefore, identification of apoptotic immune cells only based on the NADH/FAD autofluorescence ratio may be used to monitor therapeutic success in IBD patients in the future.

On the other hand, anti-TNF antibodies, such as infliximab or adalimumab, are not only regulators of T-cell apoptosis, but can also block macrophage activation in the gut mucosa [28]. Therefore, NADH and FAD signals might decrease as an effect of the non-activation of intestinal macrophages. Similar mechanisms can be discussed for other biologicals currently used in the therapy of IBD. Vedolizumab, an α4β7-integrin-specific antibody, inhibits the infiltration or so-called homing of T cells into the gut mucosa, while pro-inflammatory T cell activation can be blocked by ustekinumab, an antibody against IL12 and IL23 [28]. Both substances might lead to a measurable decrease in NADH and FAD signals in the intrastromal cells, as therapy leads to a downregulation of activated T cells. These examples illustrate the potential value of label-free diagnostics to easily assess current therapy strategies in IBD patients.

Despite this potential, certain limitations of this study must be considered. Although MPM and flow cytometry allow the evaluation of immune cell autofluorescence, flow cytometry usually achieves clearer results. A possible reason for this fact is that flow cytometry was designed for measurements at high throughput, while MPM is usually used as an imaging technology without direct quantification. The number of cells was therefore limited in MPM investigation. Furthermore, we observed that activation and cell type can lead to equivalent changes in autofluorescence. Therefore, autofluorescence signals on their own might not be enough to describe in detail immune cell types and function. A combination of different components in label-free diagnostics, including size, morphology, and granularity of cells should be established in the future.

In conclusion, our findings reveal that cell type, state and function have measurable effects on NADH and FAD autofluorescence signals of isolated murine immune cells in vitro. Such a semi-specific categorization of immune cells could allow the identification of immune cells infiltrating the lamina propria of healthy and inflamed colon tissue in the future. To make autofluorescence, as a clinical parameter, accessible to patients with IBD, application of this research to human samples, including the blood and tissue of IBD patients, is essential. As a long-term goal, the results of this research might lead to the development of automated artificial intelligence systems, able to recognize immune cell type and function based on autofluorescence signals in the diagnostics of IBD patients, paving the way to promising clinical applications.

4. Materials and Methods

4.1. Adaptive Immune Cell Isolation and Stimulation

This study was prepared and conducted within a period of 14 months between October 2020 and December 2021.

All immune cell subtypes were obtained from the spleen (CD4+/CD8+ T cells, B cells) or bone marrow (macrophages, dendritic cells, neutrophils) of wildtype C57BL/6 mice. To purify CD4+ and CD8+ T cells, as well as B cells, negative selection of the three different cell types was performed according to the respective isolation kits (Miltenyi Biotec, Bergisch Gladbach, Germany). Purity reached values of >95%. For stimulation, CD4+ and CD8+ T cells were seeded in pre-coated 24-well-plates (α-CD3/α-CD28, 10 µg/mL) and incubated for 5 days. B cells were stimulated with IL4 (10 ng/mL), LPS (5 µg/mL) and α-IgM (10 µg/mL) in 24-well-plates for 3 days.

4.2. Maturation and Stimulation of Bone Marrow Derived Cells

Macrophages and dendritic cells were both generated from murine bone marrow progenitor cells, as partly described elsewhere [29–32]. In short, the femur and tibia were flushed, and cells were resuspended in DMEM/F12 (Anprotec, Bruckberg, Germany) supplemented with 10% FCS (PAN-Biotech, Aidenbach, Germany) and 1% P/S (Sigma-Aldrich, St. Louis, USA). To obtain macrophages, cells were then plated in 6-well-plates and stimulated with M-CSF (20 ng/mL) for 7 days. On day 3, 1 mL of supplemented DMEM/F12 containing M-CSF was added to the cells. On day 7, macrophage polarization was performed: cells were resuspended in 2 mL of DMEM (Gibco, Waltham, MA, USA) supplemented with 10% FCS and 1% P/S and stimulated with either LPS (100 ng/mL) and IFN-γ (50 ng/mL) to obtain M1 macrophages or with IL-4 (20 ng/mL) to obtain M2 macrophages. To generate dendritic cells, bone marrow progenitors were seeded in 6-well-plates and stimulated with IL4 (10 ng/mL) and GM-CSF (15 ng/mL). On day 3, cells were washed and resuspended in 2 mL of supplemented DMEM/F12 containing IL4 and GM-CSF. On day 5, 2 mL of complete DMEM/F12 supplemented with IL4 and GM-CSF were added to the cells. For stimulation, dendritic cells were removed from the plate on day 7 and re-plated for 24 h in a 24-well-plate. LPS (100 ng/mL) was used as a stimulation factor.

4.3. Neutrophil Isolation and Stimulation

Neutrophils were isolated from murine bone marrow cells with a density gradient, as described previously [33]. Bones were flushed and cells were resuspended in 2 mL of PBS

(Sigma-Aldrich, St. Louis, MO, USA). Three layers of Percoll (Cytiva, Uppsala, Sweden) in different concentrations (78%, 66%, 54%) were prepared and bone marrow cells were carefully layered on top. After centrifugation (1545× g, 30 min, 20 °C, no deceleration), the neutrophil layer was collected. Cell purity was >60%. Neutrophil stimulation was performed using LPS (100 ng/mL) in a 24-well-plate for 3 h.

4.4. Flow Cytometry

Experiments were performed using a BD LSRFortessa flow cytometer (BD Biosciences, Franklin Lakes, USA) within 4 hours after isolation or collection of the cells. Autofluorescence of all samples was excited with a 355 nm UV-laser source and signals were detected with bandpass filters for NADH (BP 450/50) and FAD (BP 560/40). Additionally, samples were stained with the cell death marker Sytox Red. The cell mixes analysed in Figure 6 were stained with APC-labelled α-CD3. These two markers were chosen specifically as they do not interfere with the emission spectra of NADH and FAD and were excited by a second laser source (633 nm). The emitted signal was collected with a 670/14 bandpass filter. Data were analysed with the FlowJo software (BD Life Sciences, Franklin Lakes, USA). An example of the gating strategy can be found in Supplementary Figure S1. For reasons of simplicity and comparability, a mean value of the NADH and FAD signals was acquired for all samples and normalized to the mean value of alive, unstimulated CD4+ T-cells. These normalized signals are further referred to as NADH and FAD, respectively.

4.5. Multiphoton Microscopy

All samples were measured with an upright multiphoton microscope (TriMScope II, LaVision BioTec, Bielefeld, Germany) within 6–8 hrs after isolation or collection of the cells. A 50 µL droplet of cell suspension was placed on a glass slide and cells were allowed to settle for 5 min before covering the slide with a cover slip. Using a 25× water-immersion objective (HC Fluortar 178 L 25×/0.95 W VISIR, Leica microsystems, Wetzlar, Germany), the focal plane was adjusted and autofluorescence was excited with a mode-locked fs-pulsed Ti:Sa laser (Chameleon Vision II, Coherent, Santa Clara, USA) at 810 nm. Two bandpass filters (BP 450/70 and BP 560/40) were used to detect autofluorescence. These two bandpass filters were chosen to collect mainly the emitted light from NADH (BP 450/70) and FAD (BP 560/40). Still, other endogenous fluorophores might also contribute to cell autofluorescence to a small extent. Additionally, the DODT transmission signal, which uses scattering of the excitation laser to visualize 3D morphology of cells, was collected. In every sample, three representative positions were chosen and a 2D image was acquired. With this method, at least 30–500 cells/sample were measured.

To analyse the mixed cell suspensions shown in Figure 6, the corresponding samples were stained with APC-labelled α-CD3. A third bandpass filter (BP 675/67) was required to detect the emission of this marker. As the multiphoton microscope does not include a second laser source, the excitation wavelength was tuned to 1040 nm to evaluate the α-CD3 staining. A second image was then acquired at the same position at an excitation wavelength of 810 nm to excite natural autofluorescence as described above. Between these recordings, the focal plane was adjusted again to compensate for the different focal lengths at each wavelength. Both images were then combined for evaluation. This method is displayed in Supplementary Figure S2.

Image analysis was performed with the open-source software Fiji (v1.52s, Wayne Rasband, National Institutes of Health, Bethesda, USA). For semi-automatic evaluation, a macro was implemented. In a first step, the image was thresholded in the NADH channel by the Otsu method and a binary mask was created upon manual confirmation by the user. Background noise was subtracted, and the regions of interest (ROIs) were determined based on the mask. Finally, intensity parameters of all channels (mean and median grey value and integrated density), as well as area of the cells, were measured. A mean value of the median grey value for all cells in one sample (including the three different positions) was normalized to the mean value of alive, unstimulated CD4+ T-cells, further described as NADH and FAD.

4.6. Preparation and Analysis of Mixed Cell Samples

To analyse the mixed cell samples shown in Figure 6, four different conditions of cell samples were prepared: CD4+ T cells alone, neutrophils alone, cell mixes of 50% CD4+ T cells + 50% neutrophils and cell mixes of 80% CD4+ T cells + 20% neutrophils. The lymphocyte marker α-CD3 (APC) was used as a reference to identify CD4+ T cells. APC and NADH signals of single cells were plotted as dot plots for flow cytometry and MPM. These dot plots were divided into four quadrants by defining groups of high and low NADH and APC values. In flow cytometry, these values were chosen by visual inspection of different populations in the FlowJo software; in MPM, a cut-off value of 67 for APC raw median grey values and a cut-off value of 778 for NADH raw median grey values were identified as best thresholds by ROC curves and Youden-Index.

4.7. Statistical Analysis

GraphPad Prism 8 (GraphPad software, San Diego, CA, USA) was used for statistical analysis. Normality was tested with Shapiro–Wilk test. As some groups of samples were not normally distributed, statistical tests for non-parametric distributions were used. Two independent groups were compared with a Mann–Whitney test, and for three or more independent groups a Kruskal–Wallis test with subsequent Dunn's multiple comparisons test was performed. Boxplots represent median values, interquartile ranges, and the minimum and maximum values. Statistical significance is shown as follows: * $p < 0.05$, ** $p < 0.01$, *** $p < 0.001$, **** $p < 0.0001$.

Supplementary Materials: The following are available online at https://www.mdpi.com/article/10.3390/ijms23042338/s1.

Author Contributions: Conceptualization, S.L., O.-M.T., L.K., S.S. and M.J.W.; Data curation, S.L.; Formal analysis, S.L., O.-M.T. and L.K.; Funding acquisition, S.S. and M.J.W.; Investigation, S.L., O.-M.T., L.K. and S.V.; Methodology, S.L., O.-M.T., L.K. and S.V.; Project administration, S.S. and M.J.W.; Resources, O.F., M.F.N., S.S. and M.J.W.; Software, L.K.; Supervision, O.-M.T., L.K., S.S. and M.J.W.; Validation, O.-M.T. and L.K.; Visualization, Sarah Lemire, O.-M.T. and L.K.; Writing—original draft, S.L.; Writing—review and editing, O.-M.T., L.K., S.V., O.F., M.F.N., S.S. and M.J.W. All authors have read and agreed to the published version of the manuscript.

Funding: This research was funded by DEUTSCHE FORSCHUNGSGEMEINSCHAFT (DFG, German Research Foundation) project TRR241 (subproject C01, to Sebastian Schürmann and Maximilian Waldner). The work was supported by the Erlangen Graduate School in Advanced Optical Technologies (SAOT) within the framework of the German excellence initiative of the DFG, as well as by the Emerging Talents Initiative (ETI) of the Friedrich-Alexander-Universität Erlangen-Nürnberg (FAU) (to Lucas Kreiss).

Institutional Review Board Statement: All animal experiments were performed according to the guidelines of the Institutional Animal Care and Use Committee of the State Government of Middle Franconia.

Data Availability Statement: The data are available upon reasonable request to the corresponding authors.

Acknowledgments: We kindly thank Anabel Schmied, Carolin Reitenspieß and Alina Kämpfer for their valuable advice and technical assistance. The present work was performed in (partial) fulfilment of the requirements for obtaining the degree "Dr. med." (Sarah Lemire).

Conflicts of Interest: The authors declare no conflict of interest.

References

1. Yan, J.; Luo, M.; Chen, Z.; He, B. The Function and Role of the Th17/Treg Cell Balance in Inflammatory Bowel Disease. *J. Immunol. Res.* **2020**, *2020*, 8813558. [CrossRef]
2. Chen, M.L.; Sundrud, M.S. Cytokine Networks and T-Cell Subsets in Inflammatory Bowel Diseases. *Inflamm. Bowel Dis.* **2016**, *22*, 1157–1167. [CrossRef]
3. Seyedizade, S.S.; Afshari, K.; Bayat, S.; Rahmani, F.; Momtaz, S.; Rezaei, N.; Abdolghaffari, A.H. Current Status of M1 and M2 Macrophages Pathway as Drug Targets for Inflammatory Bowel Disease. *Arch. Immunol. Ther. Exp.* **2020**, *68*, 10. [CrossRef] [PubMed]
4. Wéra, O.; Lancellotti, P.; Oury, C. The Dual Role of Neutrophils in Inflammatory Bowel Diseases. *J. Clin. Med.* **2016**, *5*, 118. [CrossRef] [PubMed]
5. Kreiß, L.; Thoma, O.-M.; Dilipkumar, A.; Carlé, B.; Longequeue, P.; Kunert, T.; Rath, T.; Hildner, K.; Neufert, C.; Vieth, M.; et al. Label-Free In Vivo Histopathology of Experimental Colitis via 3-Channel Multiphoton Endomicroscopy. *Gastroenterology* **2020**, *159*, 832–834. [CrossRef] [PubMed]
6. Dilipkumar, A.; Al-Shemmary, A.; Kreiß, L.; Cvecek, K.; Carlé, B.; Knieling, F.; Gonzales Menezes, J.; Thoma, O.-M.; Schmidt, M.; Neurath, M.F.; et al. Label-Free Multiphoton Endomicroscopy for Minimally Invasive In Vivo Imaging. *Adv. Sci.* **2019**, *6*, 1801735. [CrossRef]
7. Monici, M. Cell and tissue autofluorescence research and diagnostic applications. *Biotechnol. Annu. Rev.* **2005**, *11*, 227–256. [CrossRef]
8. McKinnon, K.M. Flow Cytometry: An Overview. *Curr. Protoc. Immunol.* **2018**, *120*, 1–5. [CrossRef]
9. Bertolo, A.; Guerrero, J.; Stoyanov, J. Autofluorescence-based sorting removes senescent cells from mesenchymal stromal cell cultures. *Sci. Rep.* **2020**, *10*, 19084. [CrossRef] [PubMed]
10. Shah, A.T.; Cannon, T.M.; Higginbotham, J.N.; Coffey, R.J.; Skala, M.C. Autofluorescence flow sorting of breast cancer cell metabolism. *J. Biophotonics* **2017**, *10*, 1026–1033. [CrossRef]
11. Kozlova, A.A.; Verkhovskii, R.A.; Ermakov, A.V.; Bratashov, D.N. Changes in Autofluorescence Level of Live and Dead Cells for Mouse Cell Lines. *J. Fluoresc.* **2020**, *30*, 1483–1489. [CrossRef]
12. Zipfel, W.R.; Williams, R.M.; Webb, W.W. Nonlinear magic: Multiphoton microscopy in the biosciences. *Nat. Biotechnol.* **2003**, *21*, 1369–1377. [CrossRef]
13. Pathirana, W.G.W.; Chubb, S.P.; Gillett, M.J.; Vasikaran, S.D. Faecal Calprotectin. *Clin. Biochem. Rev.* **2018**, *39*, 77–90.
14. Zundler, S.; Becker, E.; Schulze, L.L.; Neurath, M.F. Immune cell trafficking and retention in inflammatory bowel disease: Mechanistic insights and therapeutic advances. *Gut* **2019**, *68*, 1688–1700. [CrossRef]
15. Gehlsen, U.; Szaszák, M.; Gebert, A.; Koop, N.; Hüttmann, G.; Steven, P. Non-Invasive Multi-Dimensional Two-Photon Microscopy enables optical fingerprinting (TPOF) of immune cells. *J. Biophotonics* **2015**, *8*, 466–479. [CrossRef] [PubMed]
16. Germic, N.; Frangez, Z.; Yousefi, S.; Simon, H.-U. Regulation of the innate immune system by autophagy: Monocytes, macrophages, dendritic cells and antigen presentation. *Cell Death Differ.* **2019**, *26*, 715–727. [CrossRef] [PubMed]
17. Germic, N.; Frangez, Z.; Yousefi, S.; Simon, H.-U. Regulation of the innate immune system by autophagy: Neutrophils, eosinophils, mast cells, NK cells. *Cell Death Differ.* **2019**, *26*, 703–714. [CrossRef] [PubMed]
18. Andersson, H.; Baechi, T.; Hoechl, M.; Richter, C. Autofluorescence of living cells. *J. Microsc.* **1998**, *191*, 1–7. [CrossRef] [PubMed]
19. Minhas, P.S.; Liu, L.; Moon, P.K.; Joshi, A.U.; Dove, C.; Mhatre, S.; Contrepois, K.; Wang, Q.; Lee, B.A.; Coronado, M.; et al. Macrophage de novo NAD+ synthesis specifies immune function in aging and inflammation. *Nat. Immunol.* **2019**, *20*, 50–63. [CrossRef]
20. Almeida, L.; Lochner, M.; Berod, L.; Sparwasser, T. Metabolic pathways in T cell activation and lineage differentiation. *Semin. Immunol.* **2016**, *28*, 514–524. [CrossRef] [PubMed]
21. Hayashi, F.; Means, T.K.; Luster, A.D. Toll-like receptors stimulate human neutrophil function. *Blood* **2003**, *102*, 2660–2669. [CrossRef]
22. Kobayashi, Y. The role of chemokines in neutrophil biology. *Front. Biosci.* **2008**, *13*, 2400–2407. [CrossRef] [PubMed]
23. Monsel, A.; Lécart, S.; Roquilly, A.; Broquet, A.; Jacqueline, C.; Mirault, T.; Troude, T.; Fontaine-Aupart, M.-P.; Asehnoune, K. Analysis of autofluorescence in polymorphonuclear neutrophils: A new tool for early infection diagnosis. *PLoS ONE* **2014**, *9*, e92564. [CrossRef] [PubMed]
24. Steinbach, E.C.; Plevy, S.E. The role of macrophages and dendritic cells in the initiation of inflammation in IBD. *Inflamm. Bowel Dis.* **2014**, *20*, 166–175. [CrossRef] [PubMed]
25. Ryter, S.W.; Kim, H.P.; Hoetzel, A.; Park, J.W.; Nakahira, K.; Wang, X.; Choi, A.M.K. Mechanisms of cell death in oxidative stress. *Antioxid. Redox Signal.* **2007**, *9*, 49–89. [CrossRef]
26. Schaefer, P.M.; Kalinina, S.; Rueck, A.; von Arnim, C.A.F.; Einem, B. von. NADH Autofluorescence-A Marker on its Way to Boost Bioenergetic Research. *Cytometry. Part. A J. Int. Soc. Anal. Cytol.* **2019**, *95*, 34–46. [CrossRef]
27. Mudter, J.; Neurath, M.F. Apoptosis of T cells and the control of inflammatory bowel disease: Therapeutic implications. *Gut* **2007**, *56*, 293–303. [CrossRef]
28. Neurath, M.F. Current and emerging therapeutic targets for IBD. *Nat. Rev. Gastroenterol. Hepatol.* **2017**, *14*, 269–278. [CrossRef]

29. Bailey, J.D.; Shaw, A.; McNeill, E.; Nicol, T.; Diotallevi, M.; Chuaiphichai, S.; Patel, J.; Hale, A.; Channon, K.M.; Crabtree, M.J. Isolation and culture of murine bone marrow-derived macrophages for nitric oxide and redox biology. *Nitric Oxide* **2020**, *100-101*, 17–29. [CrossRef]
30. Zhang, X.; Goncalves, R.; Mosser, D.M. The isolation and characterization of murine macrophages. *Curr. Protoc. Immunol.* **2008**, *83*, 14.1.1–14.1.14. [CrossRef]
31. Zhao, Y.-L.; Tian, P.-X.; Han, F.; Zheng, J.; Xia, X.-X.; Xue, W.-J.; Ding, X.-M.; Ding, C.-G. Comparison of the characteristics of macrophages derived from murine spleen, peritoneal cavity, and bone marrow. *J. Zhejiang Univ. Sci. B* **2017**, *18*, 1055–1063. [CrossRef] [PubMed]
32. Wei, H.-J.; Letterio, J.J.; Pareek, T.K. Development and Functional Characterization of Murine Tolerogenic Dendritic Cells. *J. Vis. Exp.* **2018**. [CrossRef] [PubMed]
33. Ubags, N.D.J.; Suratt, B.T. Isolation and Characterization of Mouse Neutrophils. *Methods Mol. Biol.* **2018**, *1809*, 45–57. [CrossRef] [PubMed]

MDPI
St. Alban-Anlage 66
4052 Basel
Switzerland
www.mdpi.com

International Journal of Molecular Sciences Editorial Office
E-mail: ijms@mdpi.com
www.mdpi.com/journal/ijms

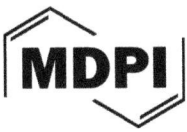

Disclaimer/Publisher's Note: The statements, opinions and data contained in all publications are solely those of the individual author(s) and contributor(s) and not of MDPI and/or the editor(s). MDPI and/or the editor(s) disclaim responsibility for any injury to people or property resulting from any ideas, methods, instructions or products referred to in the content.